Genetics in Oncology Practice: Cancer Risk Assessment

Edited by

Amy Strauss Tranin, ARNP, MS, AOCN®,
Credentialed in Familial Cancer Risk Assessment
and Management

Agnes Masny, RN, MPH, MSN, CRNP

Jean Jenkins, PhD, RN, FAAN

Oncology Nursing Society
Pittsburgh, PA

ONS Publishing Division
Publisher: Leonard Mafrica, MBA, CAE
Director, Commercial Publishing: Barbara Sigler, RN, MNEd
Production Manager: Lisa M. George
Technical Editor: Dorothy Mayernik, RN, MSN
Copy Editors: Toni Murray, Lori Wilson
Creative Services Assistant: Dany Sjoen

Genetics in Oncology Practice: Cancer Risk Assessment

Library of Congress Control Number: 2002114129

ISBN 1-890504-31-9

Publisher's Note
This book is published by the Oncology Nursing Society (ONS). ONS neither represents nor guarantees that the practices described herein will, if followed, ensure safe and
effective client care. The recommendations contained in this book reflect ONS's judgment regarding the state of general knowledge and practice in the field as of the date of
publication. The recommendations may not be appropriate for use in all circumstances.
Those who use this book should make their own determinations regarding specific safe
and appropriate client-care practices, taking into account the personnel, equipment, and
practices available at the hospital or other facility at which they are located. The editors
and publisher cannot be held responsible for any liability incurred as a consequence from
the use or application of any of the contents of this book. Figures and tables are used as
examples only. They are not meant to be all-inclusive, nor do they represent endorsement of any particular institution by ONS. Mention of specific products and opinions
related to those products do not indicate or imply endorsement by ONS.

ONS publications are originally published in English. Permission has been granted by
the ONS Board of Directors for foreign translation. (Individual tables and figures that
are reprinted or adapted require additional permission from the original source.) However, because translations from English may not always be accurate and precise, ONS
disclaims any responsibility for inaccurate translations. Readers relying on precise information should check the original English version.

Printed in the United States of America

Oncology Nursing Society
Integrity • Innovation • Stewardship • Advocacy • Excellence • Inclusiveness

Contributors

Co-Editors

Amy Strauss Tranin, ARNP, MS, AOCN®, Credentialed in Familial Cancer Risk Assessment and Management
Cancer Risk Counselor
Genetic Counseling, LLP
Overland Park, KS
Chapter 2. The Scope of Cancer Genetics Nursing Practice; Chapter 11. Ensuring Competence: Nursing Credentialing in Cancer Genetics

Jean Jenkins, PhD, RN, FAAN
Clinical Nurse Specialist Consultant
National Naval Medical Center
National Cancer Institute/CCRC
Bethesda, MD
Chapter 1. Why Should Oncology Nurses Be Interested in Genetics?; Chapter 12. Recommendations for Education

Agnes Masny, RN, MPH, MSN, CRNP
Nurse Practitioner
Fox Chase Cancer Center
Philadelphia, PA
Chapter 1. Why Should Oncology Nurses Be Interested in Genetics?

Authors

Patricia Moffa Barse, RN, MSN, AOCN®
Oncology Advanced Practice Nurse
Cooper Cancer Institute
Voorhees, NJ
Chapter 4. How to Perform a Genetic Assessment

Kathleen A. Calzone, RN, MSN, APNG(c)
Nursing Coordinator
Cancer Risk Evaluation Program
University of Pennsylvania Cancer Center
Philadelphia, PA
Chapter 2. The Scope of Cancer Genetics Nursing Practice; Chapter 12. Recommendations for Education

Eileen D. Dimond, RN, MS
Education Specialist
Office of Education and Special Initiatives
National Cancer Institute
Bethesda, MD
  Chapter 8. Establishing a Cancer Genetics Clinic

Elizabeth M. Glaser, RN, MSN
Clinical Research Coordinator
Duke University Medical Center
Durham, NC
  Chapter 10. How to Identify Appropriate Referrals and Current Resources

Karen Greco, RN, MN, ANP
Oncology Nurse Practitioner
Oregon Health & Science University
Portland, OR
  Chapter 7. How to Provide Genetic Counseling and Education

Dale Halsey Lea, RN, MPH, APNG(c)
Assistant Director
Southern Maine Genetics Services
Foundation for Blood Research
Scarborough, ME
  Chapter 9. Handling Genetic Information Responsibly

Mira Lessick, PhD, RN
Associate Professor
College of Health and Human Services
University of Toledo
Toledo, OH
Former Director of the Genetic Health Nursing Program
Rush College of Nursing
Chicago, IL

Chapter 12. Recommendations for Education

Lois J. Loescher, PhD, RN
NCI Cancer Prevention Fellow
ONS Foundation/Ortho Biotech Research Fellow
Arizona Cancer Center
University of Arizona
Tucson, AZ
  Chapter 3. The Biology of Cancer

Suzanne M. Mahon, RN, DNSc, AOCN®, APNG(c)
Assistant Clinical Professor
Division of Hematology and Oncology
St. Louis University
St. Louis, MO
  Chapter 5. Cancer Risk Assessment: Considerations for Cancer Genetics

Paula Trahan Rieger, RN, MSN, CS, AOCN®, FAAN
Director, International Affairs
American Society of Clinical Oncology
Alexandria, VA
Former Nurse Practitioner
Clinical Cancer Genetics, Clinical Cancer Prevention
The University of Texas M.D. Anderson Cancer Center
Houston, TX
  Chapter 6. The Impact of Genetic Information in the Management of Cancer

Luke Whitesell, MD
Associate Professor
Pediatric Heme/Oncology

Steele Memorial Children's Research
Center
University of Arizona
Tucson, AZ
Chapter 3. The Biology of Cancer

Rita S. Wickham, PhD, RN, AOCN®
Associate Professor
Rush College of Nursing
Clinical Nurse Specialist
Palliative Care Service
Rush-Presbyterian-St. Luke's Medical
Center
Chicago, IL
Chapter 12. Recommendations for Education

Contents

1

Why Should Oncology Nurses Be Interested in Genetics?

Jean Jenkins, PhD, RN, FAAN,
and Agnes Masny, RN, MPH, MSN, CRNP

The Human Genome Project began in 1990 as an international effort to characterize human genetic instructions (the human genome) by creating a genetic map that reflects the position of genes on chromosomes. Scientists have completed a draft map of the human genome (International Human Genome Sequencing Consortium, 2001; Venter et al., 2001). Over the next decade, work will continue with computer technology to further identify genes associated with disease and the potential for interventions in risk reduction or targeted therapeutics.

In response to these advances, the National Cancer Institute (1998) established the Genome Anatomy Project to identify all the genes responsible for cancer development and malignant transformation. In the field of oncology, this project signals a dramatic shift in the way that patients will be screened, diagnosed, and treated. Oncology nurses will be required to know about genetics to understand the basic etiology of cancer.

The most simplistic definition of cancer is uncontrolled cell growth. People familiar with the discoveries of the Human Genome Project now understand that cancer is clearly a genetic disease. Genes are units of deoxyribonucleic acid (DNA). The genes code for normal proteins, which regulate cell growth. Damage (mutation) frequently occurs during normal cell division or as a result of environmental influences. When genetic damage escapes the normal repair mechanisms of the body, the mutations accumulate, resulting in uncontrolled cell growth. Most cancers occur because of multiple mutations involving several genes at each step in the carcinogenic pathway. Oncology nurses know that the carcinogenic pathway involves five steps: initiation, promotion, progression, invasion, and metastasis. The identification of the genes related to each step in the pathway will have a dramatic impact on oncology interventions. Thus, the increasing understanding of the genetic basis of cancer and the effect that understanding will have on treatment modalities will sweep oncology nursing into a new healthcare paradigm (Engelking, 1997).

The Impact of Advancements in Genetics on the Oncology Nurse's Role

Advances in genetics will influence every aspect of the cancer continuum, from prevention and screening to treatments and palliation. Oncology nurses, because of their holistic approach to patient care, have the opportunity to incorporate these advances into their role at each point along the cancer-care continuum. They can integrate genetics concepts into counseling, education, preparation of clients for decision making, and direct caregiving. Figure 1-1 shows the carcinogenic pathway and corresponding genetic events and nursing actions. The figure suggests ways that oncology healthcare professionals can incorporate genetics principles into all aspects of patient care.

The field of cancer prevention is already focusing on the interaction of genes and environmental factors. Genetic profiles (such as blood type and

Figure 1-1. The Carcinogenic Pathway, Genetic Events, and Corresponding Nursing Actions

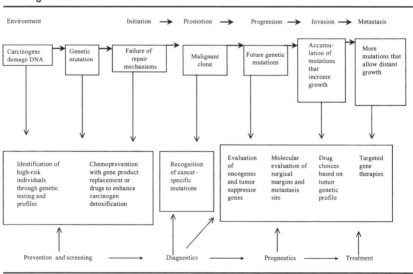

Note. Based on information from Peters, Dimond, & Jenkins, 1997.

human leukocyte antigen, or HLA, type) help to identify the individuals most susceptible to carcinogens. Genetic profiles are not profiles of mutations but of simple variations in genetic makeup. These variations, known as polymorphisms, often influence specific enzyme activity. For example, carcinogens present in tobacco are modified or detoxified by enzymes in the cytochrome P450 (*CYP*) family. Some individuals, by virtue of their genetic makeup, have a variation in one of the *CYP* genes and are unable to produce an enzyme capable of carcinogen detoxification. These individuals, both smokers and nonsmokers, are at higher-than-average risk for lung cancer (Bennett et al., 1999).

Oncology nurses working in the areas of prevention and risk reduction will routinely make use of genetic information to
- Identify high-risk populations through genetic testing or genetic profiles.
- Educate a high-risk individual about the effects of exposures based on the individual's genetic makeup.
- Recommend risk-reduction strategies that include lifestyle and behavior changes.
- Counsel individuals about the benefits and limitations of genetic testing.
- Advise individuals about the psychosocial ramifications of genetic information.

Some oncology nurses are specializing in cancer genetic-risk counseling. The technology to identify mutations in cancer-predisposition genes is clinically available for a variety of familial cancer syndromes, such as familial adenomatous polyposis (caused by an *APC* gene mutation), hereditary breast and ovarian cancer (*BRCA1* or *BRCA2*), hereditary nonpolyposis colon cancer syndrome (*MLH1, MSH2*), and multiple endocrine neoplasia 2a and 2b (*RET*) (see Chapter 6). Oncology nurses working in cancer genetic-risk assessment and counseling
- Educate individuals about the genes that predispose them to cancer.
- Provide in-depth cancer-risk assessment by evaluating family histories and statistical risk estimates.
- Guide individuals in decision making relative to genetic testing.
- Prepare individuals and families for the potential impact of genetic information.
- Address ethical concerns related to genetic information.
- Advise individuals about the benefits and limitations of risk-reduction measures, such as chemoprevention, prophylactic surgery, and lifestyle changes.

Nurses involved in the clinical arena are already using the terminology of genetics when they explain the diagnostic and prognostic features of cancer cells. As genetics continues to advance, the accuracy of diagnosis and prediction of treatment response will increase. Nurses will need to understand and explain

- Which genetic features, such as the absence or presence of a gene product or genetic changes noted histologically (Quirke & Mapstone, 1999), help to identify early cancers
- Molecular staging, which predicts which patients are at high risk for disease spread (For example, molecular staging can help to identify genetic lesions in surgical margins—lesions that are not yet malignant but are indicative of residual disease [Brennan et al., 1995].)
- How genetic markers in peripheral blood or body fluids are predictive of disease spread or relapse (Kodera et al., 1998)
- How genetic characteristics of the tumor can predict the patient's response to chemotherapy.

Innovative therapies will use replacement genes or gene products to treat cancer. Tumor cells will be genetically modified to make them more susceptible to conventional therapies. Oncology nurses will have to understand the genetics behind these soon-to-be commonplace practices.

Public interest is high regarding the use of genetic information to predict cancer susceptibility (Lerman, Daly, Masny, & Balshem, 1994; Smith & Croyle, 1995). The promise of better cancer prevention and treatment has created consumer demand for genetic information and genetic services. As a result of this demand, oncology nurses have been involved in genetic predisposition testing—that is, identifying and counseling carriers of an inherited mutation (Calzone, 1997; Giarelli, 1997). Diagnostics have always preceded therapeutics in every major paradigm shift in healthcare practice (Collins, 1997). For example, the identification of bacteria was a diagnostic discovery that was well in advance of antibiotic therapies. In the same manner, genetic testing is the diagnostic precedent to major changes in oncology practice. Figure 1-2 shows the steps from the identification of genes involved in disease to the development of therapies. Note the time gap between the detection of contributing genes and the emergence of new treatment modalities. In the field of cancer genetics, computer and DNA technology are expected to make this gap a short one. Therefore, the window of opportunity for oncology nurses to incorporate genetic information into their roles as educators, counselors, and primary caregivers is now.

Genetic Health Care and Oncology Nursing

Genetic health care is care for people whose health, wellness, or disease is caused or influenced by genes. Healthcare services must integrate genetic health care into the continuum of cancer care.

Figure 1-2. The Steps Involved From the Identification of Genes Involved in Disease to the Development of Therapies

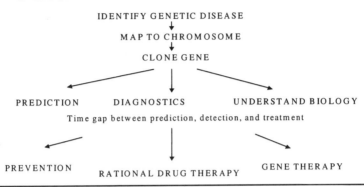

GENE-MAPPING TIMELINE

IDENTIFY GENETIC DISEASE

MAP TO CHROMOSOME

CLONE GENE

PREDICTION   DIAGNOSTICS   UNDERSTAND BIOLOGY

Time gap between prediction, detection, and treatment

PREVENTION   RATIONAL DRUG THERAPY   GENE THERAPY

Note. From "Clinical Applications of Genetic Technologies to Cancer Care," by J. Peters, E. Dimond, and J. Jenkins, 1997, *Cancer Nursing, 20,* p. 365. Copyright 1997 by Lippincott Williams and Wilkins. Reprinted with permission.

Discoveries about how genes direct the construction and operation of the human body are showing how genetic changes influence disease susceptibility and development. These discoveries offer opportunities for improvements in the care of individuals with cancer through the integration of genetic concepts into all healthcare visits.

Using genetics technology in the clinical setting creates challenges for both healthcare providers and consumers. The interest, the technology, and now the expanding applicability to all individuals with cancer provides opportunities for nurses to design new genetic health services that enhance outcomes for individuals and families. The opportunities also include different and difficult choices that accompany genetic information.

How Is Genetic Information Different?

Soon it will be possible to determine a person's individual genetic profile and his or her risk of specific disease. Information about a person's genetic makeup is very personal and reflects a permanent part of that individual. At the same time, every individual's genetic information has a familial component in the sense that genes convey traits, including cancer risk, from generation to generation. A patient's blood relative may carry the same genetic information the patient carries.

The fact that genetic information pertains to an individual and to his or her family raises issues regarding individual versus family rights to confidentiality and the right of each person to know versus the right not to know about genetic factors. Ethicists have debated whether individuals in a family have the right to be informed about genetic factors that could affect their well-being and choices (Parker, 1995; Van Leeuwen & Hertogh, 1992). For example, should healthcare providers share information about misinformed paternity? Do family members have the right not to know about cancer risk? Will knowledge of predisposing genes lead to pressure from a healthcare provider or third-party payor to modify lifestyle and screening practices? Will knowledge of genetic markers that family members share disrupt or strengthen family relationships? A better understanding of how individual uniqueness affects familial factors would help to answer these questions.

Although a person's genetic makeup is permanent, whether his or her makeup will result in undesirable consequences is uncertain (Lerman, 1997). This uncertainty affects personal decision making, which also is influenced by prior perception of risk, values, attitudes, and cultural beliefs. Identifying people who have a predisposition to developing an illness may lead asymptomatic people to question their own concept of being healthy.

Genetic information often provokes emotional and behavioral responses. It could affect insurance coverage and employability and cause discrimination.

To summarize, genetic information is different from other health-related information because it could reflect family members' risks, it does not reflect certainty about whether risk will lead to disease, it provokes unusually emotional responses that affect behavior, and it has a very high potential to affect insurance coverage and employability and expose the client to discrimination. Because of these unique features, healthcare professionals must handle genetic information with greater consideration than is applied when handling other health-related data, such as blood counts. In addition, because of the unique nature of genetic information, healthcare professionals must ensure informed consent before incorporating genetic information into general healthcare and nursing practices.

How Will Genetic Information Be Incorporated Into General Health Care?

The discovery of the contributions genetics makes to health and illness will affect the care of all clients (both adults and children) at all clinical settings and across all practice specialties.

In terms of cancer care, nurses can present information about genetics to clients during the initial assessment; during discussions of early detection, cancer prevention, diagnostics, medical surveillance, and the causes of different types of cancer; and when planning risk reduction, predicting prognosis, designing treatment options, and monitoring disease response.

What Role Will Nurses Play in Meeting the Genetic Healthcare Needs of the Future?

With some augmentation of the education they already have, nurses will be able to provide the counseling and teaching that recent genetic discoveries necessitate. Nurses must plan proactively to build on that foundation by enabling personal skill development and ensuring that they continually update their knowledge of genetics by learning about ongoing scientific discoveries that affect client care. Translating science into practical terms has always been a nursing priority. In the fast-changing field of genetics, nurses will again find ways to apply exciting scientific discoveries to the care of individual clients. This text will provide examples of responsibilities to consider in the design of a personal plan to meet these challenges.

Nurses have an opportunity to provide leadership in the design of genetic healthcare services that offer safe and ethical applications of genetic technology. Nursing's role will be important in the assessment, planning, implementation, and evaluation of cancer-genetics health services.

For oncology nurses, the integration of cancer genetics into oncology care presents countless opportunities for personal and professional growth. With these opportunities comes the obligation to ensure that genetic information and technology enhance cancer care. Another obligation is to consider the ethical, social, and legal implications of genetics knowledge along with the medical application of cancer genetics technology.

A brochure published by the American Nurses Association (ANA), *Managing Genetic Information: Implications for Nursing Practice* (Scanlon & Fibison, 1995) may help nurses to integrate ethical principles into nursing guidelines regarding genetic information.

Patient advocacy, nursing research, and legislative efforts offer additional opportunities to influence healthcare policy in regard to applying genetics to clinical care. Understanding the implications of genetic information for the individual, family, and society will enhance the ability of nurses to influence decisions that affect practice, education, and the quality of cancer care. The Oncology Nursing Society (ONS) has made the commitment to prepare its members to meet the challenges created by the Genetics Revolution (ONS, 1997). The publication of this text is one ONS-sponsored initiative designed to help to prepare nurses to incorporate genetics into practice. This text will define the education that nurses will need to accomplish this task. It will establish standards and guide practice in cancer genetics and will help to define the role of the nurse in genetic health care. This text will serve as a resource for nurses presented with genetics issues in their practice, and it will provide a model for nurses as they incorporate genetics into their practice.

Are You Using Genetic Information Yet?

You may be surprised at the extent to which you already incorporate information about genetics into your practice, even though you may have no formal training in genetics.

An ANA survey showed that only 9% of nurses in the study had genetics training. Most (68%) indicated that they were not at all or not too knowledgeable about genetics. However, most nurses reported performing some genetics-related activity at least occasionally, with a majority citing low levels of confidence in explaining genetic information (Scanlon & Fibison, 1995).

You may be performing genetics-related activities and using genetics information without recognizing it. To see how often you use or provide genetics information, take the quiz that follows. The quiz will help you to assess your knowledge of genetics. The material that follows the quiz will present the answers and direct you to the chapters in this text that will help you to develop your knowledge of specific aspects of genetics health care.

Quiz: How Frequently Do You Use or Provide Genetics Information?

Check the box beside "Yes," "No," or "Not sure" to answer the questions that follow.

1a. Have you ever told individuals to use sunscreen?
    ____Yes____No
 b. Do you know the genetic basis of this recommendation?
    ____Yes____No

2a. Has a patient ever told you about other family members with cancer?
    ____Yes____No
 b. Do you understand the genetic basis of their concern?
    ____Yes____Not sure

3a. Have you ever explained to a patient how tumor markers function in a workup or cancer follow-up?

____Yes____No

 b. Is it true that some tumor markers are genes expressed by tumors?

____Yes____Not sure

4a. Have you ever seen the term *aneuploidy* on a pathology report?

____Yes____No

 b. Did you know that *aneuploidy* refers to DNA changes?

____Yes____Not sure

5a. Have you heard of vaccines for melanoma?

____Yes____No

 b. Did you know that treatment by means of a vaccine is a form of gene therapy?

____Yes____Not sure

6a. Do you know why insurance companies ask about family history of heart disease or cancer?

____Yes____Not sure

 b. Do you know the social implications of the answer to the preceding question?

____Yes____Not sure

Scoring

To see how often you use genetics information, count the number of times you answered "yes" to questions labeled a.

0–1: You seldom use genetics information.

2–3: Like most nurses, you occasionally use genetics information.

4–6: You already use genetics information frequently in your nursing practice.

To see how much knowledge you have to explain genetics information, count the number of times you answered "yes" to questions labeled b.

0–3: Like most nurses, you have a basic understanding of genetics but are willing to incorporate new information into practice.

4–6: You already have a foundation of knowledge about genetics upon which you can build.

Quiz Answers

1. The recommendation for sunscreen has a basis in genetics. Researchers believe the pathophysiology of cancer is related to the interaction of genes and the environment. Multiple exposures to ultraviolet light cause genetic mutations that can lead to skin cancer. See Chapter 3 to learn how environmental factors figure into cancer-risk assessment and health promotion.

2. When patients tell you about family members with cancer, they may be concerned about the impact of family history on the potential for disease in themselves or a family member. The media have focused attention on the potential hereditary aspect of some cancers. From 5% to 10% of all cancers have a hereditary component. Chapters 4 and 7 provide information about familial cancer-risk assessment and the psychosocial impact of risk notification.

3. Tumor markers are proteins, antigens, enzymes, or genes expressed by the tumor or produced by normal tissue in response to the tumor. For example, the *MYC* oncogene *ERBB2* (*HER2/NEU*) is a genetic tumor marker used in the diagnosis and monitoring of cancer. Chapter 6 discusses the impact of genetic information on cancer management.

4. DNA analysis of solid tumors characterizes the DNA as normal (diploid) or abnormal (aneuploid). Aneuploidy is abnormal or disorganized DNA. DNA analysis helps to determine prognosis by assessing the proliferative potential of tumors. Chapter 6 discusses prognostic indicators.

5. Vaccines are a type of gene therapy, an approach to cancer treatment that falls into the class of immunotherapy. Vaccines stimulate the immune system's ability to mount a response against a cancer. A cancer vaccine is designed to immunize patients against their own cancers by injecting them with their own tumor cells after the cells have been modified by certain genes. The goal is to make the cancer more sensitive to chemotherapeutic agents. Chapter 6 offers information about gene therapy.

6. Family history currently is included as one of the classifications of genetic information. Potential discrimination for health or life insurance is an ongoing concern in cases in which the covered person has a family history of cancer. The Kennedy-Kassebaum legislation, enacted July 1, 1997, provides some protection against health insurance discrimination for preexisting genetic conditions for people already insured by a group plan. Federal workers are covered by an executive order that states that federal employers may not use genetic information to deny employment, make job assignments, or guide promotion decisions (National Human Genome Research Institute, 2000). The order also limits the ability of federal employers to collect or disclose genetic information about an applicant or employee. No legislation protects

individuals from genetics-based discrimination regarding life insurance. Chapter 9 discusses the uniqueness of genetic information and the handling of ethical, legal, and social aspects of cancer genetics.

Summary

Your answers to the quiz probably showed you that genetics is already part of your oncology nursing practice. Without realizing it, every nurse practicing in oncology is already using genetics information in the context of promoting healthful behaviors to prevent cancer; identifying people at risk for cancer; explaining features of cancer that affect prognosis and treatment; and addressing the legal, social, and ethical impacts of cancer.

The work of the Human Genome Project and the mapping of protein-coding genes are helping to unlock the molecular basis of the initiation, invasion, progression, and metastasis of cancer. These findings will continue to elucidate the understanding of every aspect of the cancer continuum and will initiate advances with the potential for novel interventions in risk reduction and targeted therapeutics.

This text will help oncology nurses to understand the genetic basis of cancer. Although this text focuses on assessment, it will help readers to explore how genetics will influence the entire cancer care continuum. The authors anticipate that our growing knowledge of cancer genetics will serve to further the mission of the ONS: "to promote excellence in oncology nursing and quality cancer care."

References

Bennett, W.P., Alavanja, M.C., Blomeke, B., Vahakangas, K.H., Castren, K., Welsh, J.A., et al. (1999). Environmental tobacco smoke, genetic susceptibility, and risk of lung cancer in never-smoking women. *Journal of the National Cancer Institute, 91,* 2009–2014.

Brennan, J., Mao, L., Hruban, R., Boyle, J., Eby, Y., Koch, W., et al. (1995). Molecular assessment of histopathologic staging in squamous-cell carcinoma of the head and neck. *New England Journal of Medicine, 332,* 429–435.

Calzone, K.A. (1997). Genetic predisposition testing: Clinical implications for oncology nurses. *Oncology Nursing Forum, 24,* 712–717.

Collins, F. (1997). *Proceedings of the National Coalition for Health Professional*

Education in Genetics. Bethesda, MD: National Coalition for Health Professional Education in Genetics.

Engelking, C. (1997). The applications of genetics to oncology: A new health care paradigm. *Innovations in Breast Cancer Care*, 2(4), 65, 69.

Giarelli, E. (1997). Medullary thyroid carcinoma: One component of the inherited disorder multiple endocrine neoplasia type 2A. *Oncology Nursing Forum*, 24, 1007–1019.

International Human Genome Sequencing Consortium. (2001). Initial sequencing and analysis of the human genome. *Nature*, 409, 860–921.

Kodera, Y., Nakanishi, H., Yamamura, Y., Shimizu, Y., Torii, A., Hirai, T., et al. (1998). Prognostic value and clinical implications of disseminated cancer cells in the peritoneal cavity detected by reverse transcriptase-polymerase chain reaction and cytology. *International Journal of Cancer*, 79, 429–433.

Lerman, C. (1997). Psychological aspects of genetic testing: Introduction to the special issue. *Health Psychology*, 16(1), 3–7.

Lerman, C., Daly, M., Masny, A., & Balshem, A. (1994). Attitudes about genetic testing for breast-ovarian cancer susceptibility. *Journal of Clinical Oncology*, 12, 843–850.

National Cancer Institute. (1998). *Cancer genome anatomy project*. Retrieved August 30, 2001, from http://cap.nci.nih.gov

National Human Genome Research Institute. (2000). *Background: Employment discrimination and the executive order*. Retrieved August 30, 2001, from http://www.nhgri.nih.gov/NEWS/Executive_order/fact-sheet.html

Oncology Nursing Society. (1997). *1996–1997 annual report: Expanding our horizons*. Pittsburgh: Author.

Parker, L.S. (1995). Breast cancer genetic screening and critical bioethics gaze. *Journal of Medicine and Philosophy*, 20, 313–337.

Peters, J., Dimond, E., & Jenkins, J. (1997). Clinical applications of genetic technologies to cancer care. *Cancer Nursing*, 20, 359–377.

Quirke, P., & Mapstone, N. (1999). The new biology: Histopathology. *Lancet*, 354(Suppl. 1), 26–31.

Scanlon, C., & Fibison, W. (1995). *Managing genetic information: Implications for nursing practice* [Brochure]. Washington, DC: American Nurses Association.

Smith, K., & Croyle, R. (1995). Attitudes toward genetic testing for colon cancer risk. *American Journal of Public Health*, 85, 1435–1438.

Van Leeuwen, E., & Hertogh, C. (1992). The right to genetic information: Some reflections on Dutch developments. *Journal of Medicine and Philosophy*, 17, 381–393.

Venter, J.C., Adams, M.D., Myers, E.W., Li, P.W., Mural, R.J., Sutton, G.G., et al. (2001). The sequence of the human genome. *Science*, 291, 1304–1351.

2

The Scope of Cancer Genetics Nursing Practice

Kathleen A. Calzone, RN, MSN, APNG(c), and
Amy Strauss Tranin, ARNP, MS, AOCN®, Credentialed in Familial
Cancer Risk Assessment and Management

Traditionally, knowledge of genetics has been viewed as useful but not necessary to nursing practice (George, 1992). Recently, however, cancer genetics has emerged as a medical specialty, introducing new diagnostic and therapeutic options into clinical oncology. Therefore, oncology nursing as a profession must integrate cancer genetics into general and advanced oncology nursing practice as well as recognize cancer genetics as an oncology nursing subspecialty.

Evidence of the broad implications of genetics for cancer care is clearly emerging. Genetic information is increasingly used not just to predict risk but also to understand the biology of the disease, characterize malignancies, establish tailored treatment regimens, and develop new therapeutic modalities. Traditional approaches to cancer care will not be abandoned; instead, genetic information and genetics technology will enhance and refine them (Livingston, 1997).

Thanks to the Human Genome Project and similar research, the understanding of human genetics is growing exponentially and is profoundly affecting all aspects of health care (Collins & McKusick, 2001). However, the diffusion of genetics into cancer care hinges on the ability of oncology healthcare providers, including nurses, to incorporate genetics into their practice (Holtzman, 1992). Genetics can no longer be considered nonessential to oncology nursing practice. It is instead the science that should form the basis of oncology nursing preparation and practice (Donaldson, 1997; Olsen, Baxendale-Cox, & Mock, 2000). Genetics is not coming to oncology; genetics *is* oncology.

The vast majority of oncology nurses at all levels of educational preparation have had no instruction in genetics as a basic science or preparation regarding the unique implications of genetic information (Anderson, 1996; Scanlon & Fibison, 1995). As a result, oncology nurses currently are limited in their understanding of genetics concepts and ability to incorporate genetics into their practice. Oncology nurses at both the general and advanced practice level must obtain a basic foundation in genetics to practice in the emerging healthcare environment. Oncology nurses who, in the future, will be involved in the subspecialty of cancer genetics will require extensive ongoing educational preparation and clinical experience.

Dimensions of Cancer Genetics Nursing Practice

Three levels differentiate the scope of oncology nursing practice in genetics: the general oncology nurse, advanced practice oncology nurse, and advanced practice oncology nurse with a subspecialty in genetics (see Figure 2-1). The

Figure 2-1. Three Levels of Oncology Nursing Practice in Genetics

Advanced Practice
Oncology Nurse
With a Genetics
Subspeciality

Advanced Practice
Oncology Nurse

General Oncology Nurse

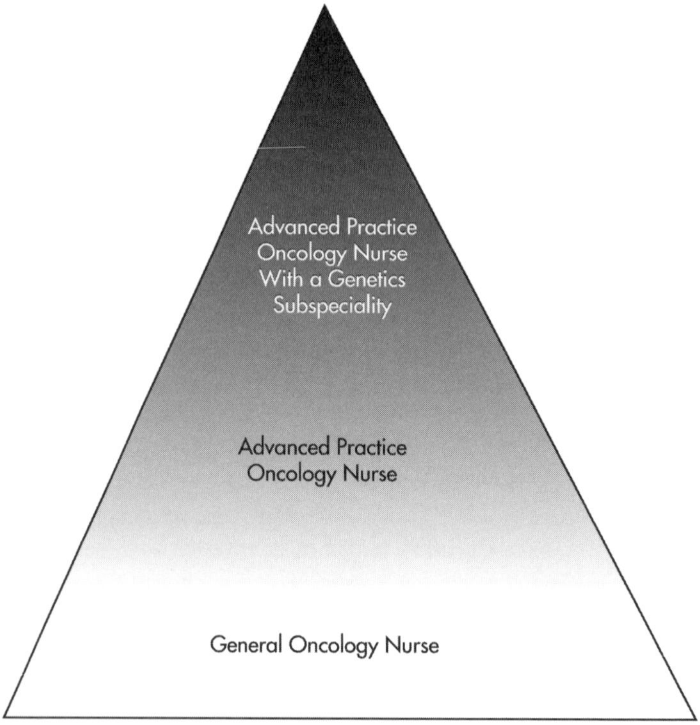

features that distinguish one level of practice from another include educational preparation, professional experience, practice specialty, and specific job roles and responsibilities. The purpose of describing each level in detail is to differentiate the requirements necessary to deliver quality and competent nursing care. As an example, the general oncology nurse may specialize in a particular area, such as radiation oncology or chemotherapy, and some tasks and job responsibilities may be the same as those of an advanced practice nurse. However, this is not equivalent to practicing at the advanced practice level, which is defined by educational preparation and overall job responsibilities.

All oncology nurses, regardless of their level of practice in genetics, are responsible for delivering care within the framework of the nursing process and the boundaries of the scope of oncology nursing practice defined by the American Nurses Association (ANA) and the Oncology Nursing Society (ONS) (1996). The scope of practice outlined in this chapter more clearly delineates the role of the oncology nurse in cancer genetics. The cancer genetic nursing role is encompassed by the scope of practice in oncology nursing. The practice of genetics oncology nursing, as in all oncology nursing, incorporates the roles of direct caregiver, educator, consultant, administrator, and researcher. Oncology nursing practice that integrates genetics extends to all care-delivery settings in which clients experiencing or at risk for developing cancer receive health care, education, and counseling for prevention, screening, early detection, treatment, and rehabilitation.

Role of the Nurse in Integrating Genetics Into Oncology Practice

At all three practice levels, the nurse incorporates theoretical knowledge of genetics into his or her roles as direct care provider, coordinator, consultant, educator, researcher, and administrator (Dimond, Calzone, Davis, & Jenkins, 1998). The general oncology nurse and the advanced practice oncology nurse use genetic information in a manner consistent with their educational preparation and the role, scope, and standards of oncology nursing as established by ONS (ANA & ONS, 1996). At both of these levels, the genetics knowledge integrated into practice has broad applicability and limited depth. Just as all oncology nurses are expected to comprehend and incorporate into their practice the basic tenets of carcinogenesis, the same expectation is applied to cancer genetics because cancer is a genetic disease. The advanced practice oncology nurse with a genetics subspecialty is prepared at the master's level with additional training in genetics.

Scope of Practice

The General Oncology Nurse

Nurses at the general level apply genetics knowledge in their practice by identifying, referring, educating, supporting, treating, and caring for clients affected by, or at risk for, cancer. The general oncology nurse requires knowledge of genetic principles as they relate to the assessment of cancer through screening, early-detection methods, prevention practices, and treatment. As clients become more aware of the genetic contribution to health and illness, general oncology nurses will need to be able to address clients' questions about genetics and be able to refer them to appropriate genetics professionals. In terms of cancer genetics practice, the general oncology nurse functions like a nurse at the beginner or advanced-beginner stage as defined by Benner (1984) and Benner, Tanner, and Chesla (1996). As Benner et al. described, these stages of practice are characterized by limited practical experience in cancer genetics and functioning directed by rules and guidelines. General oncology nurses do not have the knowledge base or experience in cancer genetics to prioritize the importance of genetic information or know what to expect in certain situations regarding genetic interventions. Practice by the general oncology nurse, related to risk assessment of genetic conditions and interventions, is focused on the accomplishment of tasks. Oncology nursing practice in genetics at the general level includes, but is not limited to, the activities described in Figure 2-2.

The Advanced Practice Oncology Nurse

The scope of practice in cancer genetics for the advanced practice oncology nurse who does not specialize in genetics is similar to that of the general nurse in oncology. However, because advanced practice nursing requires substantial theoretical knowledge and proficient use of this knowledge in providing care, the advanced practice nurse understands the role of genetics, in cancer care to a greater degree than does the general practice nurse. Although a nurse may work at the advanced practice level, in terms of genetics he or she is at the beginner or advanced-beginner stage (Benner, 1984; Benner et al., 1996). The advanced practice oncology nurse often uses theoretical knowledge uncoupled with practical experience when aspects of genetics information must be incorporated into care. Like the general oncology nurse, when presented with an atypical case, the advanced practice oncology nurse may not fully know the significance of genetic information and may not completely see the implications of a situation or know when action is needed

Figure 2-2. Scope of Oncology Nursing Practice in Genetics

General Oncology Nurse

Direct Care
- Identifies a client's significant risk factors based on personal, medical, occupational, environmental, and family risk factors
- Performs a basic cancer risk assessment that includes an assessment of the family history of cancer
- Consults with genetics experts by providing observations and individual- or family-specific data for interpretation and direction
- Serves as an advocate to ensure informed consent and voluntary autonomous decision making in regard to genetic testing and therapeutics
- Evaluates and monitors the impact of genetic conditions, therapeutics, and testing on the client
- Provides psychological support to the client and facilitates successful adaptive responses

Coordinator
- Reinforces care delivered or managed by cancer genetic specialists

Consultant
- Routinely uses an advanced practice oncology nurse as a resource regarding cancer genetic information

Educator
- Conducts an assessment of the client's learning and psychosocial needs regarding genetic services
- Answers basic questions and addresses basic concerns about cancer genetics
- Reinforces the interventions implemented by the cancer genetic healthcare team
- Evaluates individual and family outcomes with guidance from the genetics team

Researcher
- Monitors and documents the client's participation in cancer genetic clinical trials

Administrator
- Facilitates cancer genetic programs and services

Advanced Practice Oncology Nurse

Direct Care
- Identifies significant risk factors relating to a client and his or her immediate family by evaluating personal, medical, occupational, environmental, and genetic information
- Performs a basic cancer risk assessment that includes constructing a three-generation pedigree
- Relies on genetic specialists for interpretation of data about the individual and family
- Facilitates informed decision making; serves as an advocate to ensure informed consent and voluntary autonomous decision making in regard to genetic testing and therapies
- Evaluates and monitors the impact of genetic conditions, therapies, and testing on the client and his or her immediate family
- Provides psychological support to the client and his or her family and facilitates successful adaptive responses

(Continued on next page)

17

Figure 2-2. Scope of Oncology Nursing Practice in Genetics *(Continued)*

Advanced Practice Oncology Nurse *(cont.)*

Coordinator
• Facilitates genetic testing or therapeutic options

Consultant
• Routinely uses experts in cancer genetics as resources for information and for answering questions and solving problems
• Uses theoretical knowledge of basic genetics principles to guide the staff and the client and his or her immediate family

Educator
• Conducts an assessment of the learning and psychosocial needs of the client and his or her immediate family regarding genetic services
• Answers general genetic questions and addresses concerns
• Facilitates the interventions implemented by the cancer genetic healthcare team
• Integrates genetics information into education for staff, the client, and the client's family
• Evaluates clinical practice activities in terms of satisfaction and outcomes related to cancer genetic services

Researcher
• Identifies potential candidates; monitors and documents the client's participation in clinical trials

Administrator
• Participates in cancer genetic program and services development and monitoring

Advanced Practice Oncology Nurse With a Subspecialty in Genetics

Direct Care
• Conducts an in-depth personal and family assessment based on personal, medical, occupational, environmental, and family risk factors
• Performs an assessment based on prior understanding of genetic conditions and practical knowledge of what ordinarily would be expected
• Constructs a detailed pedigree expanded to the degree of reliable information but a minimum of three generations, including confirmation with medical records
• Establishes the relevancy of genetic information
• In collaboration with the cancer genetic healthcare team, uses genetics assessment data to contribute to the diagnosis of genetic risk or illness for the client and his or her family
• Evaluates eligibility for genetic testing or therapeutics
• Provides genetic counseling, which enhances voluntary and autonomous decision making
• Provides the education necessary for informed consent for genetic testing and/or therapeutics
• Remains sensitive to the ability of individuals and families to receive and understand genetic information
• Evaluates and monitors the impact of genetic conditions, therapeutics, or testing on the client and his or her extended family and intervenes as needed
• Identifies events typical of a suspected or actual genetic condition or situation and modifies the nursing plan in response to these events

(Continued on next page)

Figure 2-2. Scope of Oncology Nursing Practice in Genetics *(Continued)*

- Responds to the needs of the client and his or her extended family
- Provides psychological support to the client and his or her extended family and facilitates successful adaptive responses

Coordinator
- Coordinates and initiates the cancer genetic healthcare team's plan, including submission of genetic samples for testing, interpretation of test results, and delivery of results to the client and his or her family
- Administers and/or supervises the administration of genetic therapeutics

Consultant
- Provides consultative cancer genetic expertise to staff, the client, and the client's extended family

Educator
- Conducts an assessment of the learning and psychosocial needs of the client and his or her immediate family regarding genetic services and responds to needs that are both identified and anticipated
- Delivers genetic counseling services, answers complex genetic questions, and addresses concerns
- Develops further interventions based on typical expectations in regard to the suspected or actual genetic condition and the current situation
- Evaluates psychosocial and physical responses to genetic testing, diagnosis, and treatment
- Integrates the evaluation of responses into all aspects of care

Researcher
- Coordinates genetic clinical trials and uses research findings in care implementation
- Participates in the development of cancer genetic research trials

Administrator
- Develops and monitors cancer genetic programs and services

(Benner et al.). Nurses at both levels need other practitioners to help them to identify what they cannot recognize. Oncology nursing practice in genetics at the advanced practice level builds on the scope of practice described for the general oncology nurse and also may include, but is not limited to, the activities described in Figure 2-2.

The Advanced Practice Oncology Nurse With a Subspecialty in Genetics

Nurses at this level are advanced practice nurses whose education and clinical training in genetics extends beyond that of the advanced practice oncology nurse. The additional training, in the form of an academic degree and continuing education and experience specific to genetics or cancer genetics, prepares a nurse to

- Perform genetics-specific assessment and diagnosis.
- Conduct a physical examination from the genetic perspective.

- Develop and implement genetics-specific treatment plans.
- Monitor clients' and patients' status from the genetic perspective.
- Educate and counsel clients about genetic issues.
- Consult, collaborate with, and refer clients to other providers.

Advanced nursing practice in cancer genetics is administered by a nurse who, at minimum, has met the following three criteria.

1. Completion of an accredited graduate (master's or doctoral) program in nursing
2. Completion of graduate-level genetics course work, which includes content about human, molecular, biochemical, and population genetics; technological applications; and therapeutic modalities
3. Participation in genetic clinical training supervised by any combination of the following: genetics advanced practice nurse, clinical geneticist, and/or genetic counselor

Among the factors that distinguish advanced genetics nursing practice from basic genetics nursing practice are the complexity of decision making, leadership skills, the ability to negotiate complex organizations, and expanded practice skills and knowledge in nursing and cancer genetics (International Society of Nurses in Genetics, 1998).

Advanced practice oncology nurses with a subspecialty in genetics

- Ascertain which individuals, families, and populations need cancer genetics services.
- Provide and manage comprehensive care, which includes state-of-the-art cancer genetics counseling, screening, diagnosis, and therapy.
- Develop, evaluate, and improve cancer genetics services.
- Educate individuals, families, the general public, and healthcare professionals about cancer genetics.
- Assess, deliberate, and develop recommendations about the ethical, legal, and social consequences of new and existing genetics services and technology.

The advanced practice oncology nurse with a subspecialty in genetics practices at the proficient or expert stage as defined by Benner (1984) and Benner et al. (1996). At this level of practice, genetics is integrated into every aspect of oncology nursing care. The advanced practice oncology nurse with a subspecialty in genetics is able to establish the relevancy of information; relies on extensive practical knowledge from both oncology and genetics; and, in specific clinical situations, understands the significance of the patient's history, grasps the current situation, and modifies plans in response to events. The skills of the advanced practice oncology nurse with a subspecialty in genetics include, but are not limited to, those described in Figure 2-2.

Opportunities for Collaboration

Healthcare professionals expand their practice according to the changing needs of society and by applying new knowledge and advances in education. As a result, the changing roles of cancer genetics professionals may overlap those of other genetics healthcare providers. Comprehensive genetics nursing practice is a dynamic process that involves interdisciplinary collegiality and collaboration with genetics and other healthcare professionals to serve a shared mission: helping individuals to reach their self-defined health outcome. Nursing in cancer genetics unites nursing, medicine, and counseling with the science of oncology and genetics.

Incorporation of Cancer Genetics in Various Practice Settings

The incorporation of genetics into oncology nursing practice occurs in settings that encompass the entire spectrum of cancer care. This includes settings of health promotion, prevention, and detection; surgical, medical, and radiation oncology; and bone marrow transplantation. Cancer genetics is not simply a subspecialty; it is the scientific basis for understanding the process of carcinogenesis and the response of cancer to intervention. Therefore, genetics permeates all aspects of oncology nursing practice and has implications for the nurse in any and all oncology practice settings.

References

American Nurses Association & Oncology Nursing Society. (1996). *Statement on the scope and standards of oncology nursing practice*. Washington, DC: American Nurses Publishing.

Anderson, G. (1996). The evolution and status of genetics education in nursing in the United States 1983–1995. *Image, 28*, 101–106.

Benner, P. (1984). *From novice to expert: Excellence and power in clinical nursing practice*. Menlo Park, CA: Addison-Wesley.

Benner, P.A., Tanner, C.A., & Chesla, C.A. (1996). *Expertise in nursing practice*. New York: Springer.

Collins, F.S., & McKusick, V.A. (2001). Implications of the Human Genome Project for medical science. *JAMA, 285*, 540–544.

Dimond, E., Calzone, K., Davis, J., & Jenkins, J. (1998). The role of the nurse in cancer genetics. *Cancer Nursing, 21*, 57–75.

Donaldson, S. (1997). The genetic social revolution and the professional status of nursing. *Nursing Outlook, 45,* 278–279.

George, J.B. (1992). Genetics: Challenges for nursing education. *Journal of Pediatric Nursing, 7,* 5–8.

Holtzman, N.A. (1992). The diffusion of new genetic tests for predicting disease. *FASEB Journal, 6,* 2806–2812.

International Society of Nurses in Genetics. (1998). *Statement on the scope and standards of genetics clinical nursing practice.* Washington, DC: American Nurses Publishing.

Livingston, D.M. (1997). Genetics is coming to oncology. *JAMA, 277,* 1476–1477.

Olsen, S.J., Baxendale-Cox, L., & Mock, V. (2000). Genetics and nursing: Planning for the future. *Nursing Clinics of North America, 35,* xv–xx.

Scanlon, C., & Fibison, W. (1995). *Managing genetic information: Implications for nursing practice.* Washington, DC: American Nurses Publishing.

3

The Biology of Cancer

Lois J. Loescher, PhD, RN, and Luke Whitesell, MD

Editors' note: Learning about genes and their function means learning a new language. To help to build your genetics vocabulary, note the terms presented in boldface in this chapter. These are key terms, and their definitions appear in the glossary in the back matter of this text. Boldface key terms also appear in Chapters 5 and 6. Other ways to improve your genetics language skills are to continue reading about cancer genetics, visit Web sites about genetics, and join professional groups that have genetics as their focus. (See the resources listed in Chapter 10.) Remember that immersion—reading, practicing, and actually speaking—is the best way to learn any language. The language of cancer genetics may seem overwhelming at first. Don't be discouraged if the concepts are not clear after one reading. Comprehension of the language will increase as you build your vocabulary.

Introduction

Clinically, cancer comprises more than 100 diseases that vary in regard to age of the patient at onset and disease growth rate, differentiation, detectability, invasiveness, metastatic potential, response to treatment, and prognosis. On the molecular and cellular levels, however, cancer may actually be just a few diseases caused by similar genetic alterations and defects in cell function. Ultimately, cancer results from abnormal **gene expression** that is largely attributable to alterations in deoxyribonucleic acid (DNA) and gene **transcription** or **translation.** This chapter will present an overview of cancer biology, focusing on genetic mechanisms that may transform a normal cell into a cancer cell.

DNA and Chromosomes: Structure and Function

The **human genome,** or "master blueprint" of human genetic potential, consists of 23 pairs of chromosomes. A chromosome is a single DNA molecule that is long, intricately coiled, and composed of tightly interspersed **proteins.** The 23 pairs of chromosomes consist of 22 pairs of **autosomes,** or nonsex **chromosomes,** and one pair of sex chromosomes (XX or XY) that reside within the **nucleus** of every human cell. People inherit one chromosome of the pair from their father and the other from their mother. A chromosome has a long arm (q) and a short arm (p). Each chromosome has a unique banding pattern that identifies specific regions (see Figure 3-1). For example, a **gene** that defines susceptibility to breast and ovarian cancer, **BRCA1,** is on chromosome 17q21, or band 21 on the long arm of chromosome 17 (see Figure 3-1).

Figure 3-1. Chromosome 17

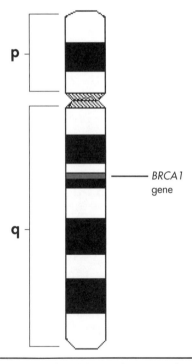

This drawing shows the petite (p) arm, long (q) arm, chromosome bands, and location of the BRCA1 gene within band 21.

If all the strands of DNA in a person's body were unwound and set end to end, they would stretch more than 5 feet but would be only 50 trillionths of an inch wide. Each DNA molecule consists of antiparallel double strands wound around each other to resemble a twisted staircase (see Figure 3-2). Each side strand is

---

Figure 3-2. The DNA Molecule

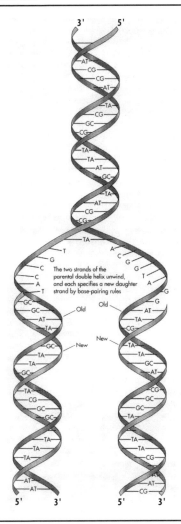

This drawing shows base pairs and daughter strands.

Note. From *Recombinant DNA* (2nd ed.) (p. 22) by J.D. Watson, M. Gilman, J. Witkowski, and M. Zollar, 1992, New York: Scientific American Books. Copyright 1992, 1983 by James D. Watson, Michael Gilman, Jan Witkowski, and Mark Zollar. Reprinted with permission.

an arrangement of units called **nucleotides,** consisting of one sugar, one phosphate, and a nitrogenous base. The nucleotides are linked together in a chain consisting of an alternating series of sugar and phosphate residues. The 5' (5 prime) position of one pentose ring is connected to the 3' (3 prime) position of the next pentose ring via a phosphate group. As a result, this "backbone" consists of 5'-3' phosphodiester linkages. The nitrogenous bases stick out from this repetitive backbone and form the "steps" of the staircase.

The steps consist of four DNA bases: the pyrimidine bases (**cytosine** and **thymine**) and the purine bases (**guanine** and **adenine**). These bases form the genetic alphabet and are abbreviated C, T, G, and A, respectively. The specific order of the bases arranged along one strand of the sugar-phosphate backbone is the **DNA sequence.** By means of weak hydrogen bonds, one strand of DNA pairs with the other strand. C on one strand always pairs with G on the other strand; similarly, T always pairs with A. This phenomenon is called complementary base pairing, and each resulting twosome is a **base pair.** The human genome contains approximately three billion base pairs. Base pairing is critical for the storage, retrieval, and transfer of genetic information, whether DNA is being copied or read (Rosenthal, 1994). In double-stranded DNA, the nucleotide sequence of the upper strand is always written and read in the 5' to 3' direction; the lower strand is written and read in the 3' to 5' direction:

<u>5' GCA</u>

3' CGT

Complementary base pairs not only ensure the structural integrity of DNA, but also are essential for its replication. Each time a **cell** divides into two daughter cells, its full genome is duplicated in the nucleus.

> Complementary DNA base pairing (A-T and G-C) is critical for the storage, retrieval, and transfer of genetic information.

Cell division in **somatic cells** (**mitosis**) results in two daughter cells with the same number of chromosomes as the parent cell (46 chromosomes). During cell division, the DNA unwinds down the middle, causing the weak bonds between the base pairs to break. Each strand serves as a template and directs synthesis of a new complementary strand (daughter strand), with free nucleotides matching up with their complementary bases on each of the separated strands (see Figure 3-2). This process allows the dividing cell to pass on its entire genetic content to its progeny.

Germ cells—also called gametes, or ovum and sperm—form during meiosis, a two-stage process of reduction and division. A reduction of the chromosome number by half (23) during meiosis is necessary so the original number of chromosomes, 46, is restored following fertilization. Without this process, the number of chromosomes in offspring would be doubled.

Genes are the smallest functional units of inherited information in DNA. Genes are segments, or regions, of DNA that occupy specific sites, or loci, on particular chromosomes. Genes consist of DNA sequences (nucleotides) that code for specific proteins. The human genome packs approximately 30,000–40,000 genes into the 46 chromosomes. Although each human gene often extends over thousands of bases, only about 10% of the genome includes protein-coding sequences of genes. These coding sequences are called exons. Sequences of genes with no coding function are called introns. Because each person inherits a set of chromosomes from each parent, alternate forms of genes, called **alleles,** may be present in the pair. A person with the same allele on both members of a chromosome pair is said to be homozygous for a particular trait; someone who has two different alleles is said to be **heterozygous.** Wild-type genes are "normal" forms of genes, meaning that the base pairs and nucleotide sequences are in the proper order. Mutant genes are abnormal forms in which the base pairs and proper nucleotide sequences have become altered.

> Genes are regions of DNA that occupy specific loci on chromosomes. Specific DNA nucleotide sequences in genes encode specific proteins, which are the primary products of gene expression.

Gene Expression

DNA has one function: to store genetic information used for the synthesis of proteins and **enzymes.** DNA stores this genetic information as a **genetic code.** The code consists of triplets of bases called **codons,** which specify the amino acid sequence of a protein. Proteins are made up of **amino acids.** Amino acids are called the body's building blocks because they are the compounds essential to body structures and chemical reactions. Of the 64 possible codons, three are stop codons. These direct termination of protein synthesis. Each of the other 61 codons codes for an amino acid. There are 20 naturally occurring amino acids; more than one codon can code for the same amino acid. This overlap may protect against the detrimental effects that could occur if a **mutation** in a codon changed the code, thereby forming the wrong amino acid. If that happened, another codon could still code for the same amino acid.

The primary product of gene expression is a protein. Protein synthesis occurs in the cytoplasm of the cell, so genetic information must travel from the cell nucleus to the cytoplasm (see Figure 3-3). This is accomplished in a process called transcription, in which **ribonucleic acid (RNA)** is synthesized from the genetic information encoded by DNA.

Figure 3-3. Gene Expression in Human Cells

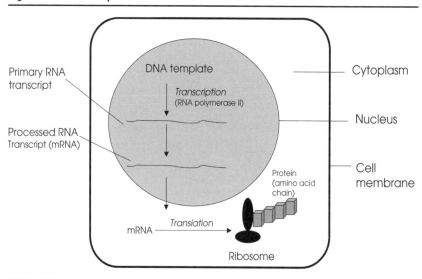

The messenger RNA (mRNA) is processed in the nucleus before transport to the cytoplasm, where it programs the translation machinery.

The enzymes that carry out transcription are called **RNA polymerases.** Certain DNA sequences tell RNA polymerase where to start transcription. During the course of transcription, one strand of DNA (the template) is copied into **messenger RNA (mRNA).** After additional processing in the nucleus, mRNA carries the genetic message into the cytoplasm to the **ribosomes,** molecular machines in which RNA directs the assembly of the amino acids that constitute proteins. The process of amino acid assembly is called translation.

In the translation process, each amino acid is carried to the ribosome by transfer RNA (tRNA). tRNA docks onto a specific coding region of mRNA. In mRNA, amino acid chains are arranged in the same order as the codons of the DNA strand. In RNA, however, uracil, U, substitutes for T. For example, the DNA sequence

5'ATGGGTGGATATCCCTAG 3'

is transcribed into the mRNA sequence

5'AUGGGUGGAUAUCCCUAG 3'

This mRNA is then translated into the amino acid chain methionine-glycine-glycine-tyrosine-proline.

Amino acid chains go through post-translational changes, such as folding upon the nucleus, assembling with other chains, or dropping off a part of a chain to form the mature protein complexes that participate in specific cellular functions. These functions include directing the duplication, replacement, and differentiation of cells.

During transcription, one strand of DNA is copied into mRNA.

During translation, RNA catalyzes the assembly of amino acids that make up proteins.

A mutation is a permanent change in the nucleotide sequence of DNA. Mutations occur frequently and can alter gene structure and regulatory sites (e.g., **exons**). Everyone has cells that have mutations in at least one gene, yet most mutations are harmless. A mutation is of concern only if it gives rise to a clonal population of cells (see Tumorigenesis, which appears later in this chapter) or affects a cell that is particularly sensitive to mutation.

Causes of Mutations

Mutations may arise during DNA replication and recombination, be caused by mutagens (environmental agents that prompt mutations), or arise spontaneously. Replication errors are rare, occurring in only one of 100 million bases. More frequently, DNA rearranges itself by recombination, a process whereby DNA is lost or may be inserted into the gene. Recombination may result in loss of control of gene expression or may disrupt the coding sequence of the gene. Mutagens that damage DNA may be made by humans (e.g., pesticides, organic chemicals, alkylating agents), occur naturally (e.g., plant toxins), or be generated during normal cellular metabolism. Chemically damaged DNA can cause incorrect base pairing during replication, resulting in a mutation being passed to daughter strands. Radiation—including gamma rays, x-rays, and ultraviolet radiation—can damage and distort DNA, impairing transcription and replication. DNA may spontaneously undergo alterations that result in self-damage. For example, one base can spontaneously change into another base, causing abnormal base pairing during subsequent replication.

Mutations may be caused by mutagens, occur during DNA replication or recombination, or arise spontaneously.

Types of Mutations Associated With Cancer

Point Mutations

Single-base substitutions, in which a single base is substituted for another base, are called point mutations. Point mutations are the most common types of mutations. Point mutations in DNA sequences that encode proteins are classified as silent, missense, or nonsense mutations (see Figure 3-4).

Figure 3-4. Point Mutations

Wild type (normal)	ATG	GCC	TGC	AAA	CGC	TGG
	Met	Ala	Cys	Lys	Arg	Trp
		↓				
Silent point mutation	ATG	GCṪ	TGC	AAA	CGC	TGG
(protein product unchanged)	Met	Ala	Cys	Lys	Arg	Trp
			↓			
Missense point mutation	ATG	GCC	ĠGC	AAA	GCG	TGG
(results in a different protein product)	Met	Ala	Arg	Lys	Arg	Trp
				↓		
Nonsense point mutation	ATG	GCC	TGȦ	AAA	GCG	TGG
(results in stop codon)	Met	Ala	–	–	–	–

The top rows in each set are DNA codons. The individual bases are A (adenine), T (thymine), G (guanine), and C (cytosine). The bottom rows in each set are amino acids encoded by the bases: Met (methionine), Ala (alanine), Cys (cysteine), Lys (lysine), Arg (arginine), and Trp (tryptophan).

Note. Used with permission of M.S. Dodson, PhD.

Silent Point Mutations

A silent point mutation is a base substitution in the third position of a codon, which usually results in the generation of a synonymous codon. In other words, the amino acid encoded by the gene does not change. Thus, the protein product of the gene is unaltered.

Missense Point Mutations

A base substitution that results in the generation of a codon specifying a different amino acid is a missense point mutation. In a missense point mutation, an amino acid in the sequence of the gene product changes. This may or may not result in a deleterious gene product, depending on the amino acid that has been substituted. If the structure and properties of the normal and substituted amino acids are similar, no deleterious gene products will result. If the structure and properties of the two amino acids are very different, a deleterious gene product may result.

Nonsense Point Mutations

A **nonsense point mutation** occurs when a base substitution results in the generation of a stop codon, meaning that the gene product will be truncated (lopped off) and, probably, nonfunctional. Nonsense point mutations are deleterious mutations.

Deletions and Insertions

A base **deletion** occurs when one or more base pairs are lost from DNA. In Figure 3-5, three DNA bases constitute each amino acid. One way to think of reading an amino acid sequence, then, is to think of a "reading frame," a window through which you always see three, and only three, bases. In Figure 3-5, brackets represent the reading frame. Deletion of one or two bases changes the reading frame of the sequence; the frame grows to allow a view of three bases, but they may not be the same three that the frame comprised before the deletion. The result is an altered message called a frameshift mutation. The gene product of such a mutation usually is nonfunctional. If a deletion of three or a multiple of three base pairs occurs, the reading frame remains intact. **Insertion** of additional base pairs also may lead to a frameshift mutation, depending on whether multiples of three base pairs are inserted.

Combinations of insertions and deletions are possible. In some cases, in fact, an insertion restores the reading frame of a gene with a deletion mutation (or vice versa). The gene product would contain a garbled amino acid sequence between the insertion and deletion, but it is otherwise correct.

Types of mutations frequently associated with cancers are point mutations (silent, missense, and nonsense mutations) and insertion and deletion mutations (frameshift mutations).

Figure 3-5. Insertion and Deletion (Frameshift) Mutations

Wild type (normal)	ATG	GCC	TGC	AAA	CGC	TGG
	Met	Ala	Cys	Lys	Arg	Trp
Frameshift (deletion of one base)	ATG Met	GC-- ⌞Ala⌟	TGC ⌞Ala⌟	AAA ⌞Asn⌟	CGC ⌞Ala⌟	TGG
Frameshift (insertion of one base)	ATG Met	GCC Ala	C TGC ⌞Leu⌟	AAA ⌞Gln⌟	CGC ⌞Thr⌟	TGG ⌞Leu⌟
Frameshift (insertion of one base and deletion of one base)	ATG Met	GCC Ala	C TGC ⌞Leu⌟	AAA ⌞Gln⌟	--GC ⌞Ser⌟	TGG Trp

The top rows in each set are DNA bases: A (adenine), T (thymine), C (cytosine), and G (guanine). The bottom rows in each set are amino acids encoded by the bases: Ala (alanine), Arg (arginine), Asn (asparagine), Cys (cysteine), Gln (glutamine), Leu (leucine), Lys (lysine), Met (methionine), Ser (serine), Thr (threonine), and Trp (tryptophan).

Note. Used with permission of M.S. Dodson, PhD.

Gene Transmission in Cancers

All cancers have a genetic component. Cancers can be simplistically categorized as two different types of genetic conditions: somatic genetic disorders and inherited genetic diseases. Most cancers are sporadic and fall under the category of somatic genetic disease. Sporadic cancers are caused by the new appearance of an abnormal form of a gene (i.e., an acquired mutation) in a somatic cell. Acquired mutations can occur throughout a lifetime and generally are not inherited.

> Most cancers are sporadic, caused by a series of acquired somatic mutations. A small percentage of cancers are genetically predisposed: The mutation is transmitted from one generation to the next via the germ cells.

A single-gene disorder occurs when an allele is mutated at a **single locus** on one or both chromosomes in a pair. If the predisposition to develop a cancer is inherited, this predisposition is thought to result from the alteration of a single gene. The pattern of single-gene disorders usually is **autosomal dominant.** In autosomal dominant inheritance, the locus of the gene is on an autosome. One allele is sufficient to transmit a trait or characteristic (**phenotype**). In other words, the allele is dominant. If a cell contains one **dominant** allele and one recessive allele, the dominant allele masks the presence of the recessive allele. However, some cancer genes transmitted through an autosomal dominant pattern at the phenotypic level may exhibit recessive characteristics at the molecular level (see Tumor Suppressor Genes, later in this chapter). Examples of cancers associated with the inheritance of a single defective gene are *BRCA1*-related breast and ovarian cancer and retinoblastoma. Cancers that develop in the context of a known inherited genetic defect account for approximately 5%–10% of all cancers.

In reality, cancer is a multifactorial disease in which gene-environment interactions play a key developmental role. These interactions are complex but can be simplistically viewed as genes acting in a specific cellular environment to generate a malignant phenotype and the environment (e.g., mutagens) acting on genetic material to produce a specific phenotype.

> Cancer is a multifactorial disease in that environmental factors and genes interact to affect its development.

Genes Implicated in Cancers

Recent studies have identified three groups of genes that mutate frequently and whose mutations cause cancer: **oncogenes,** tumor suppressor genes, and mutator genes (Vogelstein & Kinzler, 1998).

Oncogenes and Proto-Oncogenes

Oncogenes are genes that encode proteins (oncoproteins) whose action promotes cell proliferation. Oncogenes are excessively or inappropriately active versions of normal cellular genes (**proto-oncogenes**) (Strachan & Read, 1999). Almost all proto-oncogenes participate in normal transduction pathways that can be thought of as molecular bucket brigades. These brigades relay growth-stimulating signals (growth factors), via growth factor receptors, from outside to inside the cell (Hanahan & Weinberg, 2000; Weinberg, 1996). Figure 3-6 illustrates how these pathways transmit information to signal-transduction proteins and then to transcription factors in the nucleus. The transcription factors affect growth factor genes, which regulate cell behavior. Because the pathways control such essential functions as cell division, death, and motility, signaling is highly regulated. Signaling regulation is achieved through alterations in the enzymatic activity of key components in the pathways and through the assembly of large multimolecular signaling complexes within discrete cellular locations.

The complexity of these pathways results in two important implications for tumor development. First, the large number of components involved provides many potential targets that can activate oncogenes and explains the large num-

Figure 3-6. Signal Transduction by Oncogenes

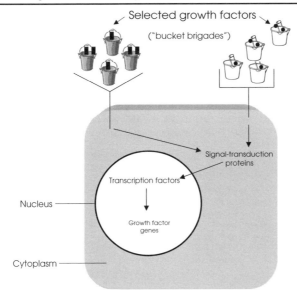

The transduction pathways are like molecular bucket brigades that deliver growth factors to the cell.

ber of proto-oncogenes that have been identified. Second, because of the intrinsic redundancy and "cross talk" within the pathways, human cancers rarely result from aberrant activation of a single proto-oncogene.

Consider an analogy to a car. A cell containing oncogenes is like a car in high gear that has its accelerator stuck to the floor: Cell growth is moving at top speed (Weinberg, 1994). Oncogenes are dominant in that only one allele of each pair needs to mutate for the gene to be activated. Oncogene-activation mechanisms result in a gain of function. In a gain of function, protein products become excessively active without appropriate regulation by the cell. Gain-of-function events increase cell proliferation and decrease cell differentiation (see Figure 3-7).

> Proto-oncogenes are normal genes that, when mutated, become oncogenes. Oncogenes cause gain of function (increased cell proliferation), largely through overactivation of signal-transduction pathways.

Figure 3-7. Mechanisms of Proto-Oncogene Activation Known to Occur in Human Tumors

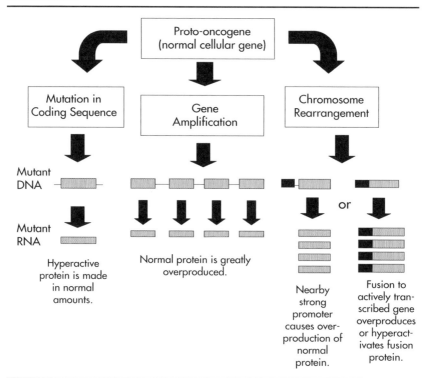

Mutations can occur in the coding sequence, through gene amplification, or by chromosome rearrangement.

Activating mutations in oncogenes usually are somatic events. Inherited mutations would likely be lethal during embryonic development. An oncogene that can be inherited, however, is the receptor tyrosine kinase (*RET*) proto-oncogene, which is associated with multiple endocrine neoplasia type 2A, 2B, and familial medullary thyroid carcinoma. These syndromes are characterized by a markedly increased incidence of medullary thyroid carcinoma, pheochromocytoma, and hyperparathyroidism.

Oncogene Classification

Oncogenes are classified according to their overall function. Broad classes of oncogenes include secreted growth factors, cell-surface growth-factor receptors, nonreceptor tyrosine kinases, membrane-associated G proteins, cytoplasmic serine threonine kinases, and transcription factors. Table 3-1 lists selected oncogenes and their cellular function.

Growth factors: Most growth factors act extracellularly as chemical signals that regulate cellular behavior. Growth factors affect cell growth, differentiation, and survival and help to determine tissue architecture and morphology. In signaling pathways, growth factors initiate signal transduction across the cell membrane. As Figure 3-6 shows, growth factors must interact with specific receptors to accomplish signaling.

The binding of a growth factor to a receptor initiates a signal that activates other cytoplasmic proteins, causing transmission of a signal to the cell nucleus. The end result of transmission is a change in the expression of certain genes that help to usher the cell through its growth cycle (Weinberg, 1996). Several growth factors, when overproduced, are associated with cancers. Vascular endothelial growth factor (VEGF) plays an important role in tumor neoangiogenesis—that is, the growth of new vessels in a tumor. VEGF is expressed in metastatic breast and colorectal cancers. Endothelial cells overexpress **fibroblast** growth factor (FGF) in hemangiomas. Overexpression of platelet-derived growth factor (PDGF) has been reported in sarcomas and gliomas. Other growth factors implicated in cancer development include epidermal growth factor (EGF), transforming growth factor (TGF), and colony-stimulating factor (CSF).

Growth factor receptors: Oncogenic growth factor receptors (GFRs) release proliferative signals into the cytoplasm (Weinberg, 1996), even in the absence of growth factors. Most GFRs possess tyrosine kinase (TK) activity, or the activity of adding inorganic phosphate to the amino acid tyrosine. Activation of TK receptors leads to biochemical reactions that stimulate mitotic cell division. As a result, TKs play a key role in regulating cell proliferation (Ruddon, 1995). Increased TK activity can cause clonal expansion of cells, a topic that will be discussed later in this chapter.

Table 3-1. Selected Oncogenes and Their Cellular Functions

Gene	Description
ABL1	• Formerly known as *ABL* (v-abl Abelson murine strain of leukemia viral homolog 1) • Codes for a nonreceptor tyrosine-specific protein kinase in the cell membrane, cytoplasm, and nucleus • Associated with 90% of cases of chronic myeloid leukemia, 25%–30% of adult cases of acute lymphoblastic leukemia, and rare cases of acute myelogenous leukemia • Located on chromosome 9q324.1
BRAF	• Homolog of v-raf murine sarcoma viral oncogene B1 • Codes for a "signal transducer" that resides in the cell membrane • Associated with gastric carcinoma • Located on chromosome 7q34
CSF1R	• Formerly known as *FMS* (McDonough feline sarcoma viral [v-fms] oncogene homolog) • Codes for a receptor of epidermal growth factor in the protein-tyrosine kinase family • Functions as a macrophage colony-stimulating factor receptor in the growth of tumors • Associated with ovarian cancer • Located on chromosome 5q33.2–q33.3
EGFR	• Formerly known as *ERBB1* (v-erb-B avian erythroblastic leukemia viral oncogene homolog) • Codes for an epidermal growth factor receptor in the protein-tyrosine kinase family • Involved in squamous cell carcinomas, astrocytoma, and melanoma • Located on chromosome 7p12.3–p12.1
ERBB2	• Also called *HER2/NEU* (v-erb-B-2 avian erythroblastic leukemia viral oncogene homolog 2) • Codes for an epidermal growth factor-like receptor protein in the tyrosine kinase family • Involved in breast, ovarian, lung, gastric, and salivary gland cancers • Overexpression of *ERBB2* increases the aggressiveness of breast cancer, inhibits paclitaxel-induced apoptosis • Located on chromosome 17q21.1
FES	• Also called *FPS* or feline sarcoma (Snyder-Theilen) viral (v-fes)/Fujinami avian sarcoma viral (v-fps) oncogene homolog • Codes for a nonreceptor tyrosine-specific protein kinase in the cell membrane • Associated with acute promyelocytic leukemia, lung cancer, and bladder cancer • Located on chromosome 15q26.1

(Continued on next page)

Table 3-1. Selected Oncogenes and Their Cellular Functions *(Continued)*

Gene	Description
FGF3	• Also called *INT2* (murine mammary tumor virus integration site [v-int-2] oncogene homolog) • Codes for a fibroblast growth factor • Associated with glioblastoma and breast cancer • Located on chromosome 11q13
FGF4	• Also called *HST* (heparin secretory transforming protein 1) or *KFGF* (Kaposi sarcoma fibroblast growth factor) • Codes for a fibroblast growth factor • Associated with glioblastoma and gastric cancer • Located on chromosome 11q13.3
FOS	• Homolog of vfos *FBJ* murine osteosarcoma viral oncogene • Codes for a factor involved in the transcription of nuclear DNA • Member of a family of proteins that have a characteristic "leucine zipper" structure • Involved in lung cancer • Located on chromosome 14q24.3
HRAS	• Homolog of v-Ha-ras Harvey rat sarcoma viral oncogene • Codes for a cellular membrane protein that functions as a GTPase • Involved in bladder, breast, lung, kidney, and colon cancers as well as melanoma • Located on chromosome 11p15.5–p15.1
JUN	• Homolog of v-jun avian sarcoma virus 17 oncogene • Also called *AP1* (activator protein 1) • Codes for a factor involved in the transcription of nuclear DNA • Member of a family of proteins that have a characteristic "leucine zipper" structure • Involved with lung cancer
KRAS2	• Homolog of v-Ki-ras2 Kirsten rat sarcoma 2 viral oncogene • Codes for a cellular membrane protein that functions as a GTPase • Involved in breast, pancreatic, thyroid, colorectal, bladder, and lung cancers as well as acute myeloid leukemia • Located on chromosome 12p12.1
LCK	• Codes for a lymphocyte-specific protein-tyrosine kinase in the cell membrane • Involved in lung cancer and colon carcinoma • Located on chromosome 1p35–p34.3
MYC	• Homolog of v-myc avian myelocytomatosis viral oncogene • Formerly known as *C-MYC* • Codes for a factor involved in activating transcription of growth-promoting genes in the nucleus

(Continued on next page)

Table 3-1. Selected Oncogenes and Their Cellular Functions (Continued)

Gene	Description
MYC (cont.)	• Member of a family of proteins that have a characteristic "helix-loop-helix" structure • Associated with Burkitt lymphoma and lung, breast, ovarian, and colon cancers • Located on chromosome 8q24.12–q24.13
MYCL1	• Homolog 1 of v-myc avian myelocytomatosis viral oncogene, lung carcinoma derived • Formerly known as L-MYC • Codes for a factor involved in activating transcription of growth-promoting genes in the nucleus • Member of a family of proteins that have a characteristic "helix-loop-helix" structure • Associated with lung cancer • Located on chromosome 1p34.3
MYCN	• Homolog of v-myc avian myelocytomatosis viral-related oncogene, neuroblastoma-derived • Formerly known as N-MYC • Codes for a factor involved in activating transcription of growth-promoting genes in the nucleus • Member of a family of proteins that have a characteristic "helix-loop-helix" structure • Associated with neuroblastoma and small-cell lung cancer • Located on chromosome 2p24.1
NRAS	• Homolog of neuroblastoma RAS viral (v-ras) oncogene • Codes for a protein that relays a stimulatory signal • Codes for a cellular membrane protein that functions as a GTPase • Involved in ovarian, rectal, and thyroid cancers, acute myeloid leukemia, and melanoma • Located on chromosome 1p13.2
RET	• RET (rearranged during transfection) proto-oncogene • Codes for a truncated, receptor-like cell-surface protein in the protein-tyrosine kinase family • Associated with medullary thyroid carcinoma and multiple endocrine neoplasia type II (MEN 2), and pheochromocytoma • Located on chromosome 10q11.2
ROS1	• Homolog 1 of v-ros avian UR2 sarcoma virus oncogene • Codes for an insulin receptor-like protein-tyrosine kinase in the cell membrane • Associated with breast cancer and glioblastoma • Located on chromosome 6q22

(Continued on next page)

Table 3-1. Selected Oncogenes and Their Cellular Functions *(Continued)*

Gene	Description
SRC	• v-src avian sarcoma (Schmidt-Ruppin A-2) viral oncogene homolog or ASV (avian sarcoma virus) • Codes for a nonreceptor protein-tyrosine kinase • Associated with colon carcinoma • Located on chromosome 20q12–q13
TCF3	• Also called *E2A* (e2-alpha immunoglobulin enhancer-binder factors E12/E47) or *ITF1* (immunoglobulin transcription factor 1) • Codes for a factor involved in the transcription of nuclear DNA • Member of a family of proteins that have a characteristic "helix-loop-helix" structure • Associated with acute lymphoblastic leukemia • Located on chromosome 19p13.3

Note. From "Oncogenes and Proto-Oncogenes" by E. Pergament and M. Fiddler (Eds.), *The Genetics of Cancer*, 2001, Melville, NY: PRR, Inc. Available at www.intouchlive.com/cancergenetics/onco.htm. Copyright 2001 by PRR, Inc. Reprinted with permission.

Examples of GFRs that are oncogenic when overexpressed are epidermal growth factor receptor *(EGFR)*, *ERBB2*, and *TGFB*. A variety of cancers express *EGFR*, including non-small cell lung cancer and breast, ovarian, and colorectal cancers. Head and neck cancers exhibit about 80%–100% overexpression of *EGFR*. Overexpression of *EGFR* in these tumors correlates with low survival. Overexpression of *ERBB2* coincides with an aggressive clinical course of certain cancers, including ovarian and breast cancers. *EGFR* and *TGFB* together are a prognostic marker for tumor relapse and decreased survival.

Nonreceptor tyrosine kinases: Some oncogenes do not require a receptor to initiate TK activity at the cell membrane. Members of the *SRC* gene family initiate TK activity that is regulated by the C terminus of the protein. Such *SRC*-initiated activity is increased in neuroblastoma, small-cell lung cancer, colon and breast adenocarcinomas, and rhabdomyosarcoma (Ruddon, 1995).

Membrane-associated G proteins: Guanine nucleotide-binding proteins (G proteins) act as signal transducers—on-off switches—for cell-surface growth-factor receptors. G proteins disrupt part of the signal cascade that occurs in the cell cytoplasm.

G proteins are members of the *RAS* superfamily, which comprises more than 50 members. The *RAS* proteins are known to act at the cell membrane to cause malignant transformation. Proteins encoded by normal *RAS* genes transmit stimulatory signals from GFRs to other proteins. Mutant *RAS* genes activate signaling pathways, even when unprompted by GFRs. Mutant *RAS* is found in virtually all types of human cancer and occurs in approximately two-thirds of all malignant tumors.

Serine threonine kinases: Oncoproteins with serine threonine protein kinase activity are important components of intracellular signal transduction. The prototype serine threonine kinase in the cytoplasm, *RAF1*, is activated by TK-associated receptors (Ruddon, 1995). In the signal-transduction pathway, *RAF1* acts as an intermediary between *RAS* on the cell membrane and the cell nucleus by activating a series of other kinases known as mitogen-activated protein (MAP) kinases. These are critical for regulating the onset of cell division.

Transcription factors: Transcription factors (TFs) are proteins that bind to DNA and cause changes in gene expression. Mutation of the transcription factors that regulate genes involved in growth and survival drives malignant transformation in many tumors. TFs have specific structures that "recognize" specific DNA sequences. Examples of oncogenic TFs are proteins with activator protein-1 (AP-1) activity (e.g., *JUN*, *FOS*), which are implicated in signal-dependent processes that control cell growth and, hence, carcinogenesis (Papavassiliou, 1995). Oncogenic TFs are associated with Ewing's sarcoma, clear-cell sarcoma, alveolar rhabdomyosarcoma, and many kinds of leukemia. All these conditions are characterized by chromosomal translocation (see Chromosomal Abnormalities, later in this chapter) (Latchman, 1996). The gene *TP53*, considered a tumor suppressor gene (see the next section) also acts as a TF. In this role, *TP53* "senses" DNA damage and halts cell division by controlling expression of other genes that directly regulate the cell cycle.

> Tumor suppressor genes normally block the action of growth-promoting proteins. In cancer cells, both alleles of a pair are mutated, or lost. Mutated TS genes cause loss of function.

Tumor Suppressor Genes

Tumor suppressor (TS) genes normally suppress or negatively regulate cell proliferation by encoding proteins that block the action of growth-promoting proteins. If cell growth is as out of control as a car with a stuck accelerator, then TS genes are the brakes, which suppress oncogenesis. At the cellular level, TS genes are recessive in that both alleles of a pair are mutated, or "lost," in cancer cells. In other words, loss or mutation of both copies of the gene is required for tumorigenesis.

Discovery and Mechanisms of TS Genes: Retinoblastoma

Studies of retinoblastoma provided initial clinical evidence of the existence and behavior of TS genes and information about their behavior. Retinoblastoma is a malignant eye tumor that occurs in children. The tumor can be either hereditary or sporadic. In the hereditary form, multiple tumors occur in early childhood and frequently involve both eyes. In the sporadic form, a single tumor forms, usually when the patient is older. A careful analysis by Knudson (1971) of families with retinoblastoma led to the "two-hit" hypothesis of cancer development.

In the hereditary form of retinoblastoma, Knudson (1971) proposed that a first mutation is transmitted in the germ line and that all cells of the body lack one normal allele of the purported *RB* gene. Eye tumors occur, Knudson continued, only when the remaining normal allele is lost or inactivated by somatic mutation. This second event could be relatively common, leading to the multifocal appearance of the hereditary form. In the sporadic form, Knudson hypothesized that all cells contain two functional copies of the putative (that is, hypothesized but not yet discovered) *RB* gene, meaning that tumors could arise only when both copies are lost or inactivated within the same target cell. Such a coincidence is rare and consistent with the unifocal presentation of sporadic retinoblastoma.

When researchers cloned the *RB* gene, they found that its mutations were highly associated with retinoblastoma. The frequent and reproducible inactivation of *RB* provided strong circumstantial evidence that an actual TS gene had been isolated. The loss of function of *RB* is now known to play a role in the development of osteosarcoma as well as in some common malignancies of adults, including lung, breast, and bladder cancers. Figure 3-8 summarizes the TS mechanisms as they relate to retinoblastoma.

Loss of Heterozygosity

Commonly, the first inherited mutation of a TS gene is a small change confined to the actual gene. Large deletions probably would be lethal if carried in every cell. Frequently, however, the second mutation involves the loss of all or part of a chromosome, resulting in allelic loss of any marker close to the TS gene. Thus, if a patient with cancer is heterozygous for a specific genetic marker located close to the TS gene, the tumor tissue loses this heterozygosity. Most tumor specimens in studies of loss of heterozygosity (LOH) contain a mixture of tumor and nontumor tissue, indicating a decreased relative intensity of tumor, rather than a total loss of the band from one allele (Strachan & Read, 1999). Investigators examining LOH have been able to identify and clone an increasing number of TS genes that, when mutated, are critical to the development of human cancers (see Table 3-2).

The gene *TP53* (located on 17p13) is one of the most well-studied TS genes. Deletions and mutations of *TP53* are common in a wide variety of cancers, including lung, breast, esophageal, liver, bladder, and ovarian carcinomas; brain tumors; sarcomas; lymphomas; and leukemias. Overall, *TP53* mutations may contribute to approximately 50% of all human cancers, making *TP53* the most

Figure 3-8. The Loss of Heterozygosity in Retinoblastoma

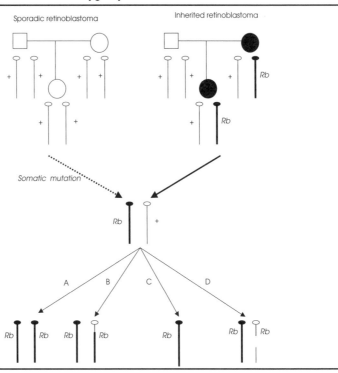

Mutations in the *RB* genes may be somatic or inherited. A second mutational event eliminates the normal allele (noted as +) by different mechanisms. Mechanism A illustrates chromosome loss followed by reduplication. Mechanism B shows recombination of *RB* and +. Mechanism C is loss of a whole chromosome. Mechanism D is deletion of the wild-type allele of the gene.

common target for genetic mutations leading to cancers (Cooper, 1995). Germline mutations of *TP53*, transmitted in an autosomal dominant fashion, are a hallmark of Li-Fraumeni syndrome.

Specific Functions of TS Genes

Some normal TS gene products are localized in the cell nucleus and act as transcription factors. For example, *MTS1*, which encodes the p16 protein, also contributes to deregulation of the cell cycle, which results in excess cell proliferation. The *TP53* gene can halt cell division and induce apoptosis (see Apoptosis, later in this chapter).

> Tumor suppressor genes play a key role in cell-cycle activity and apoptosis.

Table 3-2. Selected Cloned Tumor Suppressor Genes

Gene	Description
APC	• Adenomatous polyposis of the colon gene • Involved with familial adenomatous polyposis of the colon (FPC) • Located on chromosome 5q21–q22
BRCA1	• Familial breast/ovarian cancer gene 1 • Involved in hereditary breast cancer as well as ovarian cancer • Located on chromosome 17q21
BRCA2	• Familial breast/ovarian cancer gene 2 • Involved in hereditary breast cancer • Located on chromosome 13q12.3
CDH1	• Cadherin 1 (epithelial cadherin or E-cadherin) gene • Familial gastric carcinoma and associated with lobular breast cancer • Located on chromosome 16q22.1
CDKN1C	• Cyclin-dependent kinase inhibitor 1C gene • Beckwith-Wiedemann syndrome • Involved with Wilms' tumor and rhabdomyosarcoma • Located on chromosome 11p15.5
CDKN2A	• Cyclin-dependent kinase inhibitor 2A (p16) gene • Cutaneous malignant melanoma 2 • Located on chromosome 9p21
CYLD	• Familial cylindromatosis gene • Familial cylindromas • Located on chromosome 16q12–q13
EP300	• E1A-binding protein gene • Involved with some colorectal, breast, and pancreatic cancers • Located on chromosome 22q13.2
EXT1	• Multiple exostosis type 1 gene • Involved with some exostoses and osteosarcomas • Located on chromosome 8q24.11–q24.13
EXT2	• Multiple exostosis type 2 gene • Involved with some exostoses and osteosarcomas • Located on chromosome 11p12–p11
MADH4	• Homolog of *Drosophila mothers against decapentaplegic 4* gene • Juvenile polyposis • Involved with some gastrointestinal polyps and colorectal and pancreatic cancers • Located on chromosome 18q21.1

(Continued on next page)

Table 3-2. Selected Cloned Tumor Suppressor Genes (Continued)

Gene	Description
MAP2K4	• Mitogen-activated protein kinase 4 • Involved with some pancreatic, breast, and colon cancers • Located on chromosome 17p11.2
MEN1	• Multiple endocrine neoplasia type 1 gene • Multiple endocrine neoplasia type 1 syndrome • Involved with parathyroid/pituitary adenoma, islet-cell carcinoma, and carcinoid tumors • Located on chromosome 11q13
MLH1	• Homolog of E. coli MutL gene • Hereditary nonpolyposis colorectal cancer, type 2 • Involved with colorectal, endometrial, and ovarian cancers • Located on chromosome 3p21.3
MSH2	• Homolog of E. coli MutS 2 gene • Hereditary nonpolyposis colorectal cancer, type 1 • Involved with colorectal, endometrial, and ovarian cancers • Located on chromosome 2p22–p21
NF1	• Neurofibromatosis type 1 gene • Neurofibromatosis type 1 syndrome (von Recklinghausen disease) • Involved in neurofibromas, gliomas, and pheochromocytomas of the nervous system and myeloid leukemia • Codes for a protein that inhibits RAS, a cytoplasmic inhibitory protein • Located on chromosome 17q11.2
NF2	• Neurofibromatosis type 2 gene • Neurofibromatosis type 2 syndrome • Involved in bilateral acoustic neuromas, meningiomas, schwannomas, and ependymomas of the nervous system • Codes for a nuclear protein • Located on chromosome 22q12.2
PRKAR1A	• Protein kinase A type 1, alpha, regulatory subunit gene • Carney complex • Involved with myxoma and endocrine tumors • Located on chromosome 17q23–q24
PTCH	• Homolog of Drosophila patched gene • Nevoid basal cell carcinoma syndrome • Involved with some basal cell carcinomas and medulloblastomas and rhabdomyosarcoma • Located on chromosome 9q22.3

(Continued on next page)

Table 3-2. Selected Cloned Tumor Suppressor Genes *(Continued)*

Gene	Description
PTEN	• Phosphatase and tensin homolog gene • Cowden syndrome • Involved with some hamartomas, gliomas, and prostate and endometrial cancers • Located on chromosome 10q23.3
RB1	• Retinoblastoma gene • Familial retinoblastoma • Involved in bone, bladder, small-cell lung, and breast cancers as well as retinoblastoma • Codes for the nuclear protein pRB (p105-Rb), a major inhibitor of the cell cycle • Located on chromosome 13q14.1–q14.2
SDHD	• Succinate dehydrogenase cytochrome B small subunit gene • Familial paraganglioma • Located on chromosome 11q23
SMARCB1	• Swi/Snf5 matrix-associated actin-dependent regulator of chromatin gene • Rhabdoid predisposition syndrome • Involved with malignant rhabdoid tumors • Located on chromosome 22q11.23
STK11	• Serine threonine kinase 11 gene • Peutz-Jeghers syndrome • Involved with jejunal hamartomas, ovarian tumors, and testicular and pancreatic cancers • Located on chromosome 19p13.3
TP53	• Tumor suppressor p53 gene • Inheritance of p53 mutations through the germ line is associated with Li-Fraumeni syndrome • Involved in a wide variety of tumors • Inactive or lost in more than 50% of cancerous cells • Codes for the cytoplasmic p53 protein that regulate cell division and can induce cells to kill themselves (apoptosis) • Located on chromosome 17p13.1
TSC1	• Tuberous sclerosis type 1 gene • Tuberous sclerosis • Involved with some hamartomas and renal-cell carcinoma • Codes for hamartin • Located on chromosome 9q34

(Continued on next page)

Table 3-2. Selected Cloned Tumor Suppressor Genes *(Continued)*

Gene	Description
TSC2	• Tuberous sclerosis type 2 gene • Tuberous sclerosis • Involved with some hamartomas and renal-cell carcinoma • Codes for tuberin • Located on chromosome 16p13.3
VHL	• von Hippel-Lindau syndrome gene • von Hippel-Lindau syndrome • Involved with some renal-cell carcinomas, hemangiomas, and pheochromocytomas • Located on chromosome 3p26–p25
WT1	• Wilms' tumor 1 gene • Familial Wilms' tumor • Involved in Wilms' tumor of the kidneys (nephroblastoma) • Located on chromosome 11p13

Note. From "Tumor Suppressor Genes" by E. Pergament and M. Fiddler (Eds.), *The Genetics of Cancer,* 2001, Melville, NY: PRR, Inc. Available at www.intouchlive.com/cancergenetics/tsg.htm. Copyright 2001 by PRR, Inc. Reprinted with permission.

TS genes also can encode for proteins in the cytoplasm. The *NF1* gene encodes a protein that is similar to the proteins that modulate *RAS* oncogene function. Loss of *NF1* may keep *RAS* activated and prolong the signal for cell proliferation. Loss of other TS genes, such as *NF2* and *APC*, may cause cellular disorganization that leads to abnormal cell proliferation (Ruddon, 1995). TS genes that code for proteins with unclear cellular function include the breast-ovarian cancer genes *BRCA1* and *BRCA2* and *VHL* (the gene is associated with von Hippel-Lindau syndrome).

Mutator Genes

Unlike oncogenes or TS genes, mutator genes (DNA repair genes) are not part of cell-regulatory pathways. Instead, mutator genes prevent genetic instability. Mutator genes can be either oncogenes or TS genes. Mutator genes encode error-correction systems that check DNA for damaged or mismatched base pairs (see Defects in Mismatch Repair: Microsatellite Instability, later in this chapter). Mutations in these genes lead to inefficient replication or repair of DNA. Colon cancer studies have provided clues to the identity of genes important in stability at the DNA level (Strachan & Read, 1999).

Types of Genetic Alterations in Cancer Cells

Other than point mutations, the genetic alterations associated with cancer include chromosomal abnormalities; amplification; and defects in mismatch repair, including microsatellite instability.

Chromosomal Abnormalities

Cancer cells typically have a bizarre, unstable chromosomal structure that comprises many gains, losses, or rearrangements of chromosomes. Only a few of these abnormalities appear to be causally linked to cancer. The specific genes responsible for chromosomal instability have not yet been identified (Strachan & Read, 1999).

Recurrent structural chromosomal rearrangements are a common feature of most cancers. How these rearrangements develop may be attributed to genetic weak points or chromosomal fragile sites. Chromosomal fragile sites are regions on chromosomes that are particularly sensitive to forming nonrandom gaps or breaks when DNA synthesis is perturbed. Fragile sites are highly sensitive to low folic acid. They can be induced by a wide variety of mutagens and carcinogens that are known to act through different molecular mechanisms. Fragile sites have been implicated in a wide variety of cancers, including multiple myeloma (Krummel, Roberts, Kawakami, Glover, & Smith, 2000) and chronic lymphocytic leukemia (Auer et al., 2001).

Translocations

Chromosomal translocations are structural abnormalities that primarily affect oncogenes. Translocations cause oncogene deregulation (overexpression) and the fusion of oncogenes at the points in the chromosome where abnormal breaks occur (breakpoints). Reciprocal translocations involve exchange of genetic material between two chromosomes or within the same chromosome. Translocations are the hallmarks of leukemias and lymphomas (Solomon, Borrow, & Goddard, 1991). For example, in chronic myelogenous leukemia, the reciprocal translocation between the q arm of chromosome 9, band 34, and the q arm of chromosome 22, band 11, causes the *ABL* proto-oncogene to translocate to chromosome 22 (the Philadelphia chromosome) (see Figure 3-9). This produces the *BCR-ABL* fusion gene, which dysregulates TK activity. The abbreviated method of describing this translocation is t(9;22)(q34;q11). Eighty percent of Burkitt's lymphoma cases have a translocation of t(8;14)(q24;q32). This translocation deregulates expression of the transcription factor encoded by the *MYC* proto-oncogene, causing activation of the *MYC* oncogene (Ruddon, 1995; Solomon et al.).

Figure 3-9. Translocation of the *ABL* Proto-Oncogene on Chromosome 9

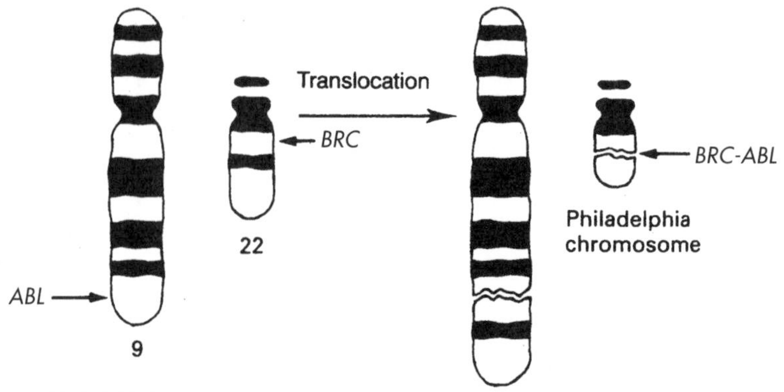

The translocation of *ABL* to the *BCR* locus on chromosome 22 forms the Philadelphia chromosome. This chromosome is activated by the *BCR-ABL* fusion oncogene.

Deletions

Chromosomal deletions are associated most often with solid tumors. The most common deletion is the deletion of specific gene sequences, which result in the loss of a chromosomal band or the LOH of a specific allele (Ruddon, 1995). Deletions, therefore, are the hallmark of TS genes. Tumors of different cellular origin exhibit the same chromosome deletions. For example, deletion of the 1p11–22 region is implicated in melanoma, breast adenocarcinoma, internal leiomyosarcoma, pleural mesothelioma, and malignant fibrous histiocytoma. Loss of the 7q21–34 region commonly occurs in uterine leiomyoma, prostate adenocarcinoma, glioma, acute myeloid leukemia, and myelodysplastic syndrome (Solomon et al., 1991).

Aneuploidy

Aneuploidy is an abnormal chromosome number. The term can refer to a gain or a loss of a chromosome. Aneuploidy is associated with malignant transformation in that gross changes in chromosome number usually occur as tumorigenesis progresses. In most colorectal cancers, for example, aneuploidy is associated with genetic instability (Lengauer, Kinzler, & Vogelstein, 1997). Aneuploidy may be random or nonrandom. In random aneuploidy, the change in chromosome number has no association with tumor type; rather, it happens late in tumor development and reflects the genetic instability of the tumor. Nonrandom aneuploidy involves a specific change in a given chromosome associated with a specific tumor. Nonrandom aneuploidy tends to occur earlier than the random form.

Amplification

Amplification, an increase in the number of gene copies, results in overexpression of the gene product without modification of the gene itself (see Figure 3-7). Amplifications can be extrachromosomal; in this case, as minichromosomes called double minutes. Amplifications also can be intra-chromosomal, appearing as homogenously stained regions (HSRs) in the chromosome—areas where chromosome regions have increased length, are stable, and remain amplified. Amplification of certain genes may be related to carcinogenesis, as in the enhancement of amplification by ultraviolet light. As tumor cells progress, they gain the ability to amplify genes as they lose cell-cycle control and TS-gene activity. Oncogenes such as *MYC* and *ERBB2* (*HER2/NEU*) often have amplified gene sequences, which may be related to tumor progression.

Defects in Mismatch Repair: Microsatellite Instability

Normal synthesis relies on a back-up signal within DNA to distinguish between a parental strand and a daughter strand that contains a replication error. In normal synthesis, specific repair proteins recognize and bind to the mismatch. The result is a process that essentially unwinds DNA in the direction of the mismatch, degrades the DNA strand, and seals the nick that degradation causes in the strand. Sometimes, however, the wrong nucleotide incorporates into the strand during DNA-strand synthesis and DNA's normal editing system fails to correct the error. Defects in genes that encode the repair proteins most often have been associated with hereditary nonpolyposis colorectal cancer (HNPCC). Most patients with HNPCC show widespread alterations in the DNA-base sequences, or **microsatellite** sequences, distributed throughout the genome. These sequences may be associated with defects in mismatch repair (Cama, Genuardi, Guanti, Radice, & Varesco, 1996; Papadopoulos et al., 1994).

Repeated microsatellite DNA sequences commonly repeated in tandem may consist of coding or noncoding DNA. In coding DNA, repeated sequences may involve different forms of large or small repeating structures. Certain sequences may be highly unstable and prone to single-nucleotide deletion or insertion. Microsatellite noncoding DNA is defined by blocks, or arrays, of tandemly repeated DNA sequences (Strachan & Read, 1999).

The length of microsatellite DNA repetitions is different in tumors than in normal tissue. Microsatellite instability (MSI) is evident in both sporadic and inherited cancers. MSI is a characteristic of autosomal-dominant HNPCC. Genes associated with HNPCC encode an error system that checks the DNA for mismatched base pairs. MSI is associated with approximately 13% of sporadic colorectal, gastric, and endometrial cancers.

> The types of genetic alterations commonly found in cancer cells include mutations; chromosomal translocations, deletions, aneuploidy; gene amplification; and defects in mismatch repair, including MSI.

The Cell Cycle

A complex molecular process in the cell nucleus, the cell cycle, regulates cell division. Normally, the cell cycle integrates the various growth-regulating signals received by the cell and "makes the decision" to allow the cell to replicate (Weinberg, 1996). In cancer, the cell cycle operates autonomously and cannot control cell proliferation.

Normal Functioning of the Cell Cycle

The cell cycle consists of four active phases (see Figure 3-10). In the first phase, gap 1 (G1), the cell readies itself to copy DNA. Late in G1 is a restriction point (R); this is the point at which the cell "decides" to commit itself to replication. After the cell makes this commitment, the cycle cannot be turned off. During the synthesis (S) phase, DNA replication occurs and the cell duplicates its complement of chromosomes. Following chromosomal replication, the cell proceeds to the gap 2 (G2) phase and prepares itself for mitosis. During the mitosis (M) phase, chromosome segregation occurs and culminates in cytokinesis (division into two daughter cells, each with a full complement of chromosomes). The daughter cells immediately enter G1. The cell cycle begins again, or it may stop cycling and enter a resting (G0) state.

Proteins called cyclins combine with and activate enzymes called cyclin-dependent kinases (CDKs). The transient activation of various cyclins and CDKs, at specific points in the cell cycle, regulates the intricate series of cell-cycle events. For example, *CDK1* is involved primarily in control of mitosis. *CDK2* is involved in G1 and in G1–S transition points. *CDK1*, *-2*, and *-3* are thought to carry out the start function of the cell cycle.

Checkpoints in the Cell Cycle

Checkpoints, specific gene products in the cell cycle, ensure that events occur in correct sequence and that one event terminates before the other begins. For example, checkpoints govern entrance into the S phase and the M phase and exit from the M phase (Ruddon, 1995). Defects in the checkpoint surveillance of DNA could account for chromosomal deletions, amplifications, and translocations. The checkpoint controlling entry into S phase prevents replication of

Figure 3-10. The Cell Cycle

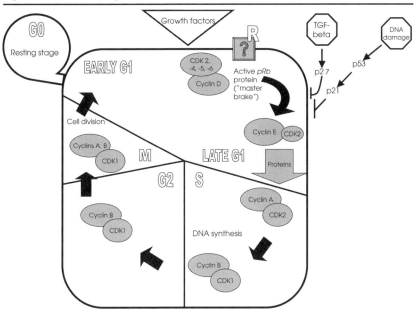

The cell cycle consists of four active stages (G1, S, G2, M) that are controlled by proteins called cyclins. The cyclins (D, E, A, B) activate upon forming complexes with enzymes called cyclin-dependent kinases (CDKs). Upon activation, the cyclin-CDK complexes allow the cell to progress through each specific cell-cycle stage. Present throughout the cell cycle, the cyclin-CDK complexes serve as checkpoints, or monitors, of the cell cycle. Inhibitory proteins—such as p21, p27, and p53—prevent progression through the cell cycle if DNA damage is present or if the nutrients or oxygen necessary to support cellular proliferation is in short supply. Inhibitory proteins, in turn, are regulated by inhibitory growth factors and *TGFB*. Cyclin-CDK complexes and pRb ("the master brake") tightly regulate the R (restriction) point. Once past R, the cell cycle "turns on," and progression through the cell cycle is inevitable. The stability of the inhibitory proteins and cyclin-CDK complexes are altered in cancer. Normal cell-cycle controls are absent and uncontrolled cellular proliferation prevails.

Note. From "Biology of Cancer" (p. 26) by J. Gibbon and L. Loescher in C.H. Yarbro, M.H. Frogge, and M. Goodman (Eds.), *Cancer Nursing: Principles and Practice* (5th ed.), 2000, Boston: Jones and Bartlett. Copyright 2000 by Jones and Bartlett, www.jbpub.com. Adapted with permission.

DNA damage. Checkpoint surveillance, therefore, plays an integral role in maintaining the integrity of the human genome (Hartwell & Kastan, 1994). Cancer cells probably have weak, or deficient, cell-cycle checkpoints (Orr-Weaver & Weinberg, 1998; Ruddon).

Currently, genetic instability in the G1/S checkpoint in human cancers is best understood. Loss of the G1/S checkpoint leads to the instability of the human genome, survival of genetically damaged cells, and clonal evolution (see Tumorigenesis). For example, mutations of *TP53* are commonly associated with several cancers, suggesting that abnormalities in the G1/S checkpoint are important in tumorigenesis.

Apoptosis

In some cases, *TP53*-induced DNA damage triggers apoptosis rather than G1 arrest. **Apoptosis** is "programmed" cell death—in other words, cell death occurs as a result of an active process that involves a distinct series of biochemical and morphologic changes. Apoptosis allows an organism to remove old, dead, or unwanted cells. Apoptosis often is a response to DNA damage. Cell-cycle progression can be arrested following externally induced damage, such as damage resulting from chemotherapeutic drugs (Hartwell & Kastan, 1994).

Loss of apoptotic signals may contribute to early tumorigenesis because of the inability to eliminate genetically damaged cells, or it may occur later in tumorigenesis and contribute to the survival of damaged cells (Hartwell & Kastan, 1994). Results of an in vivo animal study (Symonds et al., 1994) indicated that *TP53*-dependent apoptosis, in response to abnormal cell proliferation, inhibits the growth of a developing tumor. Inactivation of the *TP53* gene, either by germline mutation or expression of the *TP53*-binding domain of T cell antigen, leads to attenuation of apoptosis and rapid tumor progression. Symonds et al. also reported that loss of *TP53* function may indirectly contribute to tumor development by permitting the propagation of mutated cells. Therefore, reduced susceptibility to apoptosis may be a direct consequence of *TP53* loss rather than an accumulation of secondary mutations. These conclusions suggest that restoration of *TP53*-dependent apoptosis may provide an approach to cancer therapy.

> Several genes play a critical role in normal regulation of the cell cycle. If those genes are damaged, the cell cycle malfunctions and uncontrolled cell proliferation can occur. For apoptosis to function properly, for example, *TP53* must function properly.

Tumorigenesis

Tumorigenesis—the process of tumor development—is a complex process that has been best studied in colorectal cancer. Researchers chose colorectal cancer to study genetic mutations because most colorectal tumors arise from preexisting benign tumors (adenomas); because colorectal tumors in various stages of development, ranging from small adenomas to large metastatic lesions, can be easily accessed for study; and because colorectal cancer allowed the study of both inherited and somatic mutations. Fearon and Vogelstein (1990) proposed a model that showed the genetic basis of colorectal cancer (see Figure 3-11). Their model was among the first to suggest that tumorigenesis is a multistep process. The researchers concluded that colorectal cancers probably arise from mutational activation of oncogenes coupled with mutational inactivation of TS genes, although the latter mutations predominate. They proposed that mutations in at least four genes are necessary for tumor development. In addition, Fearon and Jones (1992) suggested that the total accumulation of mutations, not their specific sequence, is responsible for tumor formation.

The multistep model of Fearon and Vogelstein (1990) is based on the theory that all cells in all stages of tumorigenesis have a particular genetic makeup and that this homogeneity is necessary for identifying specific genes. This theory, called clonal evolution (Nowell, 1976), supports the idea that the origin of cancer lies in a single cell or a small number of cells. Initiation of clonal evolu-

Figure 3-11. A Conceptual Genetic Model for the Development of Colorectal Cancer, Illustrating Multistep Tumorigenesis

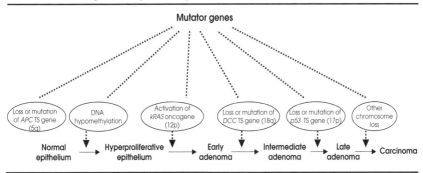

The alterations shown in this figure suggest a temporal sequence of genetic events. Not all alterations occur in individual tumors, and the order of alterations is variable. The accumulation of multiple genetic alterations in both oncogenes and tumor suppressor (TS) genes is more important than the order of events. Mutator gene mutations do not play a direct role in the multistep pathway. By increasing the overall mutation rate, however, they make each individual transition more likely. Genes shown here include the *APC* (adenomatous polyposis coli) gene and the *DCC* (deleted in colorectal carcinoma) gene.

Note. From "Biology of Cancer" (p. 19) by J. Gibbon and L. Loescher in C.H. Yarbro, M.H. Frogge, and M. Goodman (Eds.), *Cancer Nursing: Principles and Practice* (5th ed.), 2000, Boston: Jones and Bartlett. Copyright 2000 by Jones and Bartlett, www.jbpub.com. Adapted with permission.

tion likely involves a stem cell that is already dividing but increases the proportion of daughter cells in mitosis rather than proceeding to differentiation. Unrestrained proliferation may be accompanied by morphologic and biochemical changes or altered gene expression in early-stage neoplastic cells. Over time, proliferation may increase and show further evidence of escape from growth-control mechanisms. Increasingly malignant biologic characteristics during tumor progression result from acquired genetic instability in neoplastic cells and variant subpopulations produced as a result of genetic instability.

Some tumors do not behave according to the theory of clonal evolution. These include tumors of viral etiology, which may involve whole populations of infected cells, and genetically predisposed cancers, in which an inherited genetic defect involves every cell and increases susceptibility to neoplastic change.

Summary

Genetic abnormalities and instability in various forms are key features of all cancers. This chapter summarized how cancers can be traced to molecular defects in DNA, chromosomal abnormalities, and specific genes that interfere with signal transduction, enzymatic pathways, and the cell cycle. Tumorigenesis, at the molecular level, appears to be a complex, multistep process characterized by the accumulation of multiple genetic defects. Through the process of clonal evolution, these defects lead to the development of the fully malignant phenotype characteristic of clinical cancer. In other words, a single mutation may initiate a process leading to cancer, but more mutations are needed for cancer to progress. As the steps involved in cancer development are clarified, risk assessment, diagnosis, and treatment are becoming rational responses to specific cellular mechanisms.

> Cancer is the result of a complex, multistep process characterized by the accumulation of multiple genetic defects. A single genetic mutation may initiate a process leading to cancer, but more mutations are needed for cancer to progress.

References

Auer, R., Jones, C., Mullenbach, R., Syndercombe-Court, D., Milligan, D., Fegan, C., et al. (2001). Role for CGC-trinucleotide repeats in the pathogenesis of chronic lymphocytic leukemia. *Blood, 97*, 509–515.

Cama, A., Genuardi, M., Guanti, G., Radice, P., & Varesco, L. (1996). Molecular genetics of hereditary non-polyposis colorectal cancer (HNPCC). *Tumori, 82*, 122–135.

Cooper, G.M. (1995). *Oncogenes.* Boston: Jones and Bartlett.

Fearon, E.R., & Jones, P.A. (1992). Progressing toward a molecular description of colorectal cancer development. *FASEB Journal, 6,* 2783–2790.

Fearon, E.R., & Vogelstein, B. (1990). A genetic model for tumorigenesis. *Cell, 61,* 759–767.

Hanahan, D., & Weinberg, R.A. (2000). The hallmarks of cancer. *Cell, 100,* 57–70.

Hartwell, L.H., & Kastan, M.B. (1994). Cell cycle control and cancer. *Science, 266,* 1821–1828.

Knudson, A.G. (1971). Mutation and cancer: Statistical study of retinoblastoma. *Proceedings of the National Academy of Sciences, 68,* 820–823.

Krummel, K., Roberts, L., Kawakami, M., Glover, T., & Smith, D. (2000). The characterization of the common fragile site FRA 16D and its involvement in multiple myeloma translocations. *Genomic, 69,* 37–46.

Latchman, D.S. (1996). Transcription-factor mutations and disease. *New England Journal of Medicine, 334,* 28–33.

Lengauer, C., Kinzler, K.W., & Vogelstein, B. (1997). Genetic instability in colorectal cancers. *Nature, 386,* 623–627.

Nowell, P.C. (1976). The clonal evolution of tumor cell populations. *Science, 194,* 23–28.

Orr-Weaver, T.L., & Weinberg, R.A. (1998). A checkpoint on the road to cancer. *Nature, 392,* 223–224.

Papadopoulos, N., Nicolaides, N.C., Wei, Y-F., Ruben, S.M., Carter, K.C., Rosen, C.A., et al. (1994). Mutation of a mutL homolog in hereditary colon cancer. *Science, 263,* 1625–1629.

Papavassiliou, A.F. (1995). Transcription factors. *New England Journal of Medicine, 332,* 45–47.

Rosenthal, N. (1994). DNA and the genetic code. *New England Journal of Medicine, 331,* 39–41.

Ruddon, R.W. (1995). *Cancer biology.* New York: Oxford University Press.

Solomon, E., Borrow, J., & Goddard, A.D. (1991). Chromosome aberrations and cancer. *Science, 254,* 1153–1160.

Strachan, T., & Read, A.P. (1999). *Human molecular genetics* (2nd ed.). New York: Wiley-Liss.

Symonds, H., Krail, L., Remington, L., Saenz-Robles, M., Lowe, S., Jacks, T., et al. (1994). p53-dependent apoptosis suppresses tumor growth and progression in vivo. *Cell, 78,* 703–711.

Vogelstein, B., & Kinzler, K. (1998). *The genetic basis of cancer.* New York: McGraw-Hill.

Weinberg, R.A. (1994). Oncogenes and tumor suppressor genes. *CA: A Cancer*

Journal for Clinicians, 44, 160–170.

Weinberg, R.A. (1996). How cancer arises. *Scientific American, 275*(3), 62–70.

4

How to Perform a Genetic Assessment

Patricia Moffa Barse, RN, MSN, AOCN®

Most oncology nurses are adept at providing comprehensive client assessments. Now that research has provided new insight into the genetic basis of cancer, however, the definition of *comprehensive assessment* has changed. Today, in the context of oncology, a comprehensive assessment should include a genetic assessment. A genetic assessment is a tool for providing holistic care to patients and families in that a genetic assessment may reveal that a patient with cancer has a higher-than-average risk for developing other forms of cancer. In addition, it may identify family members who are at risk. It is the responsibility of the oncology nurse to identify high-risk individuals and to refer them for cancer-risk counseling.

What Is a Genetic Assessment for Cancer?

A genetic assessment for cancer determines the likelihood that an individual will develop cancer. Performing such an assessment includes gathering and evaluating information about the health history, lifestyle, cognition, and beliefs of the individual and the medical history of his or her family.

A genetic assessment for cancer also includes evaluation of noncancer genes and nongenetic risk factors.

Components of the genetic assessment:
- Comprehensive health history (personal, medical, environmental exposures)
- Lifestyle and health-behavior assessment
- Psychosocial assessment (psychiatric history, emotional state, risk perception)
- Motivation for seeking risk assessment
- Cognitive assessment
- Three-generation family history, including ethnicity
- Physical examination when appropriate

The reason: A single genetic mutation is not enough to cause a malignancy (Schatzkin, Goldstein, & Freedman, 1995). Though an individual may be born with a gene that predisposes him or her to cancer, it does not mean that the person will inevitably develop the disease. Researchers continue to focus on the complex interaction between cancer-predisposing genes and other genes in the body as well as the interactions with endogenous and exogenous factors that may initiate or modify the carcinogenic process (Schatzkin et al.). For example, a woman may be born with a mutated *BRCA1* gene, but she may not develop breast cancer. Whether she develops breast cancer is determined, in part, by the relationships among mutations and other genes, dietary factors, hormonal influences, and environmental factors. A thorough genetic assessment includes documentation and evaluation of all the factors that influence genetic predisposition.

What Is the Purpose of a Genetic Assessment?

In the context of cancer, a genetic assessment helps to determine which individuals are at genetic risk for the disease, to estimate the degree of risk, and to identify which clients might benefit from genetic testing. A genetic assessment serves as the basis for recommendations from the healthcare team about medical screening and surveillance, risk-reduction strategies, and prevention options, and it provides information that will help the client to decide whether to proceed with genetic testing.

What Are the Specific Components of a Genetic Assessment?

The specific components of a genetic assessment include
- Client's health history
- Description of the client's current health status and lifestyle, including cultural and religious beliefs
- Description of the client's psychosocial state
- Evaluation of cognitive level, style, and preferences
- Family history.

The Client's Health History

One part of assembling a client's health history is documenting his or her birth defects and past illnesses, medical conditions, and genetic disorders. This is important because, as mentioned, certain medical conditions and genetic disorders are associated with a high risk of cancer. For example, if a man's history includes undescended testes, he has a greater-than-average risk of testicular cancer.

Documenting past surgeries, using official records, also is important. The pathology report relative to a surgery may provide information about pathologic features that affect cancer risk. Such information also may prompt insights about the benefits of risk-reduction measures and prevention options. For example, collecting information about women who have had prophylactic mastectomies or oophorectomies and subsequently assessing their incidence of breast or ovarian cancer may help to answer questions about the benefits of the prophylactic measures.

A health history should include detailed biopsy information, as well. The patient probably will not be able to supply such information. Most people who have had biopsies and, as a result, learned that a growth was benign do not know the pathologic features of the growth. They recall the physician telling them that the growth was benign, but little else. For this reason, obtaining pathology reports is important. The reports will help to determine if the cells had pathologic features that affect cancer risk. For example, atypical hyperplasia and lobular carcinoma in situ are associated with an increased risk of breast cancer (Dupont et al., 1993; Page, Dupont, Rogers, & Rados, 1985).

Information about reproductive history is an important component of a health history. Such information is useful in evaluating a woman's risk of breast and ovarian cancers. In preparing a health history, document a woman's age at menarche and menopause. Record her total number of pregnancies and note whether the results were live births, terminated pregnancies, or spontaneous abortions. Note how old the woman was when her first child was born and whether she breast-fed the baby. Record whether she ever used exogenous hormones (i.e., oral contraceptives, fertility drugs, or hormone replacement therapy) and, if so, which ones, how old she was when she used them, and for how long she used them.

Also note if the client has had unusual exposures to radiation, chemicals, and/or industrial processes.

Lifestyle Assessment

A comprehensive assessment of an individual's lifestyle may provide important information about factors contributing to or modifying cancer risk. Include the client's current height and weight. These measurements are important because of the relationship between obesity and certain cancers. Individuals who weigh more than their ideal body weight have a greater-than-average risk of cancers of the colon and rectum (Potter, 1996), prostate (Kolonel, 1996), endometrium (Hill & Austin, 1996), kidney (Wolk, Lindblad, & Adami, 1996), breast (in postmenopausal women) (Hunter & Willett, 1996), and pancreas (Michaud et al., 2001).

Describe his or her diet. High-fat diets have been associated with an increased risk of cancers of the colon and rectum (Potter, 1996), prostate (Kolonel, 1996), and endometrium (Hill & Austin, 1996).

Also describe the client's exercise patterns. Exercise decreases the risk of some cancers either by preventing obesity or through other mechanisms. For example, exercise is associated with a decreased risk of cancers of the prostate and breast because of the effect that exercise has on hormone levels (Friedenreich & Rohan, 1995; Shephard, 1993). Exercise also stimulates the movement of bowel contents, reducing the time that the intestines are exposed to mutagens; this reduces the risk of colon cancer (American Cancer Society [ACS] 1996 Advisory Committee on Diet, Nutrition, and Cancer Prevention, 1996).

Note whether the client uses tobacco and alcohol and, if so, how much. It is well known that tobacco is associated with a greater risk of cancers of the lung, head or neck, bladder, and esophagus. Alcohol is associated with a greater risk of cancers of the oral cavity, esophagus, larynx (ACS 1996 Advisory Committee on Diet, Nutrition, and Cancer Prevention, 1996), and breast (Hunter & Willett, 1996).

Record whether the client is exposed to the sun on a regular basis. The effects of the sun on the risks for melanoma and nonmelanoma cancers of the skin are well established.

List the medications the client uses, and the quantities used, and do the same for vitamins. At present, little evidence exists in regard to the relationship between medication use and cancer and vitamin use and cancer. Research about these topics is under way, however, so ensure that information about medication and vitamins is in the client's history for reference in the future, when researchers may have established correlations.

Include in the lifestyle assessment a description of the client's healthcare practices and beliefs. Ask the client, for example, if he or she has had recommended screening tests. Ask if he or she is using recommended early-detection methods. If the client is not, find out why. This will allow you to clarify misperceptions and provide useful information that will help the client to understand the importance of early detection. If a woman has not been doing a monthly breast self-exam, perhaps she thinks she does not have the skills to discern an abnormality. In such a case, incorporate instruction in breast self-examination into the plan of care. Document the dates of the client's most recent screening exams and self-tests, note how frequently the client undergoes such screenings and performs self-tests, and note unusual findings.

The client's cultural and religious beliefs are an important part of a health history because they may have a profound impact on the ability to cope with risk information, willingness to share risk information with other family members, and compliance with screening measures and prevention options. For example, a characteristic of many Asian cultures is great respect for privacy. As a result, an Asian patient may not tell family members about a diagnosis of cancer. Would an Asian patient who is found to have a genetic mutation be willing to share the finding with family members? Though news of the mutation is information that would be important to family members, the client's right to privacy and autonomy are important too. Counseling the client about sharing genetic information would involve achieving a delicate balance between respecting the client's right to privacy and autonomy while advocating for the family's right to know.

Multicultural Outcomes: Guidelines for Cultural Competence (Oncology Nursing Society, 1999) is a resource that contains guidelines for delivering culturally sensitive nursing care.

Psychosocial Assessment

Gather information about the client's psychosocial state throughout the genetic assessment. Using a formal questionnaire often is helpful to ensure collection of the needed information. Keep in mind the fact that patients with cancer undergoing genetic risk assessment may have many concerns. They may, for example, be undergoing cancer treatment or coping with a fear of cancer recurrence. The psychosocial assessment should include all the relevant issues.

Motivation for Assessment

As part of the psychosocial assessment, learn the client's motivation for seeking cancer-risk information. Why does the client want to know about cancer risk, and in what form does he or she want risk information? Some clients want risk information in qualitative form (e.g., low, moderate, or high risk); others want a quantitative description of risk. For some, presenting a quantitative risk may not be feasible because limitations of quantitative risk data make the data inapplicable in some circumstances. Cancer-risk counselors need to understand how to interpret quantitative risk information so that it is used correctly.

If genetic testing may be an appropriate option for the client, assess the client's interest in pursuing genetic testing and the reasons for his or her interest. Ask clients how they think genetic test results would affect them and their families (Daly et al., 2001). Role playing may be a way to help the client to express anticipated reactions. Ask the client to pretend that he or she has received a positive test result and then a negative test result. In addition to helping you to learn about the client's response, the exercise may prompt discussion of pertinent issues.

History of Anxiety or Depression

Assess the client's history of anxiety or depression. If the client has such a history, document the interventions used to treat each condition. An assessment by a social worker, psychologist, or psychiatrist may be advisable to ensure a comprehensive evaluation.

Present Emotional State

Does the client appear anxious? Anxiety may be demonstrated by excessive talking or an inability to provide information. Or a client may verbalize anxiety by saying how he or she feels overwhelmed when discussing family history. For some people, the decision to pursue risk assessment may have been triggered by a specific event, such as the recent diagnosis of cancer in the family or the anniversary of the death of a relative who had cancer. Similarly, an event in the family history may prompt a client to discuss memories of a relative's illness or death. These memories may evoke a myriad of emotions. Be sensitive to the client's feelings and, in the course of taking the family history, note the insights into his or her psychosocial state that the client's recollections provide. Note whether the history suggests life stressors that may affect the client's ability to cope with risk information.

Risk Perception

Assess the client's perception of his or her risk of developing cancer. In many cases, the client's perception has been influenced by a personal experience with cancer or the experiences of family members. Asking the client to quantify his or her risk perception and to describe beliefs about factors contributing to cancer development may be helpful. For example, one client reported that she had two sisters. Both were diagnosed with breast cancer at the age of 36, six months after each had given birth for the second time. The client and her family believed that the second birth had triggered the development of the cancer. The client had recently given birth to her second child and was considering having a prophylactic mastectomy because of her fear of developing breast cancer. This client's family experience had had a profound impact on her perception of risk.

Effects of Risk Perception on Choices and Behaviors

Determine how the client's perception of cancer risk affects his or her lifestyle choices and health behaviors. This evaluation may provide clues regarding the client's response to risk information. For example, a client who has declined cancer screenings may be even less apt to have such tests if the client discovers that he or she actually is at risk for cancer.

How the Client Copes With Perceived Risk

To assess the client's past responses and coping strategies in dealing with cancer risk and other life stressors, determine his or her use of social support and professional help. Ask the client if he or she uses self-implemented strategies, such as exercise, relaxation, or meditation. This information will help you to assess the client's ability to cope with risk information as well as to determine coping strategies that are effective and ineffective for the client. Encourage the client to use coping mechanisms that have been helpful in the past and discuss with the client new coping strategies that may be effective. In addition, explore the client's family dynamics and assess how genetic information will affect the client's relationships with his or her spouse or significant other, children, siblings, and other family members. Sharing information of such a sensitive nature may be difficult, especially if the client does not have close relationships with family members, if relatives are not interested in learning about cancer risk, or if relatives do not understand the implications of genetic information. Inviting family members to attend a genetics education session with the client may be helpful.

Cognitive Assessment

The cognitive-assessment component of a genetic assessment begins with an evaluation of how much the client knows about cancer-risk factors, the effectiveness and limitations of screening measures, prevention options, and the influence of family history on cancer risk. (Many clients have the false assumption that they are only at risk for cancer if they have a family history of the disease.) Also document the client's literacy level, cultural background, language skills, and learning style and the resources the client has used in the past (e.g., written materials, audio or visual aids, the Internet) to get cancer and cancer genetics information.

By knowing what the client needs to learn and in what form information will be most effective, a nurse will be able to tailor the intervention to the client's needs. Begin the education efforts at the client's level of understanding, and explain hereditary cancer syndromes (HCSs), genetic information, and genetic testing. Simple analogies and pictures can help clients to understand this complex information.

To facilitate holistic care, ask clients if they would like their physicians to be informed of the recommendations about cancer surveillance, risk-reduction measures, and prevention options that the genetic assessment will yield. As you conduct the educational session, identify the client's misperceptions and clarify information as needed.

Family History

Only 5%–10% of all cancers are hereditary, with most following an autosomal-dominant inheritance pattern. The majority of families who have experienced an excess of cancer do not have an HCS. Complex gene-environment interactions may be causing the cancers in these families. HCS is characterized by

- **Early age of the client at onset of the disease:** If a cancer is an HCS, it usually occurs 10–15 years earlier than it would if it were a sporadic cancer. For example, colon cancer is a disease that usually occurs at ages 60–70; the occurrence of this disease in a man in his 30s suggests the possibility of an HCS.
- **Bilateral disease:** In an HCS, paired organs often are involved. Bilateral breast cancer involves both breasts. Bilateral retinoblastoma involves both eyes.
- **Multiple affected family members:** If many individuals in the same family are affected with the same cancer or a cluster of certain cancers, often within the same generation, the cause may be an HCS. For example, an HCS is the likely cause if a 30-year-old woman has breast cancer and her 40-year-old sister has ovarian cancer.
- **Transmission across three generations:** Typically, if cancer is present in three generations of a family, the cause is an HCS. For example, a family in which the grandfather, daughter, and grandson have early-onset colorectal cancer probably has an HCS. So does a family in which the daughter develops breast cancer in her 20s; her mother, ovarian cancer in her 40s; and the grandmother, breast cancer in her 50s. If cancer is hereditary, it typically appears earlier than expected in the normal population and in each successive generation.
- **Unique tumor-site combinations:** Certain types of hereditary cancers tend to cluster within one individual or one family. For example, if a person has hereditary nonpolyposis colorectal carcinoma (HNPCC), also known as

Lynch II syndrome, he or she is at greater-than-average risk for cancers of the colon, uterus, and ovary. Individuals with a mutated *BRCA1* gene may have family members with cancers of the breast, ovary, colon, and prostate. Additionally, multiple primary cancers in the same individual raise suspicion of hereditary cancer.

- **Rare cancers:** Certain cancers (e.g., retinoblastoma, medullary thyroid carcinoma) are so rare that their presence in more than one individual in a family suggests an HCS.

- **Precursor lesions or syndromes:** In cases of HCS, family members may manifest precursor lesions or syndromes—that is, lesions or syndromes that evolve into invasive cancers. For example, the colon and rectum of an individual with familial adenomatous polyposis (FAP) typically are carpeted with hundreds of thousands of polyps. In most cases, these polyps evolve into an invasive carcinoma. (Some clients undergo colectomies as a way to prevent disease progression.) If a genetic disorder or medical condition is associated with cancer, it may be indicative of a premalignant syndrome (e.g., dysplastic nevi, numerous polyps in FAP).

In conducting a genetic-risk assessment, document precursor lesions, biopsy results, and pertinent physical findings associated with heritable diseases. Record the presence of all genetic disorders and health problems within the family. For example, clients with Cowden's disease, a rare genetic autosomal-dominant skin disorder, have a greater risk of breast cancer than do people without the disease. Similarly, some cancer-predisposing genes may increase one's risk of developing other diseases, so documenting all genetic disorders and health problems in the family is very important.

An in-depth family history is a powerful tool for evaluating the presence of a hereditary cancer pattern. The assessment begins with an evaluation of the client and then proceeds to the maternal and paternal relatives. The family history assessment includes at least three generations. First-degree relatives, who share 50% of the client's genes, include parents, siblings, and children. Second-degree relatives, who share 25% of the client's genes, include aunts, uncles, grandparents, nieces, and nephews. Third-degree relatives, who share 12.5% of the client's genes, include cousins, great-aunts, great-uncles, and great-grandparents.

Hallmarks of hereditary cancers:
- Early age of disease onset
- Multiple affected family members
- Transmission across three generations
- Specific tumor-site clusters
- Multiple primary cancers in the same individual
- Bilateral disease
- Presence of rare cancers in multiple family members
- Precursor lesions

Documentation of the family history must
- State the race and ethnicity of the family.
- Define consanguineous relationships.
- Provide the ages of all living relatives.
- Provide pertinent medical and surgical histories for all members described.
- List the cause of death and age at death of all members considered.
- Cite the types of cancer members experienced, with the family member's age at diagnosis; the number of primary cancers and the presence of metastases; and whether disease was unilateral or bilateral.
- List significant environmental exposures for those with and without cancer.

Ethnicity

Information about a client's maternal and paternal ethnicity may be an important part of a genetic assessment because certain mutations in cancer-predisposing genes are specific to certain ethnic groups. For example, specific mutations of the *BRCA1* and *BRCA2* genes are unique to the Ashkenazic (eastern European) Jewish community (Fitzgerald et al., 1996; Struewing et al., 1995). Researchers are now trying to determine the cancer risks associated with these genetic mutations. Other investigators have identified mutations specific to the Dutch (Peelen et al., 1997; Petrij-Bosch et al., 1997) and Finnish populations (Vehmanen et al., 1997), in *BRCA1* and *BRCA2*, respectively.

Mutations specific to a certain ethnic group are the result of the founder effect. This occurs when one individual in an isolated community develops a mutation that is rare to the population as a whole. Because the community is small and isolated from other communities, the mutation stays within the community and is passed down from one generation to the next. Mutations carried by earlier members of a segregated community result in later generations having a higher frequency of the mutation than the population outside the community.

Assessment of ethnicity may facilitate the identification of an HCS and help to determine appropriate options for genetic testing. As genetics research evolves, investigators will surely find more links between specific ethnicities and particular genetic mutations. Therefore, recording ethnicity in a file today may, in the future, facilitate insight about a genetic manifestation.

Follow-Up Regarding a Known Mutation

A client may request a genetic assessment because a family member has been identified as having a cancer-predisposing genetic mutation. In this instance, request documentation of the relative's genetic mutation and family history. If the relative with the known mutation provides authorization, a healthcare professional may be able to obtain the documentation and family history from the institution that produced them.

Review the family history with the client to ensure its accuracy and to educate the client about inheritance patterns. Assess the information to determine if genetic testing would be appropriate for the client and, if so, which kind would be most appropriate. For most clients, testing for the known mutation within the family is all that is required. If the client is of Ashkenazic Jewish descent, however, testing the client for all three genetic mutations of *BRCA1* and *BRCA2* that are specific to that population is prudent.

The Assessment Process

A genetic assessment may take several visits to complete. A questionnaire can facilitate the process by helping the client to gather and submit information before the first consultation.

The Questionnaire

A questionnaire, completed and submitted by the client before the first assessment visit, presents information about the client's health record, lifestyle, occupational exposures, and personal risk factors. It also provides information about the medical history of the client's family members. Completing the questionnaire at home allows the client the opportunity to find answers to questions that he or she does not know, providing time to contact family members or check family records. If the completed questionnaire is submitted before the first visit, the nurse who will complete the genetic assessment is able to use the information on the questionnaire to prepare a preliminary pedigree. The client and the nurse, working together, will correct, clarify, and expand the pedigree during consultations.

The Pedigree

A pedigree is a symbolic representation of family members, social and biologic relationships, lines of descent, and reproductive scenarios. Analysis of the family pedigree results in identification of inheritance patterns, HCSs, and high-risk individuals. Standardized nomenclature for human pedigrees was developed in 1994 to facilitate correct interpretation of the pedigree and communication between healthcare professionals providing genetic services and researchers involved in genetic studies (Bennett et al., 1995; Schutte & Bennett, 1998). Figure 4-1 presents pedigree symbols and their definitions. Some nurses hand-draw pedigrees; others use computer software to create the drawings and store relevant data.

Figure 4-1. Pedigree Symbols

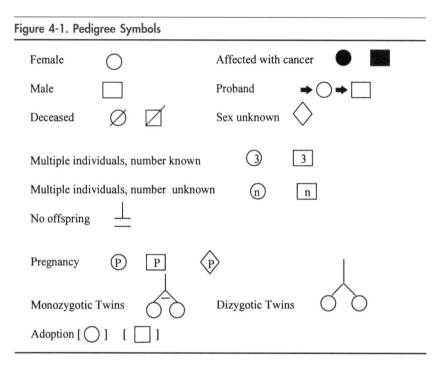

Review the preliminary pedigree with the client. Ensure that the family history is properly represented. Clients often, by mistake, provide inaccurate information; seeing the mistake on the pedigree often prompts them to identify and correct the error. Be particularly careful to verify biologic relationships. Ask the client if her offspring and those of her relatives share the same mother and father. Do not make assumptions about paternity. If biologic relationships are inaccurately documented, the result could be a misdiagnosis.

The Environment

Preferably, the environment for conducting a genetic assessment is private and conducive to client interaction, typically an area such as a small conference room or consultation room. Such a setting provides a therapeutic environment for counseling, as opposed to a clinical atmosphere, such as that of an examination room. A table facilitates the discussion of family history because it enables the nurse and client to see the pedigree as it is developed. Keep interruptions to a minimum—they are distracting and may upset the client, who may be talking about confidential and personal matters.

The Sequence

Begin the assessment with a discussion of the client's motivation for seeking cancer-risk counseling. Ask the client to describe his or her expectations in regard to the consultation. Describe the assessment process and tell how the pedigree will be used to prompt questions and clarify information.

A genetic assessment does not proceed in any standard format, but it may be helpful to obtain family history last. Getting the family data is the most time-consuming task and the most likely to spill over into subsequent sessions. Psychosocial evaluations can be made throughout the genetic assessment as the client shares information about family dynamics, cancer experiences, and the impact of these experiences.

Solicitation and Verification of Family History

A study of the accuracy of clients' reports of family history (Love, Evans, & Josten, 1985) found that information about first-degree relatives was 83% accurate, information about second-degree relatives was 67% accurate, and information about third-degree relatives was only 60% accurate. An inaccurate family history may result in misdiagnosis of the presence, absence, or type of hereditary pattern (Kerber & Slattery, 1997). In addition, misdiagnosis may affect recommendations about screening and prevention (Douglas, O'Dair, Robinson, Evans, & Lynch, 1999; Katballe et al., 2001).

One way to prompt accurate responses is to ask the client specific questions. For example, when questioning the client about family members, ask about specific symptoms experienced or treatment received. Direct questions may help the client to remember. Clients often become frustrated when they cannot provide information. Reassure the client by saying that many clients have limited information. Express appreciation for the information the client is able to provide, and explore with the client the feasibility of obtaining further information by contacting family members or obtaining official records. This may be difficult if family members have had little contact, are estranged, are uncomfortable discussing family history, or have moved to unknown locations.

The documents needed to verify clients' reports include medical records, pathology reports, death certificates, and autopsy reports. These documents are not always helpful in verifying a cancer that may not have caused a person's death (Novakovic, Goldstein, & Tuker, 1996). If family members are deceased, the next of kin with legal authority must sign authorization papers to permit release of the necessary documents. Study the documents carefully to verify that the client has supplied accurate information about the age of the family member at the onset of cancer, the types of cancer in the family, and biopsy results and surgeries.

The examples that follow illustrate the importance of obtaining documentation.

- A client reported that an aunt had breast cancer in both breasts and that the cancer was treated by means of bilateral mastectomy. The aunt's medical records, however, showed that she had unilateral breast cancer and that surgeons performed a contralateral mastectomy for prophylactic reasons.
- A client reported that her grandmother died from "stomach problems"; the medical records show that the woman died of ovarian cancer.

If the medical records had not been obtained, the result could have been an inaccurate genetic diagnosis.

Confidentiality and Genetic-Risk Assessment Records

The issue of confidentiality often is raised in regard to the placement of the genetic risk assessment in the medical record. Traditionally, family history data have been part of the medical history. Currently, family history information is defined as genetic information and therefore requires due concern for confidentiality and secure storage (Scanlon & Fibison, 1995). All records documenting family history require confidential handling. In the cancer risk assessment setting, the genetic team should enlist administrative and legal advice in making the decision whether to keep the genetic risk assessment as part of the medical record. Chapters 7 and 8 will further discuss the storage of genetic information.

Common Problems of Genetic Evaluation

This chapter has already shown how inaccurate client-supplied information can be problematic in a genetic assessment. One of the best defenses against misinformation is thorough knowledge of the cancers being reported: the usual age at onset, the natural history of the disease, treatment methods, and survival rates. This knowledge may lead a nurse to question the accuracy of a client's report. For example, if a client reports that her father had pancreatic cancer in his 40s and lived to his 60s, a knowledgeable nurse will question the report or the diagnosis. Similarly, if a client reports that her mother had ovarian cancer in her 30s and is still alive at 90, a knowledgeable nurse will seek verification.

Family characteristics may prove to be limitations. For example, if the client has a small family and if individuals died young, not living long enough to be affected by cancer, or if the client was adopted, the family history, though accurately reported, may not tell the nurse what he or she needs to know.

Suppose a patient had breast cancer in her 20s; no siblings; a mother who had breast cancer in her 40s; and a maternal uncle who died, without offspring, of influenza at the age of 24. The patient has no information about her grandparents. In such a case, the maternal family history is limited. Assuming the paternal family history is negative for cancer, hereditary breast cancer syndrome may be suspected because two generations were affected with breast cancer and the patient was diagnosed while young. Thus, the nurse may recommend that the patient consider having genetic testing to determine her risk. If the patient does not want testing, she should be screened as a high-risk individual.

Models to Facilitate Risk Assessment

Among the models available to assess the risk of certain HCSs or inheriting mutations in cancer-predisposing genes are the Claus (Claus, Risch, & Thompson, 1994) and Gail (Gail et al., 1989) models. These models help to assess the risk of breast cancer; however, they may underestimate the risk of mutation carriers and overestimate the risk of noncarriers.

The Amsterdam criteria (Vasen, Mecklin, Khan, & Lynch, 1991) and the Bethesda guidelines (Rodriguez-Bigas et al., 1997) are used to assess families with a history of colon cancer for their risk of HNPCC. Models also are available to estimate a woman's risk of having a mutation in *BRCA1* (Couch et al., 1997; Frank et al., 1997; Shattuck-Eidens et al., 1995) and *BRCA2* (Frank et al.). See Chapter 5 for risk-model discussion.

A Sample Assessment

The Case

Sarah is a patient seeking counseling about her risk of breast cancer. She is 36 years old and has had two breast biopsies, both of which were significant for atypical hyperplasia. She is married and has never been pregnant. She experienced menarche at age 14 and is premenopausal. She does not smoke and reports rare alcohol use, approximately two glasses of wine per month. Her mother had bilateral breast cancer at the ages of 39 and 56; she currently is without evidence of disease at age 69. Her maternal aunt had ovarian cancer at age 53 and died at 54. Her maternal uncle had prostate cancer at 62, and he had a daughter who had breast cancer at age 43 and died at 45. Her maternal grand-mother died at age 91 of natural causes. Her maternal grandfather died of a heart attack at the age of 54. She is of Ashkenazic Jewish heritage both mater-nally and paternally.

The Assessment

Figure 4-2 shows Sarah's pedigree. This patient's family history suggests a hereditary breast-ovarian cancer syndrome. Hereditary risk factors identified in this family include

- Mother with bilateral breast cancer and early age at onset at the time of the first diagnosis
- Maternal aunt with early-onset ovarian cancer
- Maternal uncle with prostate cancer (increased prostate cancer risk is asso-ciated with breast-ovarian cancer syndrome)
- Maternal first cousin with early-onset breast cancer.

Other risk factors include the patient's ethnicity and the fact that she is 36 and nulliparous and has had two breast biopsies with atypical hyperplasia. In terms of ethnicity, it is estimated that one in 40 Ashkenazic Jewish individuals has a mutation in *BRCA1* or *BRCA2*. Nulliparity and atypical hyperplasia are associated with a higher-than-average risk of breast cancer; however, the inter-

Figure 4-2. Sample Pedigree

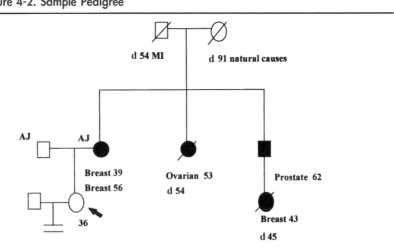

action between genetic mutations and these personal risk factors is not well understood.

Based on this assessment, the patient is offered the option of genetic testing to determine her risk. If she is not interested in testing, she should be considered a high-risk individual and appropriate screening and prevention measures discussed.

Conclusion

Clients are asking questions about genetic testing. They are seeking answers to explain the burden of cancer in their families. Oncology nurses will encounter these questions from patients in all clinical areas. Nurses have a duty to answer these questions and provide support and referrals to cancer-risk evaluation services. As part of their role in delivering holistic care to patients, oncology nurses must incorporate genetic assessment into general patient assessment, and they must maintain their knowledge of cancer genetics to perform the assessment competently. As genetic diagnostics and genetic therapies advance, the nurse's role in performing a genetic assessment will expand beyond that of assessing a client's risk of cancer. The nurse's new role will include assessment of the implications of genetic information on the diagnosis and treatment of cancer.

References

American Cancer Society 1996 Advisory Committee on Diet, Nutrition, and Cancer Prevention. (1996). Guidelines on diet, nutrition, and cancer prevention: Reducing the risk of cancer with healthy food choices and physical activity. *CA: A Cancer Journal for Clinicians, 46,* 325–341.

Bennett, R., Steinhaus, K., Uhrich, S.B., O'Sullivan, C.K., Resta, R.G., Lochner-Doyle, D., Markel, D.S., Vincent, V., & Hamanishi, J. (1995). Recommendations for standardized human pedigree nomenclature. *American Journal of Human Genetics, 56,* 745–752.

Claus, E., Risch, N., & Thompson, W. (1994). Autosomal dominant inheritance of early-onset breast cancer. *Cancer, 73,* 643–651.

Couch, F., DeShano, M., Blackwood, M.A., Calzone, K., Stopfer, J., Campeau, L., et al. (1997). BRCA1 mutations in the women attending clinics that evaluate the risk of breast cancer. *New England Journal of Medicine, 336,* 1409–1415.

Daly, M., Barsevick, A., Miller, S., Buckman, R., Costalas, J., Montgomery, S., et al. (2001). Communicating genetic test results to the family: A six-step, skill-building strategy. *Family Community Health, 24*, 13–26.

Douglas, F., O'Dair, L., Robinson, M., Evans, D., & Lynch, S. (1999). The accuracy of diagnoses as reported in families with cancer: A retrospective study. *Journal of Medical Genetics, 36*, 309–312.

Dupont, W., Parl, F., Hartmann, W., Brinton, L., Winfield, A., Worrell, J., et al. (1993). Breast cancer risk associated with proliferative breast disease and atypical hyperplasia. *Cancer, 71*, 1258–1265.

Fitzgerald, M.G., MacDonald, D.J., Krainer, M., Hoover, I., O'Neil, E., Unsal, H., et al. (1996). Germline BRCA1 mutations in Jewish and non-Jewish women with early-onset breast cancer. *New England Journal of Medicine, 334*, 143–149.

Frank, T., Manley, S., Thomas, A., McClure, M., Ward, B., Shattuck-Eidens, D., et al. (1997). BRCA1 and BRCA2 sequence analysis of 335 high-risk women. *American Journal of Human Genetics, 61*(Suppl. A65).

Friedenreich, C., & Rohan, T. (1995). A review of physical activity and breast cancer. *Epidemiology, 6*, 311–317.

Gail, M., Brinton, L., Byar, D., Corle, D., Green, S., Schairer, C., et al. (1989). Projecting individualized probabilities of developing breast cancer for white females who are being examined annually. *Journal of the National Cancer Institute, 81*, 1879–1886.

Hill, A., & Austin, H. (1996). Nutrition and endometrial cancer. *Cancer Causes and Control, 7*, 19–32.

Hunter, D., & Willett, W. (1996). Nutrition and breast cancer. *Cancer Causes and Control, 7*, 56–68.

Katballe, N., Juul, S., Christensen, M., Orntoft, T., Wilkman, F., & Laurberg, S. (2001). Patient accuracy of reporting on hereditary non-polyposis colorectal-cancer related malignancy in family members. *British Journal of Surgery, 88*, 1228–1233.

Kerber, R., & Slattery, M. (1997). Comparison of self-reported and data base-linked family history of cancer data in a case-control study. *American Journal of Epidemiology, 146*, 244–248.

Kolonel, L. (1996). Nutrition and prostate cancer. *Cancer Causes and Control, 7*, 83–94.

Love, R., Evans, A., & Josten, D. (1985). The accuracy of client reports of a family history of cancer. *Journal of Chronic Disease, 38*, 289–293.

Michaud, D., Giovannucci, E., Willett, W., Colditz, G., Stampfer, M., & Fuchs, C. (2001). Physical activity, obesity, height, and the risk of pancreatic cancer. *JAMA, 286*, 921–929.

Novakovic, B., Goldstein, A., & Tucker, M. (1996). Validation of family history of cancer in deceased family members. *Journal of the National Cancer Institute, 88*, 1492–1493.

Oncology Nursing Society. (1999). *Oncology Nursing Society multicultural outcomes: Guidelines for cultural competence.* Pittsburgh: Author.

Page, D., Dupont, W.D., Rogers, L.W., & Rados, M.S. (1985). Atypical hyperplastic lesions of the female breast: A long-term follow-up study. *Cancer, 55*, 2698–2708.

Peelen, T., van Vliet, M., Petrij-Bosch, A., Mieremet, R., Szabo, C., van den Ouweland, A., et al. (1997). A high proportion of novel mutations in BRCA1 with strong founder effects among Dutch and Belgian hereditary breast and ovarian cancer families. *American Journal of Human Genetics, 60*, 1041–1049.

Petrij-Bosch, A., Peelen, T., van Vliet, M., van Eijk, R., Olmer, R., Drusedau, M., et al. (1997). BRCA1 genomic deletions are major founder mutations in Dutch breast cancer clients. *Nature Genetics, 17*, 341–345.

Potter, J. (1996). Nutrition and colorectal cancer. *Cancer Causes and Control, 7*, 127–146.

Rodriguez-Bigas, M.A., Boland, C.R., Hamilton, S.R., Henson, D.E., Jass, J.R., Khan, P.M., et al. (1997). A National Cancer Institute workshop on hereditary nonpolyposis colorectal cancer syndrome: Meeting highlights and Bethesda guidelines. *Journal of the National Cancer Institute, 89*, 1758–1762.

Scanlon, C., & Fibison, W. (1995). *Managing genetic information: Implications for nursing practice.* Washington, DC: American Nurses Association.

Schatzkin, A., Goldstein, A., & Freedman, L. (1995). What does it mean to be a cancer gene carrier? Problems in establishing causality from the molecular genetics of cancer. *Journal of the National Cancer Institute, 87*, 1126–1130.

Schutte, J., & Bennett, R. (1998). Lessons in history: Obtaining the family history and constructing a pedigree. In D. Baker, J. Schutte, & W. Uhlman (Eds.), *A guide to genetic counseling* (pp. 27–51). New York: Wiley-Liss.

Shattuck-Eidens, D., McClure, M., Simard, J., Labrie, F., Narod, S., Couch, F., et al. (1995). A collaborative survey of 80 mutations in the BRCA1 breast and ovarian cancer susceptibility gene: Implications for presymptomatic testing and screening. *JAMA, 273*, 535–541.

Shephard, R. (1993). Exercise in the prevention and treatment of cancer: An update. *Sports Medicine, 15*, 258–280.

Struewing, J., Abeliovich, D., Peretz, T., Avishai, N., Kaback, M., Collins, F., et al. (1995). The carrier frequency of the BRCA1 185delAG mutation is approximately 1 percent in Ashkenazi Jewish individuals. *Nature Genetics, 11*, 198–200.

Vasen, H., Mecklin, J., Khan, P., & Lynch, H. (1991). The International Collaborative Group on Hereditary Nonpolyposis Colorectal Cancer (ICG-HNPCC). *Disorders of the Colon and Rectum, 34,* 424–425.

Vehmanen, P., Friedman, L., Eerola, H., Sarantaus, L., Pyrhonen, S., Ponder, B., et al. (1997). A low proportion of BRCA2 mutations in Finnish breast cancer families. *American Journal of Human Genetics, 60,* 1050–1058.

Wolk, A., Lindblad, P., & Adami, H. (1996). Nutrition and renal cell cancer. *Cancer Causes and Control, 7,* 5–18.

5

Cancer-Risk Assessment: Considerations for Cancer Genetics

Suzanne M. Mahon, RN, DNSc, AOCN®, APNG(c)

Editors' note: The terms that appear in boldface in this chapter are defined in the glossary. Glossary terms also are highlighted in Chapters 3 and 6.

Introduction

By collecting and interpreting cancer-risk information, healthcare professionals can help clients to make informed decisions about participation in cancer-prevention and surveillance programs as well as to decide whether genetic testing is appropriate. Applied research about communicating cancer-risk information is sparse, and very little is known about effective communication when multiple risks exist.

In one of the few articles about cancer-risk communication, Weinstein (1999) noted that the goals of risk communication should not be limited to helping people understand the risks they face. Other goals should include building trust, influencing public policy, and fulfilling legal obligations.

In addition to guiding screening decisions, risk assessment should guide treatment decisions. If risk is known, then those who stand to gain the most from preventive treatment, such as chemoprevention or prophylactic surgery, can undergo it. Accurate risk assessment is vital to responsible decision making.

Genetic testing, the most recent addition to the tools used for risk assessment (Weitzel, 1999), has brought new prominence to cancer-risk assessment in the last few years (Kelly, 1999). Many people seek cancer-risk assessment to determine if they should undergo genetic testing, but much can be gained from the assessment process regardless of whether genetic testing is ever done. Genetic testing is just one of the tools used in comprehensive cancer-risk assessment. Nurses who counsel about cancer risk must remember that risk assessment is as important for people who decline genetic testing as for those who decide to have it. People who decline testing need to understand their risk of developing cancer and the inherent strengths and weaknesses associated with screening tests. Risk-factor assessment should be a component of the cancer-screening process for all individuals. Furthermore—because families share a pool of genes and, therefore, similar risks—genetic risk assessment must include not only individuals, but also entire families.

This chapter will discuss types of risk and risk-prediction models; methods of communicating risk information to clients; psychosocial and ethical concerns in risk-factor assessment; clinical issues of risk assessment, including documentation; and issues involved in following up on risk assessment. Clinical examples involving breast cancer and colon cancer will clarify discussion. The concepts the examples show are applicable to the other cancers for which risk-factor assessment commonly is performed.

Terms Commonly Used in Risk Assessment

Literature about cancer-risk assessment, cancer screening, and cancer genetic counseling typically uses a variety of epidemiologic and statistical terms. Nurses who provide genetics services must know how to use the terms and explain them to clients.

A **risk factor** is a trait or characteristic associated with a statistically significant increased likelihood of developing a disease (Mahon, 2000). Note, however, that having a risk factor does not mean a that a person will develop the disease, such as a malignancy, nor does the absence of a risk factor make the person immune to developing the disease.

Basic elements of a cancer-risk assessment include a review of medical history, a history of exposures to carcinogens in daily living, and a detailed family history. The goals of risk-factor assessment and counseling are to provide accurate information about the genetic, biologic, and environmental factors related to an individual's risk of developing cancer, formulate appropriate recommendations for primary and secondary prevention, and offer emotional and psychosocial support to facilitate adjustment to the information regarding risk and promote adherence to recommendations for prevention and early detection.

Although cancer-risk assessment often is applied to the process of cancer screening, assessment has clinical applications in all phases of the cancer trajectory. After a risk factor is identified, cancer-prevention measures can be implemented.

Primary cancer prevention includes measures to avoid carcinogen exposure and improve health practices, and, in some cases, includes the use of chemopreventive agents. Primary prevention also may include the use of prophylactic surgery to prevent or significantly reduce the risk of malignancy development.

Secondary cancer prevention includes identifying people at risk of malignancy and implementing appropriate screening recommendations.

Tertiary cancer prevention is aimed at people with a history of malignancy. It includes monitoring for and preventing recurrence of the originally diagnosed cancer and screening for second primary cancers. In many cases, those who have been diagnosed with cancer and who carry a mutated cancer-susceptibility gene are at significantly higher risk for developing a second malignancy. Tertiary cancer prevention is particularly important for this group of individuals.

The results of genetic testing ultimately guide primary, secondary, and tertiary cancer-prevention efforts.

The **prevalence** of cancer is the actual number of cancers in a defined population at a given time. The prevalence rate is commonly expressed as the number of cancers per 100,000 individuals in the population. Estimates of the prevalence of various cancers are available from the American Cancer Society (ACS) and the National Cancer Institute (NCI).

The **incidence** of cancer is the number of cancers that develop in a population during a defined period, such as a year. For example, ACS (2001) estimated that 192,200 women would be diagnosed with breast cancer during 2001. Incidence numbers can be helpful when trying to understand cancer risks for the general population.

The **mortality rate** is the number of people who die of a particular cancer during a defined period. The estimated mortality for breast cancer for women in 2001 is 40,200 deaths (ACS, 2001). Compare that mortality estimate to the mortality estimate for small-intestine cancer: 1,100 deaths annually (ACS).

Population is the number of people in a defined group who are capable of developing a disease. It may refer to the general population or a specific group of people defined by geographic, physical, or social characteristics. For example, nurses who provide genetic-risk assessment and counseling about cancer ask if a client is a member of the Ashkenazic Jewish population. This specific group is at high risk for three specific mutations associated with hereditary breast cancer (Struewing et al., 1997).

Outcomes are the health and economic results that occur related to screening or genetic testing. Outcomes may include the benefits, harms, and costs of screening or testing and the diagnostic evaluations that result from screening or testing (Clark & Reintgen, 1996). Short-term outcomes include the number of people screened or tested, the number of cancers detected, or the cost per cancer detected. Long-term outcomes include site-specific cancers detected in the screened population, total costs of treatment in the entire population, and the stage distribution of detected cancers (Lai & Hardy, 1999). Nurses who provide genetic-risk assessments should be familiar with outcome measures because they must be able to give clients detailed information about the risks and benefits of testing, screening, detection, and prevention strategies.

Validity is a measure of how well a test measures what it is supposed to measure. To be able to make recommendations about screening, for example, nurses must be able to compare the validity of various screening tests. Table 5-1 lists six characteristics that define the validity of mammography, x-ray imaging of the chest, and pelvic examination. Being able to compare validity in such

Table 5-1. Comparison of the Validity of Various Screening Tests

Characteristics of Disease	Breast Cancer	Lung Cancer	Ovarian Cancer
# of new cases	192,200	169,500	23,400
# of deaths annually	40,600	157,400	13,900
Effective treatment for early stage of disease	Five-year survival rate for localized disease is 92%	Five-year survival rate for localized disease is less than 50%	Five-year survival rate for localized disease is 95%

Characteristics of Screening Tests	Mammography	Chest X-Ray	Pelvic Examination
Able to detect pre-clinical disease	Can detect micro-calcifications and in situ disease	Lesion must be at least 1 cm	Lesion must be at least a 4- x 6-cm mass
Sensitivity	80%	Less than 50%	67%
Specificity	95%	89%	4% (24 false positives for each case detected)
Safety	Minimal radiation exposure	Minimal radiation exposure	Minimal risks
Acceptable to the client	Some find it uncomfortable, embarrassing	Generally acceptable	Some find it uncomfortable, embarrassing
Cost	$70–$150	$70–$100	Bundled with standard exam cost—very low

Note. Based on information from American Cancer Society, 2001; Clark, 1996; Florica & Roberts, 1996; Wolpaw, 1996. From "Principles of Cancer Prevention and Detection," by S.M. Mahon, 2000, *Clinical Journal of Oncology Nursing, 4,* p. 174. Copyright 2000 by the Oncology Nursing Society. Adapted with permission.

a way is important because recommendations regarding a specific test may vary according to the organization that issues them. ACS, the United States Preventive Services Task Force (USPSTF), and NCI may have different recommendations about the same test, for example. These differences result from the fact that each organization uses different criteria to formulate recommendations. The result is that screening information often is very confusing to the general public. Being able to speak in terms of validity provides a means of cutting through the confusion. The concept of validity also may help clients to understand that screening recommendations for those of average risk, which are issued by groups such as ACS, may be inadequate for those with higher risk.

The **accuracy** of a screening test is the degree to which a measurement represents the true value of the characteristic being measured. In the context of cancer screening, results fall into one of the following categories of accuracy.

- **True positive (TP):** TP results indicate that the person tested has cancer and he or she actually does. In Table 5-2, the number of TP tests is 85.
- **True negative (TN):** TN results indicate that the person tested does not have cancer and, indeed, that person neither has nor develops cancer within a defined period. In Table 5-2, the number of TN tests is 775.
- **False negative (FN):** A person has an FN result if the test says the client does not have cancer but he or she actually does. In Table 5-2, the number of FN results is 15.

Table 5-2. Results From a Screening Test

Results of the Screening Tests	Characteristics in the Population (N = 1,000)	
	Number of Individuals Who Actually Have Cancer	Number of Individuals Who Actually Do Not Have Cancer
Positive test	85 true positive (TP)	125 false positive (FP)
Negative test	15 false negative (FN)	775 true negative (TN)
Total	100	900

$$\text{Sensitivity} = \frac{TP}{TP+FN} = \frac{85}{85+15} = 0.85$$

$$\text{Specificity} = \frac{TN}{TN+FP} = \frac{775}{775+125} = 0.86$$

Note. From "Principles of Cancer Prevention and Early Detection," by S.M. Mahon, 2000, *Clinical Journal of Oncology Nursing, 4*, p. 174. Copyright 2000 by the Oncology Nursing Society. Reprinted with permission.

- **False positive (FP):** An FP result occurs when the screening test says a person has cancer but he or she does not. In Table 5-2, the number of FN results is 125.

Information about accuracy categories is necessary to calculate sensitivity and specificity.

The **sensitivity** of a screening test is its ability to detect those individuals with cancer. It is calculated by taking the number of TPs and dividing it by the total number of cancer cases (TP + FN). Using the data in Table 5-2, the calculation for sensitivity is $85 \div (85 + 15) = 0.85$

Most people are unwilling to accept a test with a high FN rate because the test will miss many cancers.

The **specificity** of a test is its ability to identify individuals who actually do not have cancer. It is calculated by dividing the TN by the sum of the number of TN and FP results. Using the data in Table 5-2, the calculation for specificity is $775 \div (775 + 125) = 0.86$

A high FP rate can result in unnecessary follow-up testing and anxiety for clients who receive FP results.

Understanding the principles of sensitivity and specificity helps clients realize the strengths and limitations of the screening test they are considering. Nurses and clients must recognize that the perfect screening test does not exist. Even mammography fails to detect 6%–10% of all breast cancers (Bilimoria & Morrow, 1995). Failure rates regarding the detection of breast cancer may even be higher in women under age 50 (Rosenberg et al., 1998). Many individuals choose to undergo screening even if the test has a relatively low sensitivity and specificity in the hope that the test will be effective for them. Screening for ovarian cancer is an excellent example. No highly specific and sensitive screening test that allows early detection of ovarian cancer currently is available. Many women, however, still want an annual pelvic examination in which a clinician assesses her for ovarian masses, despite the fact that some clinicians are much better at detecting ovarian masses than others and that many ovarian cancers cannot be detected in a pelvic exam, even when performed by a skilled clinician. On the positive side, the test is relatively inexpensive and well tolerated by most women. As long as a woman realizes that the test may fail to detect ovarian cancer and is willing to accept this limitation, deciding to have a pelvic exam is an appropriate choice for a woman at average risk for ovarian cancer. A woman at higher risk may choose to undergo CA-125 antigen testing and a transvaginal ultrasound. Research has never proved either of these tests effective in reducing the morbidity and mortality associated with ovarian cancer, yet high-risk women continue to undergo them at their physicians' recommendation.

General Limitations of Risk Assessment

Newell and Vogel (1988) discussed two important reasons for identifying and quantifying cancer risks: The identification of risk factors contributes to the understanding of the biology of cancer, and, when identified, such risk factors can be altered to decrease the number of new cases of or deaths from cancer. Not all risk factors are amenable to change, however, as is the case with many risk factors for breast cancer (see Table 5-3). An individual cannot change her gender, age, history, and some of the other cited factors. In such a case, a nurse should recommend secondary cancer-prevention efforts.

The second limitation of risk assessment relates to the assessment models, which are based on assumptions and epidemiologic studies. If these assumptions and studies are weak or deficient, the resulting assessment can be inaccurate or inappropriate. Most studies are epidemiologic; they identify an association between exposure or no exposure to an agent and the subsequent occurrence of disease. If a statistically significant correlation is found, researchers can make one conclusion only: that an association (not necessarily a cause-and-effect relationship) exists between the substance and cancer.

Sometimes researchers suspect an etiology, or cause of disease. Table 5-3 lists the common etiologies relative to specific risk factors for breast cancer. As with many cancers, the etiology of breast cancer appears to be multifactorial, with endogenous and exogenous risk factors contributing to risk. No model can include all the risk factors that may apply to each individual. Therefore, another general limitation of risk assessment is that no model completely and accurately explains an individual's risk for developing a particular cancer (Leventhal, Kelly, & Leventhal, 1999).

On the topic of the weakness of models, note that, in regard to most cancers, a portion of the cancer diagnoses cannot be explained by recognized risk factors. For example, in a study of 7,508 women, approximately 41% of breast cancer cases were attributable to the usual risk factors (i.e., later age at first birth, nulliparity, and a family history of breast cancer) (Madigan, Ziegler, Benichou, Byrne, & Hoover, 1995). The researchers noted that, ideally, knowledge of risk factors should guide primary prevention efforts. However, in the case of breast cancer, the inability to alter most risk factors limited their relevance for primary prevention. In some cancers, such as breast cancer, the central role of risk-factor identification is to identify women at higher-than-average risk, particularly those with a genetic susceptibility to breast cancer, and to screen them more aggressively. For example, women from families prone to breast cancer may be advised to undergo mammographies at a younger age than usually recommended or have a clinical breast examination more than once a year, depending on the clinician.

Table 5-3. Risk Factors for Breast Cancer

Risk Factor	Possible Etiology
Female	Females have a greater proportion of breast tissue than do males.
Age	Higher cumulative exposure to carcinogens
Personal history of breast cancer	Role not entirely clear but especially true with premenopausal women and lobular carcinoma in situ
Family history	The cancer-susceptibility genes BRCA1 and BRCA2 may predispose a woman to developing breast cancer because the initial genetic mutation has occurred and fewer mutations are needed for the breast cancer to develop.
Personal or family history of ovarian, endometrial, or colon cancer	Possible genetic predisposition (including disposition to hereditary nonpolyposis colorectal cancer, Lynch syndrome type I or II)
Early menarche Nulliparity First pregnancy after age 30 Late menopause (after age 50)	The breast tissue of a woman prior to pregnancy may be more sensitive to carcinogens than breast tissue that has gone through its complete hormonal development. This also may be related to the total number of ovulatory cycles a woman has completed.
Diet	High-fat diet may change the metabolism of estrogen. An abundance of estrogen could increase risk of breast cancer.
Biopsy-proven atypia	Increased proliferation of tissue may lead to cellular abnormalities.
Alcohol consumption	Mechanisms are poorly understood.
Contraceptive use	Long-term use of contraceptives prior to first pregnancy may increase risk slightly.
Hormone replacement	Long-term use may increase risk, but actual influence is largely unknown.

Note. Based on information from Bilmoria & Morrow, 1995; Kelly, 1991; Love, 1989. From "Cancer Risk Assessment: Conceptual Considerations for Clinical Practice," by S.M. Mahon, 1998, *Oncology Nursing Forum, 25,* p. 1536. Copyright 1998 by the Oncology Nursing Society. Adapted with permission.

Each risk-assessment model has inherent strengths and weaknesses; these will be discussed later in this chapter. Nurses need to be aware of these and provide each client with a balanced discussion that incorporates an understanding of each model's characteristics.

Major Types of Risk

Most risk discussions include, at minimum, a discussion of absolute risk, relative risk, and attributable risk.

Absolute Risk

Absolute risk is a measure of the occurrence of cancer, either incidence (new cases) or mortality (deaths), in the general population. Absolute risk can be expressed either as the number of cases for a specified denominator (e.g., 50 cases per 10,000 people annually) or as a cumulative risk up to a specified age (e.g., one in eight women who live to age 85 will develop breast cancer). Another way to express absolute risk is to discuss the average risk of developing breast cancer at a certain age. Table 5-4 illustrates why risk always should be discussed in light of an individual's current age. Risk estimates for a 40-year-old woman are much different from those for a 70-year-old woman; approximately 50% of the cases of breast cancer occur after age 65 (Ries et al., 1999).

Clients who present for screenings must understand the assumptions involved in reaching an absolute risk figure. For example, in Table 5-4, "1 in 8" in the "Birth to Death" column for breast cancer describes the average risk of breast cancer in white American women and takes into consideration other causes of death over the life span. The 1-in-8 estimate overestimates breast cancer risk for some women with no risk factors and underestimates the risk for women with several risk factors (Love, 1995). What 1 in 8 actually means is that the average woman's breast cancer risk is just 2% to age 50; 6% from 50 to 70; and 3% from age 70 to 85 (Kelly, 2000). The estimate of an 11%, or 1 in 8, risk is obtained by adding the risk in each age category (2% + 6% + 3% = 11%).

When a woman who has average risk reaches age 50 without a diagnosis of breast cancer, she has passed through 2% of her risk, so her risk to age 80 is 11% minus 2%, or 9%. When she reaches age 70 without a diagnosis of breast cancer, her risk to age 80 is 11% minus 2% minus 6%, or 3%. For a risk figure to be meaningful, time must be considered. For example, the average 50-year-old woman's risk is 6% to age 70 but 9% to age 80 (Kelly, 2000) (see Figure 5-1).

Relative Risk

The term *relative risk* (**RR**) refers to a comparison of the incidence of a risk factor or the number of deaths among those with a risk factor compared to those without the risk factor. RR should not be confused with absolute risk: Absolute risk is calculated on the basis of all individuals in the population who have the disease, regardless of risk.

Table 5-4. Probability of Developing Invasive Cancers Over Selected Age Intervals, by Sex, United States, 1995–1997[b]

		Birth to 39 (%)	40–59 (%)	60–79 (%)	Birth to Death (%)
All sites[b]	Male	1.56 (1 in 64)	8.25 (1 in 12)	33.13 (1 in 3)	43.48 (1 in 2)
	Female	1.96 (1 in 51)	9.37 (1 in 11)	22.39 (1 in 4)	38.34 (1 in 3)
Bladder[c]	Male	0.03 (1 in 3,437)	0.44 (1 in 226)	2.39 (1 in 42)	3.40 (1 in 29)
	Female	—(< 1 in 10,000)	0.14 (1 in 699)	0.68 (1 in 146)	1.18 (1 in 85)
Breast	Female	0.44 (1 in 225)	4.15 (1 in 24)	7.02 (1 in 14)	12.83 (1 in 8)
Colon and rectum	Male	0.07 (1 in 1,531)	0.87 (1 in 115)	4.00 (1 in 25)	5.78 (1 in 17)
	Female	0.05 (1 in 1,855)	0.69 (1 in 146)	3.04 (1 in 33)	5.55 (1 in 18)
Leukemia	Male	0.15 (1 in 654)	0.21 (1 in 467)	0.84 (1 in 119)	1.42 (1 in 70)
	Female	0.11 (1 in 900)	0.15 (1 in 671)	0.50 (1 in 199)	1.05 (1 in 95)
Lung and bronchus	Male	0.4 (1 in 2,499)	1.24 (1 in 80)	6.29 (1 in 16)	8.09 (1 in 12)
	Female	0.03 (1 in 2,997)	0.92 (1 in 108)	4.04 (1 in 25)	5.78 (1 in 17)

(Continued on next page)

Table 5-4. Probability of Developing Invasive Cancers Over Selected Age Intervals, by Sex, United States, 1995–1997[a] (Continued)

		Birth to 39 (%)	40–59 (%)	60–79 (%)	Birth to Death (%)
Melanoma of the skin	Male	0.13 (1 in 744)	0.53 (1 in 190)	0.94 (1 in 106)	1.68 (1 in 60)
	Female	0.22 (1 in 453)	0.40 (1 in 249)	0.48 (1 in 207)	1.25 (1 in 80)
Non-Hodgkin's lymphoma	Male	0.19 (1 in 513)	0.50 (1 in 198)	1.21 (1 in 83)	2.11 (1 in 47)
	Female	0.08 (1 in 1,296)	0.32 (1 in 312)	0.97 (1 in 103)	1.74 (1 in 57)
Prostate	Male	< 1 in 10,000	2.06 (1 in 49)	13.42 (1 in 7)	15.89 (1 in 6)
Uterine cervix	Female	0.17 (1 in 576)	0.30 (1 in 332)	0.26 (1 in 387)	0.78 (1 in 129)
Uterine corpus	Female	0.05 (1 in 2,142)	0.74 (1 in 136)	1.67 (1 in 60)	2.73 (1 in 37)

[a] For those free of cancer at beginning of age interval. Based on cancer cases diagnosed during 1995–1997. The "1 in" statistic and the inverse of the percentage may not be equivalent because of rounding.
[b] Excludes basal- and squamous-cell skin cancers and in situ carcinomas except those of the urinary bladder.
[c] Includes invasive and in situ cancer cases.

Sources: DEVCAN Software, Version 4.0, Surveillance, Epidemiology, and End Results Program, 1973–1997, Division of Cancer Control and Population Sciences, National Cancer Institute, 2000. American Cancer Society, Surveillance Research, 2001.

Note. From "Cancer Statistics, 2001," by R.T. Greenlee, M.B. Hill-Harmon, T. Murray, and M. Thun, 2001, *CA: A Cancer Journal for Clinicians, 51,* p. 13. Copyright 2001 by Lippincott Williams & Wilkins. Reprinted with permission.

Figure 5-1. Age-Specific Risk of Developing Breast Cancer

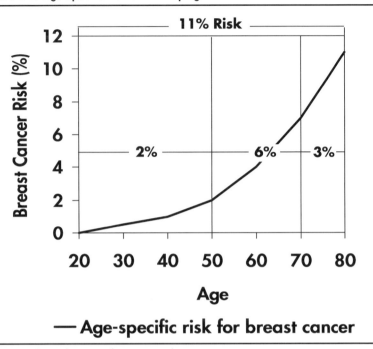

— Age-specific risk for breast cancer

Note. Based on information from Ries et al., 1999.

By using risk factors, a woman can determine her risk by using RR figures and thus gain a better understanding of her personal chances of developing breast cancer as compared to women without such risk factors. When looking at RR figures, the reference point is 1.0. An RR > 1.0 indicates a risk factor associated with disease. An RR < 1.0 is not a risk factor in that population. As Table 5-5 shows, the RR for a woman whose mother (first-degree relative) had bilateral breast cancer diagnosed at age 40 (premenopausal) is 8.5–9.0. This means that her risk of developing breast cancer is 8.5–9.0 times higher than the risk of a woman with no known risk of developing breast cancer.

RR factors can be confusing to some clients. For them, viewing information in table format, such as the format shown in Table 5-5, may be helpful. When giving a client information about RR, healthcare professionals must specify exactly what comparison is being made.

Percentages also can be the basis of confusion. If a news report states that there is a 30%–50% increase in breast cancer risk because of a particular hormone therapy used after menopause, the report means, in numeric terms, that

Table 5-5. Relative Risk of Developing Breast Cancer

Factor	Relative Risk
First-degree relative with breast cancer	1.2–3.0
Premenopausal	3.1
Premenopausal and bilateral	8.5–9.0
Postmenopausal	1.5
Postmenopausal and bilateral	4.0–5.4
Menstrual history	
Age at menarche < 12	1.3
Age at menopause < 55	1.5–2.0
Pregnancy	
First live birth from ages 25–29	1.5
First live birth after age 30	1.9
First live birth after age 35	2.0–3.0
Nulliparous	3.0
Benign breast diseases	
Proliferative disease	1.9
Proliferative disease with atypical hyperplasia	4.4
Lobular carcinoma in situ	6.9–12.0

Note. From "The Woman at Increased Risk for Breast Cancer: Evaluation and Management Strategies," by M.M. Bilimoria and M. Morrow, 1995, *CA: A Cancer Journal for Clinicians, 45*, p. 265. Copyright 1995 by Lippincott Williams & Wilkins. Reprinted with permission.

there will be 0.3–0.5 more cases of breast cancer per 100 women. Similarly, if a study reports a 49% decrease in risk for women who take a particular chemopreventive agent, 0.49 fewer cases of breast cancer per 100 women will occur. However, the absolute risk reduction may not be as great as the percentage, 49%, might suggest. The only way to be able to accurately convert the percentage figure to an absolute risk is by looking at the actual study data. Kelly (2000) provided a thorough analysis of the tamoxifen prevention trial results, explaining the differences in the derivation of risk figures.

RR sometimes is expressed as a ratio. Ratios can create problems because people fail to consider the relevant sample size. For example, individuals may respond differently to a ratio when it is expressed as 1:10 rather than 10:100, even though both ratios express the same probability (Rothman & Kiviniemi, 1999). People may rate a health problem as riskier if informed that it kills 1,275 of 10,000 people (12.75%) when compared with 12.75 of 100 people (12.75%).

RR statistics are only helpful if everyone understands what the baseline group is. If the baseline is unclear, a statement of RR can be misleading (see Figure 5-2).

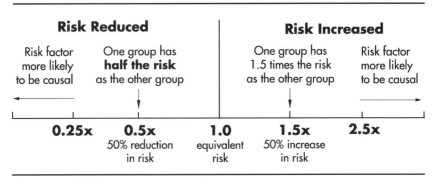

Figure 5-2. Relative Risk That a Specific Factor Is Causal in the Development of Cancer

Attributable Risk

Attributable risk is the amount of disease within a population that could be prevented by altering a risk factor. Although historically this component of risk assessment has not received much attention, attributable risk carries important implications for public health policy. A risk factor could convey a very large relative risk but be restricted to a few individuals; changing it would benefit a small group only. Conversely, altering a risk factor such as cigarette smoking could decrease cancer-related morbidity and mortality across the population.

The package insert for the contraceptive medroxyprogesterone acetate (Depo-Provera®, Pharmacia & Upjohn, Peapack, NJ) provides an example of attributable risk. For women younger than age 35 whose first exposure to the contraceptive is within the previous four years, the insert reports a relative risk of breast cancer of 2.19. Because the annual incidence rate (absolute risk) for women ages 30–34 is 26.7 per 100,000, a relative risk of 2.19 increases the possible risk from 26.7 to 58.5 cases per 100,000 women. The attributable risk of breast cancer is 3.18 per 10,000 additional women per year. This slight increase in the number of cases may be associated with the use of the contraceptive.

Prediction Models and Criteria

Model and Method Selection

Several factors can influence the selection of a risk-prediction model or method. Different models and methods are appropriate for different purposes (Armstrong, Eisen, & Weber, 2000). To decide whether to use mammography screening, for example, simply considering a woman's age may be sufficient if she is 40 to 49 years old. Using a woman's age to determine if tamoxifen may be effective in reducing breast cancer risk in a 45-year-old woman is probably inappropriate. Chemoprevention is best used for those with a moderate to high risk for developing a particular cancer, and age alone does not necessarily constitute a high-enough risk to consider taking a chemopreventive agent. Some decisions about prevention require specific and detailed risk assessments. Decisions about whether to undergo a prophylactic surgical procedure are best made after genetic testing. Prophylactic surgery involves too many physical and psychological risks to be used in those at average or moderate risk for cancer (Vogel, 2000). It is reserved only for those with a high risk that is probably best identified through genetic testing.

Genetic heterogeneity affects model selection. Genetic heterogeneity occurs in regard to breast and colorectal cancer. Both *BRCA1* and *BRCA2* mutations are associated with hereditary breast and ovarian cancer. Hereditary breast cancer also may be the primary manifestation of Cowden's disease or Li-Fraumeni syndrome because of mutations of the *PTEN* or *TP53* gene. Colorectal cancer may be the primary manifestation of familial adenomatous polyposis (FAP) syndrome or hereditary nonpolyposis colorectal cancer (HNPCC). Knowledge of differentiating clinical features is important in identifying the correct syndrome. Such cases highlight the need for both physical examination and a thorough family history in interpreting risk assessment data (Weitzel, 1999). If genetic testing is being considered, one must consider all appropriate cancer syndromes and their respective risk-assessment models, if available.

The type of information the nurse or client wants from the model influences model choice. At present, risk-assessment models exist primarily for hereditary breast, ovarian, and colon cancers (Stopfer, 2000). (For the purpose of model use, breast and ovarian cancers are usually combined.) In general, these models generate two types of risk information. The first type describes a client's chance of developing a particular cancer. This information usually is presented as an estimated chance of developing breast cancer both in the next five years and over the client's lifetime. The second type of risk information usually is produced for a client with a family history that suggests hereditary susceptibility. The information is an assessment of the client's chance of carrying a mutation in a particular cancer-susceptibility gene. This sometimes is referred to as the prior probability of carrying a gene mutation (Stopfer), or prior-probability risk. This risk figure is important for those who are considering genetic testing. Many groups, such as the American Society of Clinical Oncology (ASCO) (1996), state that a client should have a prior probability of at least 10% before undergoing genetic testing.

Specific Models

The Gail Model

The Gail model is based on a sample of women who were undergoing mammography as part of the Breast Cancer Detection Demonstration Project (Gail, Brinton, & Byar, 1989). Researchers used the Gail model to estimate cancer risk in the National Surgical Adjuvant Breast and Bowel Project, the P1 chemoprevention trial, and revised the model (Constantino et al., 1999). A validation study showed that the Gail model overpredicted absolute breast cancer risk by 33% among women ages 25–61 who did not receive annual screening (Spiegelman, Colditz, Hunter, & Hertzmark, 1994).

A breast cancer-risk assessment tool modified from the Gail model is available on NCI's Web site at http://bcra.nci.nih.gov/brc/. Many physicians use this model (see Figure 5-3) before making recommendations about using tamoxifen for chemoprevention.

Some of the risk factors for breast cancer are well known—early menarche, late age at first childbirth, late menopause, previous breast biopsies, and first-degree relatives with breast cancer. These factors have been included in the Gail model for cancer risk. The Gail model also considers a woman's current age and makes a risk calculation for the next five years and lifetime.

The Gail model excludes some well-known predictors. It does not include family history of ovarian cancer, ages at which relatives were diagnosed with

---

Figure 5-3. The Gail Model

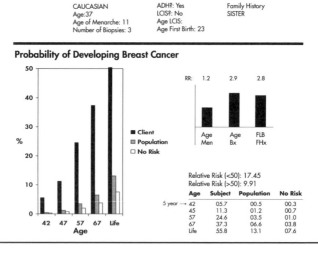

breast cancer, affected second-degree relatives, and paternal family history. Because of these limitations, the model underestimates risk for women who have *BRCA1* or *BRCA2* mutations and overestimates risk for women who have some family history of breast cancer but do not have a *BRCA1* or *BRCA2* mutation.

The Gail model is best used for women with a minimal to moderate family history of breast cancer.

The Claus Model

The Claus model provides useful age-specific risk estimates based on the number and age of first- and second-degree relatives with breast cancer (Claus, Risch, & Thompson, 1994; Claus, Schildkraut, Thompson, & Risch, 1996). This model uses only family history to calculate risk (see Figure 5-4). The Claus model is based on the Contraceptive and Steroid Hormone Study, which included approximately 5,000 women (ages 20–54) with breast cancer and an equal number of age-matched controls.

The major strength of the Claus model is that it includes both maternal and paternal family histories. Also, it considers the age at which an individual is

---

Figure 5-4. The Claus Model

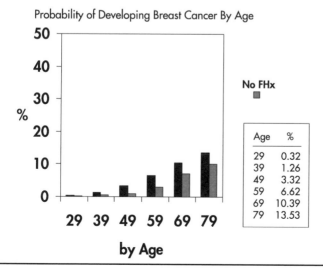

Claus Family History Model
The Claus table used in this calculation is:
One first-degree relative

Probability of Developing Breast Cancer By Age

No FHx

Age	%
29	0.32
39	1.26
49	3.32
59	6.62
69	10.39
79	13.53

by Age

---

diagnosed; these data are key in hereditary breast cancer. The model calculates risk in 10-year increments, which can be helpful for younger women who are trying to keep their risk in perspective.

The Claus model is not without disadvantages. Like the Gail model, it can significantly underestimate breast cancer risk for women who carry a *BRCA1* or *BRCA2* mutation, and it can overestimate risk for women who do not have a *BRCA1* or *BRCA2* mutation but do have a family history of breast cancer. The model does not consider a family history of ovarian cancer.

The Claus model, because it does not consider ethnicity, does not reflect the increased risk of breast cancer for women of Ashkenazic Jewish descent.

The Couch Model

The Couch model is a method of estimating the chance of carrying a *BRCA1* mutation (see Figure 5-5). It does not calculate a woman's immediate or life-time risk of developing breast cancer. The Couch model, sometimes called the University of Pennsylvania model, is based on logistic regression statistics (Couch et al., 1997).

Figure 5-5. The *BRCA* Prediction Models

BRCA Mutation Probability Models

BRCA1	Individual	Family
U. Penn	0.286	0.572
Myriad I	0.390	0.779
Myriad II	0.434	0.867
BRCAPRO	0.300	■■■

BRCA2	Individual	Family
Myriad II	0.011	0.022
BRCAPRO	0.193	■■■

BRCA*	Individual	Family
Myriad II	0.445	0.890
BRCAPRO	0.487	■■■

Pedigree Information

Ashkenazi family: Yes
Number of family members: 20
Number with breast cancer only: 3
Number with ovarian cancer only: 1
Number with both breast and ovarian cancer: 0
Number with bilateral breast cancer: 1
Mean age breast cancer: 46
Mean age ovarian cancer: 64

* Either *BRCA1* or *BRCA2*
Values expressed as probabilities, not percents
■■■ means no calculation possible

Researchers based the Couch model on a population of 263 women diagnosed with breast cancer who were members of families with a history of breast cancer. The women were receiving care at an academic cancer center. The Couch model considers the average age at which breast cancer has been diagnosed in an individual's family. It also considers Ashkenazic Jewish background and family history of ovarian cancer.

One of the limitations of the Couch model is that it is based on families with an average of 3.5 cases of breast and/or ovarian cancer. It is fairly useful for families with multiple affected members but may be less useful for smaller families or families with fewer numbers of cancers. Care must be taken to select the proper table to use and to read the table correctly. Furthermore, the data that contributed to model development reflected white women, for the most part. This fact may limit the model's applicability to other populations. The Couch model predicts *BRCA1* mutations only.

The Shattuck-Eidens Model

The Shattuck-Eidens model calculates the possibility of carrying a *BRCA1* mutation (Shattuck-Eidens, Oliphant, & McClure, 1997). It is sometimes referred to as the Myriad I model. The model is based on data derived from 798 women who had risk factors associated with *BRCA1* carrier status, including early-onset breast cancer, bilateral breast cancer, ovarian cancer, and Ashkenazic Jewish heritage. This model is compared with other *BRCA* mutation-probability models in Figure 5-5.

The Berry Model

The Berry model is a mathematical model that uses principles of Mendelian inheritance and Bayes' theorem to calculate the probability that a woman with a family history of breast and/or ovarian cancer carries a *BRCA1* or *BRCA2* mutation (Berry, Parmigiani, Sanchez, Schildkraut, & Winer, 1997). It sometimes is called the Duke or BRCAPRO model (see Figure 5-6).

The model considers family history, including first- and second-degree relatives as well as age at diagnosis and age at death of affected family members. The distinct advantage of this model is that it takes into account multiple variables, such as data regarding the uncertainty of family members' genetic status, uncertainty about the prevalence of the mutation in the population, and uncertainty about the cancer rate for carriers.

The Frank Model

The Frank model estimates the probability that a woman with breast cancer diagnosed before age 50 carries a *BRCA1* or *BRCA2* mutation (Frank et

Figure 5-6. The BRCAPRO Model

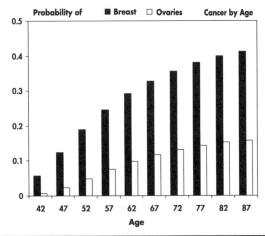

BRCAPRO: The Duke University Model
Carrier Probabilities

BRCA1:	*0.300*
BRCA2:	*0.193*
BRCA 1 or 2:	*0.487*

Age	Breast	Ovaries
42	0.057880	0.006886
47	0.124085	0.023587
52	0.189654	0.049027
57	0.246300	0.075536
62	0.292006	0.098193
67	0.327833	0.116486
72	0.356184	0.131461
77	0.380382	0.143420
82	0.399621	0.151892
87	0.412389	0.156957

al., 1998). It is sometimes called the Myriad II model (see Figure 5-5). This model relies on family history (see Tables 5-6 and 5-7). It predicts the probability of finding a mutation in family members by determining their relationships to the proband. Unaffected first-degree relatives have half the probability of the affected member, and second-degree relatives have a quarter of the probability.

Clinical Criteria Regarding Colorectal Cancer

Decisions about whether to test for a mutation that suggests a hereditary predisposition to developing HNPCC usually are based on clinical criteria, such as the Amsterdam Criteria or the Bethesda Guidelines. One model, the Wijnen model, provides probability ranges for the risk of carrying a *MSH2* or *MLH1 mutation.*

The Amsterdam Criteria

In 1991, an international group developed, as research criteria, the first set of criteria for the diagnosis of HNPCC. The criteria are now known as the

Table 5-6. Prevalence of Mutations in *BRCA1* in *BRCA2* by Personal and Family History of Cancer in 4,518 Women (Excluding Women of Ashkenazic Jewish Ancestry)

Client's History	Family History (%)					
	No breast cancer under age 50 or ovarian cancer in anyone	Breast cancer under age 50 in one relative; no ovarian cancer in anyone	Breast cancer under age 50 in more than one relative; no ovarian cancer in anyone	Ovarian cancer at any age in one relative; no breast cancer under age 50 in anyone	Ovarian cancer in more than one relative; no breast cancer under age 50 in anyone	Breast cancer under age 50 and ovarian cancer at any age
No breast cancer or ovarian cancer at any age	41.0	4.0	11.1	2.7	7.3	16.8
Breast cancer at age 50 or older	2.4	9.6	10.7	4.8	5.6[a]	24.7
Breast cancer under age 50	9.7	18.9	37.6	16.3	18.4	48.2
Ovarian cancer at any age, no breast cancer	6.4	34.1	40.7	28.0	37.9	47.8
Breast cancer at age 50 or older and ovarian cancer at any age	20.8	10.0[a]	36.4[a]	16.7[a]	33.3[a]	40.0[a]
Breast cancer under age 50 and ovarian cancer at any age	18.2	46.2[a]	66.7[a]	66.7	66.7[a]	78.9[a]

[a] N < 20

Note. From "Mutation Prevalence Tables," by Myriad Genetic Laboratories, retrieved July 20, 2001, from http://www.myriad.com/med/brac/mutptables.html. Copyright 2001 by Myriad Genetic Laboratories. Adapted with permission.

Table 5-7. Prevalence of Mutations in *BRCA1* and *BRCA2* by Personal and Family History of Cancer in 2,262 Women of Ashkenazic Jewish Ancestry

Client's History	Family History (%)					
	No breast cancer under age 50 or ovarian cancer in anyone	Breast cancer under age 50 in one relative; no ovarian cancer in anyone	Breast cancer under age 50 in more than one relative; no ovarian cancer in anyone	Ovarian cancer at any age in one relative; no breast cancer under age 50 in anyone	Ovarian cancer in more than one relative; no breast cancer under age 50 in anyone	Breast cancer under age 50 and ovarian cancer at any age
No breast cancer or ovarian cancer at any age	5.5	13.5	18.9	17.5	23.7	131.9
Breast cancer at age 50 or older	4.5	9.7	12.5	13.0	37.5ᵃ	37.0
Breast cancer under age 50	12.3	26.6	43.4	44.6	66.7	58.6
Ovarian cancer at any age, no breast cancer	22.6	15.4ᵃ	71.4ᵃ	47.4	70.0	82.4ᵃ
Breast cancer at age 50 or older and ovarian cancer at any age	33.3ᵃ	0ᵃ	100ᵃ	33.3ᵃ	None tested	50.0ᵃ
Breast cancer under age 50 and ovarian cancer at any age	77.8ᵃ	83.3ᵃ	50.0ᵃ	50.0ᵃ	None tested	None tested

ᵃ N < 20

Note. From "Mutation Prevalence Tables," by Myriad Genetic Laboratories, retrieved July 20, 2001, from http://www.myriad.com/med/brac/mutptables.html. Copyright 2001 by Myriad Genetic Laboratories. Adapted with permission.

Amsterdam I Criteria (Vasen, Mecklin, Khan, & Lynch, 1991). A client meets Amsterdam I Criteria when

- A family contains three or more relatives with a histologically verified colorectal cancer (with one relative being a first-degree relative of the other).
- The colorectal cancer involves at least two generations.
- One or more colorectal cancers were diagnosed before the client reached age 50.
- FAP is ruled out.

In 1999, the Amsterdam Criteria were modified to recognize the extracolonic manifestations of HNPCC (Vasen, Watson, Mecklin, & Lynch, 1999). Extracolonic manifestations include gastric cancers and cancers of the ovary, brain, endometrium, small bowel, ureter, and renal pelvis. These additional cancers, along with Amsterdam Criteria, are known as Amsterdam II.

The Bethesda Guidelines

Researchers developed the Bethesda Guidelines because genetic testing revealed that the Amsterdam I Criteria failed to recognize at least one-third of the families with a *MSH2* or *MLH1* mutation (Rodriguez-Bigas et al., 1997). Published in 1997, the Bethesda Guidelines consider clinicopathologic factors and can be used to help to identify clients at highest risk of HNPCC who might benefit from further evaluation (see Figure 5-7). The Bethesda Guidelines focus primarily on an individual, rather than an entire family. The Bethesda Guidelines require a client to meet only one criterion, not multiple criteria as in the Amsterdam Criteria.

The Wijnen Model

The Wijnen model, a logistic probability model published in 1998, considers the risk of carrying a *MSH2* or *MLH1* mutation (Wijnen, Vasen, & Khan, 1998). Nurses often use this model before offering genetic testing for these mutations, which are the two mutations most commonly associated with HNPCC. The Wijnen model is available in a software package called BRCAPRO (see Figure 5-8). Most nurses use the Wijnen model with clinical criteria such as the Amsterdam Criteria or the Bethesda Guidelines. In some cases, microsatellite instability (MSI) testing should be used as well.

Genetic-risk assessment for colorectal cancer, specifically HNPCC, is not as refined as risk assessment for hereditary breast cancer. Those who provide risk counseling must carefully consider the selection of clinical criteria, explain why MSI testing may be indicated, and specify the limitations of the Wijnen model.

Figure 5-7. The Bethesda Criteria

Client may meet ANY ONE of the following:
- Individuals with cancer in families who meet the Amsterdam Criteria
- Individuals with two HNPCC-related cancers, including synchronous and metachronous colorectal cancers or associated extracolonic cancers; endometrial, ovarian, gastric, hepatobiliary, small-bowel cancer or transitional-cell carcinoma of the renal pelvis or ureter
- Individuals with colorectal cancer and a first-degree relative with colorectal cancer and/ or HNPCC-related extracolonic cancer and/or a colorectal adenoma; one of the cancers diagnosed when the client is younger than 45 years, and the adenoma diagnosed when the client is younger than 40 years.
- Individuals with colorectal cancer or endometrial cancer diagnosed at an age younger than 45 years
- Individuals with right-sided colorectal cancer with an undifferentiated pattern (solid/ cribiform) on histology diagnosed at age younger than 45 years. The solid/cribiform pattern is defined as poorly differentiated or undifferentiated carcinoma composed of irregular, solid sheets of large eosinophilic cells and containing small glandlike spaces.
- Individuals with signet-ring cell type colorectal cancer diagnosed at age younger than 45 years. The signet-ring cell type is defined as a tumor composed of more than 50% signet-ring cells.
- Individuals with colorectal adenomas diagnosed at an age younger than 40 years

---

Figure 5-8. The Wijnen Model

Hereditary Nonpolyposis Colorectal Cancer

HNPCC: *MSH2* or *MLH1* Mutation Probability

Information used in this calculation:

Proband: Brother

Proband age at colorectal cancer diagnosis: 31

Mean age colorectal cancer diagnosis: 31

Endometrial cancer? Yes

Amsterdam criteria met? No

Probability that this family carries a mutation:

0.5

MSI Testing

MSI testing usually is recommended in cases in which HNPCC is suspected but the first three Bethesda criteria do not apply. MSI testing can be conducted on a resected colorectal cancer specimen. MSI is present in 90% of HNPCC-related colorectal cancers but in only 15%–20% of sporadic cancers. Clinicians must remind clients that finding MSI does not, by itself, mean that the cancer is caused by a mutation associated with HNPCC. A positive MSI test only indicates that offering genetic testing for HNPCC-associated mutations is appropriate.

Different Models and Methods, Different Results

As Stopfer (2000) noted, different models and methods can produce different risk assessments for the same individual. For example, in a study using the Claus model, the Murday method (which uses Bayes' formula, a mathematical tool that combines prior knowledge with current data to produce a risk assessment) and a qualitative method based on the number of affected relatives produced vastly different results: The two methods placed only 54% of the women with a family history of breast cancer in the same risk category (Murday, 1994; Tischkowitz, Wheeler, France, Chapman, & Lucassen, 2000). Conflicting information often leads to increased stress for clients and families.

Different models produce different results because each model is based on different and unique combinations of information. To minimize confusion, those providing genetic-risk assessment and counseling must explain why they chose the model they did and what the results mean. They should distinguish between risk models that produce information about risk of disease and those that produce information about the risk of carrying a specific mutation. Rosser, Hurst, and Chapman (1996) recommended using one model consistently and explaining its inherent strengths and weaknesses to the client and family.

Figures 5-3 through 5-8 demonstrate how different models, applied to one family history, can produce different results. The differences result from the fact that the risk of cancer and/or the probability of carrying a mutation are calculated from different data sets. Each figure highlights the fact that healthcare providers must choose an appropriate model and explain its strengths and weaknesses to the client and family.

The Importance of Knowledge to Risk Assessment

Risk assessment demands that healthcare professionals know the risk factors for the major cancers and their significance. Because risk factors guide screening recommendations, healthcare professionals also must understand various guidelines for cancer prevention and early detection. These guidelines—usually endorsed by an organization such as ACS, National Comprehensive Cancer Network, or NCI—are revised periodically (ACS, 2001; Daly, 1999; Leitch et al., 1997), so continually staying up-to-date on this information is important. All healthcare professionals should tell clients which guidelines they follow and why (Foltz, 2000).

In applying prevention and screening guidelines, healthcare professionals must bear in mind the fact that the guidelines require a comprehensive risk assessment. For example, the ACS guidelines for the early detection of endometrial cancer (ACS, 2001) recommend that women who are at high risk for developing endometrial cancer (including women on tamoxifen therapy and those with a history of infertility, obesity, anovulatory menstrual cycles, and abnormal uterine bleeding) undergo endometrial tissue sampling at menopause and thereafter at the discretion of the examiner. Similarly, ACS recommends a colonoscopy instead of a 60-centimeter sigmoidoscopy for the early detection of colorectal cancer if the client has a genetic susceptibility for colon cancer, so the clinician must consider family history before making a recommendation (Byers, Levin, Rothenberger, Dodd, & Smith, 1997). If a risk assessment does not include information about infertility or tamoxifen exposure, the correct screening procedure, which includes endometrial sampling, may not be included.

Communication of Risk Assessment

Transmitting risk information is a central component of all screening and genetic-risk assessment counseling programs, and the task is much more difficult than it appears. As Slovik (1986) noted, healthcare professionals often fail to understand the complexity of risk assessment; the lay public understands it even less. Love (1989) stated that many healthcare professionals have difficulty educating and counseling clients because they do not have the epidemiologic background needed to interpret data and understand the epidemiologic reports published in scientific journals. The difficulty is compounded by the fact that, at the technical level, professionals are in a continual debate about terminology and techniques.

Figure 5-9 provides an overview of information to be discussed in a risk-assessment interview.

Professional judgment, in the form of standards of practice and position statements, may affect the way healthcare professionals communicate risk information (Fischhoff, Lichtenstein, Slovic, Derby, & Keeney, 1983). Such statements include the ASCO guidelines for genetic testing (ASCO, 1996), which state that genetic testing should be offered when the results will influence the management of care, and adequate pre- and postcounseling services are available. Similar guidelines are available from the Oncology Nursing Society (ONS); see the ONS Position on the Role of the Oncology Nurse in Cancer Genetic Testing and Risk Assessment Counseling (ONS, 2000). (Chapter 10 discusses the ONS position.)

Figure 5-9. Cancer-Risk Assessment and Counseling Using Breast Cancer as a Clinical Example

Information to Obtain in a Cancer-Risk Assessment
(The rationale for collecting this information should be explained at the beginning of the session and then again when the factors are interpreted.)
- Family history (to include at a minimum parents, siblings, grandparents, aunts, and uncles). Whenever possible, obtain information about the age at diagnosis, if cancer occurred bilaterally in paired organs, and any information about histology.
- Personal history (to include information about past medical history specific to the cancer-risk assessment, such as reproductive history)
- Lifestyle factors (to include amount and duration of exposure to carcinogens, whenever possible)
- Information on beliefs about cancer risk and causation

Information to Include When Communicating Risk
- Incidence
- Types of risk (e.g., absolute, relative)
- Ramifications and appropriateness of genetic testing
- Etiology
- Prognosis if detected early

Information About Cancer Prevention
- Diet, alcohol consumption, exercise
- Use of exogenous hormones
- Environmental exposure
- Prophylactic surgical procedures

Information About Early Detection
- Strengths and limitations of screening tests and how tests are performed, including a basic discussion of anatomy and physiology of the at-risk organs
- Program of recommended early detection for the individual
- Signs and symptoms that should be addressed immediately

Psychosocial Concerns
- Provide an opportunity to share fears or concerns.
- Check for signs of distress that may require further follow-up.

Note. From "Cancer Risk Assessment: Conceptual Considerations for Clinical Practice," by S.M. Mahon, 1998, *Oncology Nursing Forum, 25,* p. 1538. Copyright 1998 by the Oncology Nursing Society. Reprinted with permission.

Communication about cancer risk is challenging because it usually includes both a qualitative and a quantitative component (Fischhoff, 1999). Many experts in risk communication believe that all discussions of risk should include both components (Rothman & Kiviniemi, 1999). The quantitative component usually is the more straightforward of the two. It involves explaining figures about absolute or relative risk and the probability of having a mutation in a cancer-susceptibility gene. Fischhoff stated that qualitative information should follow the presentation of quantitative data. The qualitative presentation involves discussion of the meaning of the quantitative data and often touches on emotionally charged issues, such as genetic testing. No matter how nonjudgmental the healthcare professional tries to be, he or she is likely to communicate personal biases (Fischhoff). The nurse needs to acknowledge these biases to the client and family and make a conscientious effort to be nonjudgmental. Communicating risk information properly is labor-intensive and takes time. Most clinicians agree that collecting, interpreting, and communicating genetic information to a client and family takes from one to three 60- to 90-minute visits (Weitzel, 1999). The process can take even longer if problems in verifying family history arise, and they often do. In such cases, clinicians must request, receive, and interpret pathology reports.

To communicate information about risk to clients, healthcare professionals must be fully aware of the strengths and limits of the methods used to generate the information. Kelly (1996) noted that, unless healthcare professionals appreciate the complexities involved in providing information about risk in a clinically useful manner, organized programs for cancer-risk assessment may only appear to provide informed consent. However, the programs may lack the time, structure, and skilled personnel needed to provide the information that would make true informed consent possible.

Love (1989, 1995) emphasized that, before communicating any numbers regarding cancer risk to a client, the healthcare professional must clearly explain how the numbers were derived. Numbers have great potential to confuse and mislead. For example, consider a headline stating that drinking five alcoholic beverages a week increases breast cancer risk by 50%. Someone may think the meaning is that an individual who drinks five glasses of wine per week has a 50/50 chance of getting breast cancer. In actuality, the glasses of wine increase the relative risk of developing breast cancer by 50%. If a woman's lifetime risk is 3.3% and she drinks five glasses of wine per week, her lifetime risk increases to 5%.

Furthermore, risk factors do not necessarily increase in a simple mathematical fashion (Love, 1995). For example, if one risk factor gives a woman a 12%

risk of developing breast cancer and another gives the woman an 18% risk, the two numbers cannot be assumed to mean the woman now has a 30% chance of developing breast cancer. The interaction of risk factors is complicated. Breast cancer is a disease that has many causes that interact in ways that researchers do not fully understand. In fact, some researchers estimated that 70% of breast cancers occur in women without any of the classic risk factors (Madigan et al., 1995). Healthcare professionals must be aware of the strengths and limitations of risk factors and communicate all these considerations to clients.

Consideration also should be given to the client's ability to understand risk information. An individual's likelihood of seeking cancer-risk assessment may be related to his or her education level and ability to understand complex technical concepts. Risk information should be presented in accord with how much the client or family wishes to know (Hopwood, 1997). Timing also may be important. Messages suggesting increased susceptibility to breast cancer may be less effective if delivered too soon after the diagnosis of breast cancer in a close relative. Several months after the diagnosis, such messages might be appropriate (Rimer, Schildkraut, Lerman, Lin, & Audrain, 1996).

Techniques for Communicating Cancer-Risk Assessments

The list that follows cites some of the guidelines that apply to communicating cancer-risk information (Arkin, 1999; Kelly, 2000; Maibach, 1999; and Walker, 1997).

- Identify the risk-communication goal. Determine what audience or individual is to be informed about risk, and choose a strategy that is appropriate.
- Determine what the group needs to know. Clearly, large public groups may need to know something different about a cancer risk or genetic susceptibility than a small family with limited resources.
- Consider the audience's perception of risks. This is extremely difficult to do when the audience is a large group in the general public. When working with individuals and families, an understanding of personal beliefs can offer much insight and set the stage for providing more in-depth education and, when needed, correcting misconceptions.
- Explain the risks in different formats, including numerically, visually, and with verbal explanations. Principles of autosomal transmission can be demonstrated using a pedigree. Choose the best visual means to present the information necessary to communicate the risk. Some visual aids are more appropriately used with large public groups, whereas individuals receiving

cancer-risk counseling may benefit from different visual aids and, in some cases, tailored print pieces.

- Explain risks in context. An appropriate amount of background information must be included to facilitate decision making. Be sure to explain that cancer risks are multiple and cumulative in nature and that the interaction of risks is not completely understood.
- When possible, use absolute terms to explain risk.
- Explain the risk clearly, using the appropriate statistics. When using relative-risk statistics, give the comparison, or anchor. Relative-risk figures tend to be difficult for individuals to understand. Avoid framing the risk to persuade an individual to make a decision. The purpose of risk communication is to give enough balanced information to allow an individual to make a decision about risk management—a decision that is best for that individual.
- Define and explain the consequences of the risk.
- Remember that cancer genetics counseling also includes a discussion of the risks and benefits associated with screening; chemoprevention; and, in some cases, prophylactic surgery. This means that people receiving cancer genetics counseling must not only understand their possible risk of developing cancer and the implications and risks associated with testing, but also the risks and benefits associated with screening and prevention.
- Acknowledge the uncertainty that exists when communicating cancer risks. When appropriate, discuss the limitations of existing research. Point out what gaps in information exist. When discussing research findings, include a discussion of any conflicts that could arise because of funding and any significant limitations of the study.

Promoting Effective Communication

Northouse and Northouse (1992) noted that communication tends to be more effective if the healthcare professional considers several variables.

- Empathy (i.e., feeling with the other person and observing the world from the other's point of view)
- Personal control (i.e., the perception that a person can control his or her circumstances)
- Trust (i.e., accepting others without evaluating or judging them)
- Self-disclosure (i.e., any message about one's self that is communicated to others)

What Is the Best Format for a Risk Discussion?

Schoenbach, Wagner, and Beery (1987) noted that a health-risk assessment with the purpose of motivating the client to improve health behaviors or undergo appropriate screening may be best communicated through a personal counseling approach. Furthermore, counseling may be most effective if conducted as part of an ongoing client-provider relationship. Clearly, the professional should augment the sessions by providing written materials about the cancer of concern. The materials should reinforce education about risk signs and symptoms and recommended screening and prevention measures. Such materials must be suitable to the educational and cultural background of the population being served (Lerman, Rimer, & Engstrom, 1991).

What Is the Best Format for Presenting Risk Data?

After risk-assessment data are collected, the nurse must choose the best method to communicate the significance of the data. Risk can be presented as a numeric risk, a statistical comparison to an anchor risk, a risk category (i.e., low, average, or high), or a graph or some other pictorial presentation. Risk also can be expressed in qualitative terms (e.g., a smoker is more likely to develop this disease than a person who does not smoke).

A numeric result, such as an absolute- or relative-risk figure, can appear highly scientific and be difficult for many clients to understand. Conversely, using verbal terms, such as *high risk* or *low risk*, can be equally confusing. A high risk to one woman might mean a 100% chance of developing breast cancer; for another, it might mean a 25% chance.

Those who communicate cancer-risk assessments to clients must be aware of the clients' perception of risk and remind clients of the fundamental purposes of risk assessment: determining appropriate cancer-prevention strategies, when known, and developing a reasonable schedule for cancer screening. Individuals with significantly higher risks, such as individuals with a potential genetic susceptibility to breast cancer, may choose to participate in a chemoprevention trial or an aggressive screening schedule.

What Is the Best Way to Frame Information?

The manner in which the information is communicated, in terms of attitude and context, is called framing. Framing can have a significant effect on how the client perceives the information (Salovey, Schneider, & Apanovitch, 1999).

If risk information is presented in a negative fashion, the client may assume the risk is more than it actually is. If the discussion is too positive, the client may underestimate or minimize risk. The same is true in discussions of options. Consider a woman who tests positive for a *BRCA1* mutation. Her nurse tells her that a screening procedure fails to detect 60% of ovarian cancer cases. The client is unlikely to think that taking the test is worth the effort. The healthcare professional might do better to frame the information differently, to emphasize the fact that the screening detects ovarian cancer 40% of the time and stress the importance of early detection.

Statistical context can constitute framing. If a healthcare professional tells a client that he or she has a 1.3 in 10,000 chance of developing a particular cancer, compared to the general population's risk of 1 in 10,000, the client probably will not be concerned. If the professional communicates the same risk by saying that the client's risk is 30% higher than average, the client probably will be concerned (Bottorff, Ratner, Johnson, Lovato, & Jaob, 1998).

Clearly, framing statistical information appropriately is one of the most challenging aspects of cancer-risk assessment communication. The goal is not to frighten a client unnecessarily; however, if the risk is underplayed too much, the client may not see the value in recommended cancer prevention and screening activities (Meyerowitz & Chaiken, 1987).

What Is a Typical Information-Presentation Sequence?

The list that follows shows the typical risk-communication sequence.

1. Remind the client of the purpose, strengths, and limitations of a cancer-risk assessment. Clients must understand that life is filled with inherent risks and that no guarantee of good health exists. The goal of risk assessment is to help clients understand how they can maximize chances for good health and long life.

2. Provide basic information about the cancer for which the person is at risk (e.g., the number of people affected annually, the average age at diagnosis, the clinical characteristics of the disease). Review basic anatomy and physiology, using diagrams and models when they are helpful. Provide information about the general population that can serve as a baseline against which the client can measure the magnitude of his or her risk. Allow the client adequate opportunity to ask questions and express concerns. Only if the client can initiate comments will the interview be an effective information-sharing session. Expand the discussion according to the magnitude of the risk and the ability and desire of the client to understand content. If the client needs and wants a large amount of information, you may want to provide facts such as those in Tables 5-4 and 5-5. Distinguish between absolute and relative risk, and reinforce the fact that risk factors do not combine in a simple mathematical fashion.

3. Talk about lifestyle factors that are amenable to change. For example, women with a strong family history of breast cancer may need to weigh the benefits

and risks of taking oral contraceptives or estrogen replacement therapy. A discussion of these risks is critical to informed decision making for each client.

4. Provide information about the strengths and limitations of screening tools (see Tables 5-1, 5-2, and 5-8), including information about the recommended time interval for using each tool. For most clients, the standard recommendations endorsed by an organization such as ACS (2001) are appropriate. People with significantly higher risk may need more aggressive screening and should understand the rationale, strengths, and limitations of such a schedule, as well as the strengths and limitations associated with chemoprevention agents and prophylactic surgery.

5. Discuss signs and symptoms that need immediate attention. In regard to breast cancer, for example, augment information about breast self-examination (BSE) with personal instruction; use models, pictures, and videos as appropriate to increase the woman's proficiency and confidence in performing BSE.

Table 5-8. Strengths and Limitations of Screening Tools for Breast Cancer

Tool	Strengths	Limitations
Breast self-examination (BSE)	Notes interval changes Convenient Inexpensive May note a subtle change	Lump must be large enough to palpate. Women forget to do BSE. Women may be afraid of finding a lump. Women may lack confidence in their ability.
Clinical breast examination	Locates abnormalities for radiologist Locates tumors not detected on mammography Provides an opportunity to teach BSE	Dependent on the skill of the examiner Lump must be large enough to palpate.
Mammography	Finds abnormalities before palpable May offer better possibility for conservative surgery	Cannot detect all abnormalities May be considered uncomfortable May be too costly for some women

Note. From "Cancer Risk Assessment: Conceptual Considerations for Clinical Practice," by S.M. Mahon, 1998, *Oncology Nursing Forum, 25,* p. 1540. Copyright 1998 by the Oncology Nursing Society. Reprinted with permission.

Tools for Communicating Risk

Computer Software

A few programs relating to cancer risk are available for the public and healthcare professionals. An advantage of using computer software and multimedia technologies is that they tend to involve clients actively rather than passively (Strecher, Greenwood, Wang, & Dumont, 1999). In addition, they can be used to deliver a consistent message to a large number of people at a relatively low cost. A disadvantage of these technologies is that ensuring comprehension of the material and the implications of the risk assessment is difficult. Also, research has not yet established the effectiveness of these programs.

Rohwer and Wandberg (1997) studied the use and effectiveness of an interactive cancer-risk assessment program called Right Choices, which was designed to be used in grades 7 through 12 in conjunction with a cancer-prevention program delivered in school health classes and pediatricians' offices. At the end of the study, which included 722 young people, the authors concluded that the computer program resulted in no significant change in student knowledge or behavior. However, the program may have raised consciousness about the changes needed to decrease cancer risk. Awareness of what must change certainly is the first step to change.

Software developers recently have developed office-based risk-assessment tools in response to the time constraints of primary care providers (Emery et al., 2000; Schwartz, Woloshin, & Welch, 1999). Programs even exist for handheld personal data assistants. A face-to-face interview to gather family history can be a lengthy process. Obtaining family history by telephone prior to the visit also is time-consuming. An office-based tool allows a client to enter family data directly into a computer. Many view such a tool as the most efficient means of gathering risk information (Westman, Hampel, & Bradley, 2000).

NCI's Risk Assessment Tool is probably the best known breast cancer risk assessment tool. It requires the clinician to ensure that data are collected; the tool generates and communicates a pictorial rendition of the results. Many of these tools are disease-specific and do not ensure a comprehensive cancer-risk assessment. Likewise, such programs do not interpret information, and they do not provide recommendations about prevention, detection, or evaluation.

Visual Aids

Graphics can be a very effective means to communicate risk—especially in communicating numeric risk (Lipkus & Hollands, 1999). Graphics often can reveal data patterns that may otherwise go undetected, and they hold attention longer than does text, leading to an increased understanding of the data being presented. To be useful, graphics must communicate magnitude of risk, relative risk, cumulative risk, uncertainty, and interactions among risk factors. Despite the popularity of using graphics, few researchers have studied their impact on the communication of risk information. Many nurses use a combination of formats to present numeric, visual, and explanatory data (Press, Fishman, & Koenig, 2000).

Pictorial Elements

Bar graphs: A bar graph should decrease the number of mathematical computations that the user must make. The data-to-ink ratio should be high—that is, the graph should not contain extra pictures, busy backgrounds, and patterned fills (see Figure 5-10). Graphs should not be used to communicate a low-probability event (Lipkus & Hollands, 1999), such as an event with a 0.0003 chance. Although most people can understand the probability that accompanies a high-probability event, such as the probability of a flipped coin coming up heads (which represents a 0.50 or 50% chance), understanding a low-probability event, such as a 0.0003 chance, is much more difficult. A solution to this problem is to change the probability to a frequency (i.e., 3 out of 10,000).

Figure 5-10. Confusing Graph With Low Data-to-Ink Ratio

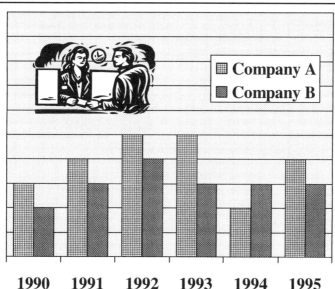

Line graphs: Line graphs effectively communicate trends and changes in data. They are commonly used to show changes in incidence or mortality over time, and most clients have experience reading them. Figure 5-11 shows a line graph.

Pie charts: Pie charts effectively communicate information about proportions. Pie charts can be combined to explain subcategories of data (see Figure 5-12).

Risk ladders: A risk ladder can be used to portray the relative risk associated with environmental hazards. The higher up the ladder the hazard is, the greater the risk it represents (see Figure 5-13). The position on the ladder helps the viewer to conceptualize risks in relation to each other, "anchoring" risk perception to highest and lowest reference points.

Stick figures: Stick figures often are used to communicate relative risk or to show how many people out of a certain number may develop a particular disease (see Figure 5-14). When a small number of figures is used, the viewer may perceive the risk to be higher (Lipkus & Hollands, 1999). If the number of figures is increased, the impact may not be as strong, and some will find the presentation busy and difficult to understand.

Histograms: Figure 5-15 presents a histogram, a type of representation that most clients have some experience reading. Lipkus and Hollands (1999) noted that histograms often convey the magnitude of the risk more clearly than do numbers alone.

Figure 5-11. A Line Graph

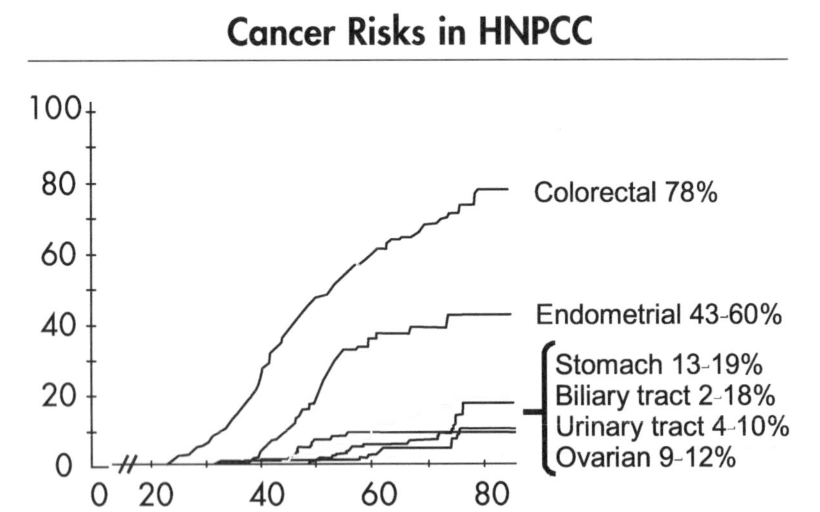

Cancer Risks in HNPCC

Colorectal 78%

Endometrial 43–60%

Stomach 13–19%
Biliary tract 2–18%
Urinary tract 4–10%
Ovarian 9–12%

Figure 5-12. A Pie Chart

Contribution of Gene Mutations to HNPCC Families

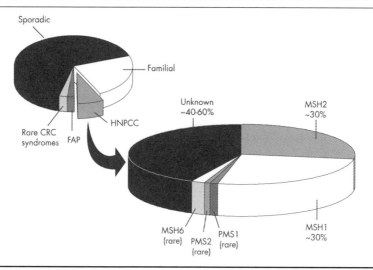

Figure 5-13. A Risk Ladder

This ladder shows the chance that women who have a family history of breast or ovarian cancer, and are themselves diagnosed with cancer, carry a *BRCA* mutation.[a]

Location of Cancer	Chance of *BRCA* Mutation (%)
One breast	31
Both breasts	51
Ovary	45
Ovary and breast	88

[a] Breast cancer diagnosed before age 50; ovarian cancer diagnosed at any age.

Note. Based on information from Frank, 1998.

The Impact of the Client's Beliefs

A counselor may do his or her best to present clear, comprehensive, unbiased information. The client does not make decisions about risk that are based on information alone, however (Weinstein, 1999). Other factors may exert a powerful influence on decision making. These include emotions, personal values, experience, social pressures, environmental barriers, and economic constraints.

Figure 5-14. Use of Stick Figures

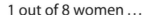

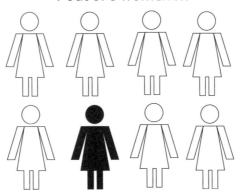

will develop breast cancer if they live to age 85.

Figure 5-15. A Histogram

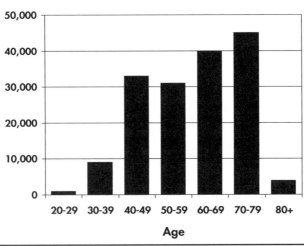

Perception of Risk

Figure 5-9 shows some of the factors that influence the perception of risk. If risk were unaffected by individual beliefs, the United States would be a nation of health-conscious adults who exercise, eat a healthful diet, never use tobacco products, limit exposure to ultraviolet light, and have regular cancer-screening examinations. Personal beliefs and perceptions of risk are so strong that they prevent many individuals from adopting healthful behaviors (Rodgers, 1999). Smokers can always describe a relative who smoked three packs per day for 60 years and never developed lung cancer. A man may think he does not need a colonoscopy because he does not have the symptoms of colon cancer or because he has no relatives with the disease. Given the personal nature of risk perception, genetic counselors often have trouble determining which risks a client will deem acceptable or unacceptable (Rowan, 1996).

People often have an inaccurate perception of their risk of cancer (Kelly, 1996; Kreuter, 1999; Slovik, 1986). Perception of risk often is inaccurate even in families who are aware of their high risk of cancer (Hopwood, 1997). Misperception of risk may be one reason individuals are not screened regularly for malignancy (Newell & Vogel, 1988). In addition, a client's anxiety can limit his or her ability to comprehend risk information. Perception of risk may be based on inaccurate memories, the need to cope, personality-related bias, and prior experience with cancer.

Common Bases of Inaccurate Perceptions

Misperception based on inaccurate memories: Memories of past events can affect perception of risk. Studies suggest that, in some cases, these memories may be inaccurate. Researchers in one study found that family reports were accurate 83% of the time for first-degree relatives, 67% accurate for second-degree relatives, and 60% accurate for third-degree relatives (Love, Evans, & Josten, 1985). Accuracy of self-reports may not be adequate in cancers of similar organs (Kerber & Slattery, 1997). Nurses must order pathology reports, mammograms, and other documentation to verify the accuracy of client-supplied material. If the client misremembers a diagnosis, for example, the risk assessment could be significantly inaccurate. For example, there is a big difference between breast cancer risk in a woman with a biopsy-proven fibroadenoma and biopsy-proven ductal hyperplasia with atypia.

Misperception as a coping mechanism: Information about risk may frighten, frustrate, and confuse a client. One way for a client to avoid such feelings is to misconstrue the information. Such misperception, which occurs on the unconscious level, is a coping mechanism.

Similarly, a cancer-risk assessment may remind a client that his or her behavior is unwise (Gerrard, Gibbons, & Reis-Bergan, 1999). If the client is unwilling to hear this message, his or her unconscious may render the client unable to understand it. Though intellectually capable of comprehending the assessment, the client uses avoidance to shield him- or herself from what the client does not want to hear.

Optimistic or pessimistic bias: Some people underestimate their risk or impart to it what is called an optimistic bias. Those who overestimate their risk are said to have a pessimistic bias. People with a pessimistic bias often suffer unnecessary anxiety and concern. They may have difficulty accepting a lower, more accurate risk assessment because their strong beliefs are difficult to modify. Optimistic and pessimistic biases occur because of personality, the inability to comprehend complex information, or a psychological inability to cope with accurate risk information.

Previous experience with cancer: Perception of cancer risk can be greatly influenced by a client's previous experience with cancer (Weitzel, 1999). A woman who helped to care for her mother as she died from ovarian cancer may perceive even a small or modest increased risk for developing ovarian cancer as intolerable, even though the risk may be lower than average. Weitzel stressed that, for this reason, healthcare professionals should assess and appreciate the client's motivations and previous experiences. A client may request genetic testing after achieving a significant milestone, such as the birth of a child or achieving the same age at which a parent was diagnosed with cancer.

Lack of trust in the healthcare professional: Sachs (1999) explained that, to perceive risk accurately, clients and families must trust the professional who provides risk information. The degree of trust is probably influenced by previous experiences with healthcare providers. One way the healthcare professional can build trust, however, is to respond empathetically when the client discloses family history.

When listening to a family history, a healthcare provider wants to hear the story of the disease. When disclosing family history, a client is telling a story about real people who are very similar to him- or herself. By listening to the human story, the healthcare provider can gain insight about the cultural background of the family and the client's personal beliefs and coping mechanisms.

Inaccurate Information or Beliefs

In addition to misperceptions about risk, people who seek cancer-risk assessment may have inaccurate information or beliefs about the causes of cancer.

Such inaccuracy may prevent them from seeking or understanding risk information, treatment options, or the advantages of early detection (Kelly, 2000). People may incorrectly assume that they have a genetic predisposition for breast malignancy because of a physical resemblance to a close relative diagnosed with breast cancer. Many women with a family history of breast cancer incorrectly assume that the issue is not whether they will be diagnosed with breast cancer, but when. Kelly (1991) stated that, as women approach the age at which their mothers were diagnosed with breast cancer, their anxiety often increases. As they pass that age, they may begin to feel their risk is sufficiently different and believe they might not get breast cancer after all. Unfortunately, some become overconfident and fail to get adequate screening. Healthcare professionals must understand how clients' beliefs about cancer will influence their understanding of the information they receive as part of risk assessment.

Kelly (1991) stressed that such an understanding can seldom be obtained quickly or in a straightforward way because individuals usually are unaware of their beliefs. A nurse can gain insight by listening carefully as a client describes past experiences with cancer. Although the client may realize intellectually that improved treatments are now available, he or she may continue to remember, and dread, the disease as experienced by a friend or relative. For example, a woman whose mother was treated with a Halsted radical mastectomy may fear the same treatment for herself; therefore, she ignores a breast lump despite the availability of more cosmetically acceptable forms of treatment. Such fears must be addressed before they can be corrected.

Socioeconomic and Cultural Factors

Socioeconomic and cultural differences affect beliefs about disease (Huerta & Macario, 1999; Marcus, 1999). Some cultures and ethnic groups have specific beliefs about cancer and what occurs during a cancer screening. Some groups are more trusting of healthcare professionals than others. These beliefs, whether accurate or not, influence perceptions of cancer risk.

Motivation

Knowing the client's motivation for genetic-risk assessment and counseling or testing can be important. Kash et al. (2000) reported that breast cancer anxiety, not evidence of breast cancer risk, motivates clients to request genetic testing. As a result, the researchers concluded, the clients most likely to request genetic testing were the clients most likely to be psychologically vulnerable. They wondered if offering genetic testing to this group could cause more harm than good.

The Challenge of Uncertainty

Although predisposition testing helps to quantify risk, much uncertainty still exists for most tested clients (Bottorff, Ratner, Johnson, Lovato, & Joab, 1998).

Uncertainty and Risk Factors

Uncertainty exists about some of the risk factors for many cancers. For example, experts disagree in regard to the extent that hormonal therapy after menopause increases the risk of breast cancer.

The best way to assess the association would be to do a prospective, randomized study in which a large group of women with similar risks of breast cancer were randomly assigned to either take or not take hormone replacement therapy. Researchers would assess these women for a number of years, to see what differences in the number of breast cancer cases arose. If the groups were large enough, factors other than hormone replacement therapy would be evenly distributed between the two groups; any differences in breast cancer rates would probably be a result of the therapy. Randomized studies can be very expensive, however, and years pass before the results are available.

Currently, most of what is known about hormone replacement therapy and breast cancer risk is based on observational studies. Such studies usually do not establish a strong causal relationship between a risk factor and a disease. Therefore, when risk-factor assessments based on observational studies are completed, the clients who receive the assessments must live with the fact that all the risk factors for a particular cancer may not be known. Other risk factors, such as the risk of using hormone replacement therapy after menopause, may not be fully understood. Those who conduct risk assessments must educate clients about these gaps in knowledge and the uncertainty associated with them.

The Uncertainty of Test Results

If clients test positive for a mutation, they know that their chance of developing one or more malignancies is very high, but they do not know when they will develop a malignancy. A negative test result does not completely eliminate risk for clients who receive one. These clients have the same risk of developing a sporadic cancer as the general population. For clients whose results reveal a change of "indeterminate significance," the uncertainty is very large. These clients have not gained any new or helpful information from genetic testing.

Uncertainty and Screening Recommendations

Uncertainty also accompanies recommended prevention and detection strategies. This may be the most serious limitation of genetic testing (Kash et al., 2000). No screening strategy is completely effective in detecting cancer early. The sensitivity and specificity of screening tests are widely variable. Further, many of the prophylactic measures, and sometimes the chemoprevention recommendations, are not based on scientific studies of people with mutations. Often, data are extrapolated from other studies and information. This means that the certainty with which healthcare professionals can make screening recommendations may be limited at best.

Variable Penetrance

Nurses also must address the issue of variable penetrance (Cornelisse & Devilee, 1997). Penetrance is the proportion of a population that has a particular genotype or mutation that actually expresses the corresponding phenotype or cancer. In many of the mutations associated with hereditary cancer, penetrance is incomplete. Some mutations are associated with higher risks of cancer than are others. Penetrance can change with age and specific mutation it can vary considerably from family to family. Genetic factors associated with different mutations probably modify the risks of gene carriers. To date, these additional factors are unknown. Thus, clients who test positive trade the uncertainty of not knowing if they are at significant risk for the uncertainty of knowing when, if at all, the cancer will develop.

Uncertainty Associated With Clinical Vignettes

Much of the clinical knowledge healthcare professionals use is stored, not in tables or graphs, but as clinical vignettes. Clinicians often make diagnoses by comparing the case at hand to these clinical stories (Worthen, 1999). This works well in some cases. It works less well, as a rule, when trying to determine genetic predisposition for disease. The enormous variability of genetic disorders, penetrance, family size, and the resemblance between many hereditary and sporadic cancers make constructing a classic case difficult. If a classic case exists, it is not always useful because it refers to a pedigree, not an individual (Worthen).

Navigating Statistics

Statistical Significance Versus Clinical Significance

Those providing genetic-risk assessment and counseling must help clients to understand that statistical significance is not the same as clinical significance. Statistical significance is a measure of the likelihood that a result was not caused by chance alone.

Sometimes a statistically significant finding may mean little clinically. Consider, for example, a woman who has a *BRCA2* mutation. A nurse, in counseling the woman about chemoprevention, tells her that, in a study, participants who took a specific chemopreventive agent for 12 years developed breast cancer 60 days later than participants who did not; the result was statistically significant. The nurse should explain that, despite statistical significance, a 60-day onset delay may not make the agent worth using if it causes bothersome or dangerous side effects. In other words, the 60-day onset delay, in light of side effects, may be clinically insignificant. Another reason not to take an agent is high cost. Clients need to know all the factors involved to make informed decisions.

The Inequality of Statistics

Those providing genetic-risk assessment and counseling must help clients to understand that statistics from some studies are more important than others. Clients should give more weight to statistics generated by studies that are well designed and executed than to statistics from poorly designed studies. Healthcare professionals can help clients to identify sound statistics from sound studies and explain to them the evaluation criteria, which include adequacy of sample size, appropriateness of the statistical tests used, and whether the study used random sampling. Also important is whether the characteristics of the group studied are similar to the client's characteristics.

Promoting Screening and Prevention

Research continues to suggest that the single most important factor in whether an individual has ever had a screening test or has recently had a screening test is a recommendation from a healthcare provider (Smith, Mettlin, Davis, & Eyre, 2000).

Focusing on Wellness

When providing clients with information about cancer control, healthcare professionals should focus on wellness. Focusing on the negative aspects—

disease and treatment—may distress some clients to such a degree that they decline screening and prevention efforts.

The emphasis, in education about cancer control, should be the advantages of early detection—that, when cancer is detected early, morbidity and mortality decrease and quality of life increases. Written materials that focus on nutrition, participation in chemoprevention trials, self-examination techniques, and Pap smears are available through NCI and ACS. Other examples of printed materials that focus on wellness are available in the professional literature (Mahon, 1995, 1996; Mahon & Casperson, 1991; Mahon, Casperson, & Wolf, 1994).

Helping Clients to Understand Their Own Degree of Motivation

Healthcare professionals can help clients to understand how willing they are to accept the risk of potential side effects and the need for additional health monitoring. For example, using tamoxifen, a breast cancer preventive, can cause changes in the endometrium. Some clients who take tamoxifen need to undergo endometrial sampling to ensure that the changes do not signal endometrial hyperplasia, endometrial thickening, or cancer (Fisher et al., 1998). This test is somewhat uncomfortable. The client needs to understand the risks and discomforts associated with the preventive in the context of her risk of, in this case, breast cancer.

Some preventives and treatments require a client to take a medication, which may have side effects, for many years. The nurse should help the client decide whether he or she is willing to do this, stressing that taking the medication will require continued follow-up to determine if the medication is effective and safe.

The nurse also must ensure that the client understands that no preventive is a guarantee against cancer.

The Media's Role in Risk Information

Trends in Media Coverage of Cancer Risk

Today, many sources provide health-related information to the public: radio, television news, talk shows, commercials, newspapers, magazines, and the Internet. The media often needs more than numbers or complex research to make a story. A reporter usually is looking for human interest and an emotional component (Russell, 1993). Stories seem to have more impact if children or celebrities are involved. The subtleties of risk and technical points often get lost in these pieces of the story (Levine, 1999).

Russell (1999) discerned trends in how the media has covered stories about cancer risk. During the 1970s and early 1980s, the focus often was on environmental carcinogens and risks. During the mid-1980s, the focus shifted to individual behaviors and lifestyle risks. With the isolation of the breast cancer susceptibility genes and the widespread use of tumor markers, such as prostate-specific antigen, the focus of news stories changed again in the 1990s. The stories about early developments in cancer genetics often reported very preliminary findings and relied on abstracts as the basis of content. Conflicting information, controversy, and confusion were the results in many cases. Recently, the trend has been to provide in-depth reporting. A reporter may take the time to do solid, in-depth research and wait to publish the story until findings can appear in proper perspective (Brody, 1999).

Despite recent improvements, Kelly (1996) noted that media coverage about cancer risks in general does not address individual concerns about risk or provide sufficient detail to resolve conflicts. Many reports fail to emphasize the uncertainty involved in assessing cancer risk (Russell, 1999). Similarly, many reports fail to distinguish between absolute and relative risks.

Research suggests that, when faced with differing opinions and incomplete information about risk and etiology, even highly educated people may become anxious, realizing that they lack sufficient information to make informed decisions. Superficial media coverage that does not offer a way of receiving in-depth information can cause emotional and physical concerns to individual members of the public.

McCall (1988) noted that scientists and journalists often disagree about how to convey information about risk because their goals differ. Scientists, McCall said, tend to be interested in abstract principles, tentative conclusions, and a complete report; journalists seek concrete applications, certain conclusions, and a summary.

Initial reports about the isolation of the breast cancer susceptibility genes *BRCA1* and *BRCA2* provide an example of how journalists' focus has sometimes resulted in misleading coverage. The early reports gave little attention to the fact that such genes explain only a small percentage of cases of breast cancer.

How to Work Effectively With Media Reports and the Media

Reports of newly discovered cancer risks can conjure fear among members of the public. Healthcare providers need to be aware of news reports so they can be prepared to address their clients' concerns. Going to the primary source to check the accuracy of the reports can enable providers to present the issues accurately and answer clients' questions.

When communicating with the media, healthcare professionals also consult with primary sources to ensure the accuracy of the information. ACS and NCI are trustworthy sources, especially in regard to statistics.

Each year, ACS publishes *Cancer Facts and Figures* (ACS, 2001). This helpful resource presents estimates about cancer cases, including the estimated mortality and the number of new cases of a specific cancer per year (incidence). Incidence rates are given by state. *Cancer Facts and Figures* also offers detailed data about primary and secondary prevention of the major tumors and projected survival data by stage. The publication is free and available from local ACS units.

Another resource is the Surveillance, Epidemiology, and End Results (SEER) Program (Ries et al., 1999). Currently, SEER provides incidence, mortality, and survival data from 1973 through 1996. Data from the nine SEER geographic areas represent an estimated 9.5% of the U.S. population. Currently, the SEER database contains information about 2.3 million cancer cases diagnosed since 1973. Approximately 125,000 new cases are added yearly. SEER data are available on the NCI Web site (www-seer.ims.nci.nih.gov) or by ordering the *SEER Cancer Statistics Review 1973–1996* through NCI by calling 800-4CANCER (800-422-6237) and requesting publication number 00-2789.

The Long-Term Impact of Risk Communication

Kelly (1996) reported that, after risk information has been communicated, the client may have difficulty remembering it. Healthcare professionals can reinforce communication about risk and recommended screenings by sending clients a postvisit letter that summarizes important information. In fact, postvisit letters are a standard expectation in clinical care. However, including the client as a receiver of such a letter is not routine, although doing so improves communication.

Of great concern is the effect of information on health-related behaviors. Postvisit letters to the client's referring physician, discussing the risk assessment and medical management recommendations, also may be routine in some settings. Contact with the primary or referring physician, with appropriate client consent, may assist the client in screening and risk-reduction behaviors.

Individuals who are distressed because their cancer risk is high may be less likely than those with less anxiety to follow reasonable health programs. This distress may explain the less-than-adequate healthcare behaviors of clients having one or more affected first-degree relatives with breast cancer. These clients may not follow guidelines suggested for the general population, let alone submit to the closer follow-up that their circumstances usually warrant. Kelly (1996) stressed that a realistic perception of risk does not appear to be "straightforward," nor is it usually formed in one short educational session.

Risk-factor assessment is an ongoing part of oncology nursing practice. Each client's risk-factor profile should be reviewed at least annually. Clients should be questioned about changes in family history since the last assessment, any new risk-associated health problems have developed (e.g., abnormal Pap test, a diagnosis of hypertension), and if the client has started new medications (e.g., increased estrogen replacement therapy) that may have changed the risk profile. If significant changes have occurred, screening recommendations may need modification. Even if no significant changes have occurred, the annual review of the risk-factor assessment offers an excellent opportunity to reinforce information about cancer prevention and early detection. In addition, it communicates an ongoing concern for the client and identifies the nurse as a source of further information if a problem develops.

Risk-Assessment Documentation

Few published reports describe documentation of risk-factor assessment. White (1986) described a checklist of major risk factors for the various cancers that can be completed after an interview. This format does not allow space or encourage documentation specific to the risk factor, such as the number of years the client used estrogen replacement therapy or the number of packs of cigarettes the client smokes per year.

Trying to find risk factors by category or anatomic site can be confusing to the client, result in a disjointed interview, and may not be as thorough as a comprehensive health history. Researchers have noted that structuring the interview in a traditional medical-history format, however, facilitates a smooth process (University of Texas M.D. Anderson Cancer Center Cancer Prevention and Detection Programs Staff, 1988). A comprehensive cancer-risk assessment is more likely than a site-specific assessment to ensure that the client has the information he or she needs to make informed decisions. For example, if a woman comes in for breast screening and a site-specific risk assessment is completed, the nurse may overlook a significant risk for colon or ovarian cancer.

To conduct a comprehensive interview, the clinician must document cancer-prevention and early-detection recommendations somewhere on the chart. For that reason, specially designed forms that encourage comprehensive interviews and documentation and make information easy to retrieve, update, and interpret are helpful.

The Face Sheet

A face sheet can provide quick access to demographic information and allow space to document previous surgeries and health problems. Figure 5-16 lists the possible elements of such a form. This information may or may not be pertinent to cancer screening, but it provides information about the client's overall health. Blank space at the bottom is useful for documenting all types of information, such as where mammograms are stored and information about further evaluation or follow-ups. The face sheet can be placed on the front of one side of the chart.

The Family History Form and Pedigree

A family history form must focus on first- and second-degree relatives. It should include at least three generations. The completed form should include an assessment of both paternal and maternal sides, because many autosomal-dominant syndromes are passed through either the father or mother. First-degree relatives include parents, siblings, and children. Because first-degree relatives share 50% of their genes, these will be the relatives most likely to inherit similar genetic information. Information about second-degree relatives also can be helpful. Second-degree relatives include grandparents, aunts, and uncles. Second-degree relatives have 25% of their genes in common. Older second-degree relatives can provide important information about genetic risk because they would manifest an early-onset cancer if a hereditary trait were present in the family. The history also should include nieces and nephews. Information about these family members can provide information about childhood cancers, which has implications for the client's genetic risk. Third-degree relatives (cousins, great-aunts and great-uncles, and great-grandparents) also can be included, although the accuracy of reports on these relatives is not always high. These relatives share 12.5% of the same genes.

After all this information is documented, it should be arranged in standard pedigree format. A pedigree is a graphic representation of family medical history (see Figure 5-17). Pedigrees can be helpful in teaching concepts of genetics, clarifying relationships, and providing a quick reference, especially when the family includes multiple malignancies. The recent availability of software to draw these pedigrees has made updating the information quite simple.

Figure 5-16. Suggested Elements in a Cancer-Screening Form

Face Sheet
- Name
- Social Security number
- Address
- Occupation
- Telephone number(s)

- Primary physician
- Date of birth
- Sex
- Past surgery and medical problems

Family History
- Father
- Mother
- Sisters
- Brothers
- Maternal
  - Grandmother
  - Grandfather
  - Aunts
  - Uncles

- Paternal
  - Grandmother
  - Grandfather
  - Aunts
  - Uncles
- Children
- Grandchildren

Male Risk Assessment
- Family history of cancer
  - Prostate
  - Colon/polyps
  - Testicle
  - Skin/melanoma
  - Breast/gynecology
- Medical history
- Lifestyle history
  - High-fat diet

  - Chemical exposure
  - Light/fair complexion
  - Previous skin cancer/nevi removal
  - Previous x-ray exposure
  - Sun exposure
  - Tanning parlor use
  - Tobacco use
  - Alcohol use

Female Risk Assessment
- Family history of cancer
  - Breast
  - Colon/polyps
  - Ovary
  - Uterus
  - Skin/melanoma
- Reproductive history
  - Menarche
  - Menopause
  - Hormone history
  - Pregnancy history
  - Early parity
  - Previous breast biopsies
  - Early first coitus multiple partners
  - History of cervical dysplasia

  - Exposure to diethylstilbestrol
  - Infertility
- Medical/lifestyle history
  - Hypertension
  - Diabetes
  - Obesity
  - High-fat diet
  - Light/fair complexion
  - Previous skin cancer/nevi removal
  - Previous x-ray exposure
  - Sun exposure
  - Tanning parlor use
  - Chemical exposure
  - Tobacco use
  - Alcohol use

Note. From "Cancer Risk Assessment: Conceptual Considerations for Clinical Practice," by S.M. Mahon, 1998, *Oncology Nursing Forum, 25,* p. 1544. Copyright 1998 by the Oncology Nursing Society. Reprinted with permission.

Figure 5-17. A Sample Pedigree

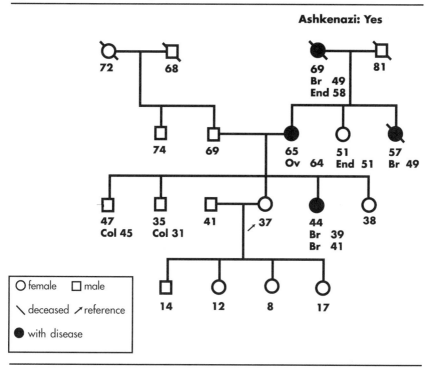

The pedigree provides an organized way to document the risk factors related to family history, such as if a relative is alive or dead, age at death if applicable, significant medical diagnoses, or a diagnosis of cancer. Space can be provided to detail the specific type of cancer, age at diagnosis, and other characteristics, such as if a breast cancer was premenopausal or bilateral. Specific knowledge may influence recommendations for screening.

Using a family history form and pedigree is useful for identifying families with a possible hereditary predisposition to malignancy and other illnesses. Healthcare providers should ask clients about specific relatives and their health individually rather than asking a more general question, such as "Have any of your relatives been diagnosed with cancer?" Figure 5-16 presents a useful review of the cancers that tend to have a hereditary predisposition. After gathering the family history, it is important to ask again whether any of the client's relatives have been diagnosed with these cancers. Clients forget to provide this information surprisingly often, and reiterating this question provides valuable information.

Documentation of History Assessment

Assessment of medical history and personal-history factors that may increase the risk of developing cancer should be documented. Many of these risk factors are not within an individual's control and are not amenable to primary prevention efforts (e.g., age at menarche). Lifestyle factors, often within the control of the individual, complete the risk-factor assessment and provide a framework for providing education about primary prevention efforts.

After all the risk data are collected, the clinician must assimilate the risk factors mentally and provide information about them to the client for each of the major cancers. For example, early menarche, nulliparity, and late menopause are risk factors for both breast and endometrial cancer. The communication of risk should include a discussion of the risk for developing both these cancers.

Consent Forms and Waivers

Each client should sign a consent form that summarizes all the screening and/or testing procedures the client intends to undergo. The consent form should state who will provide each screening or test and state that the procedure may not detect all cancers. If the client declines any recommended screening, the client should sign a waiver that lists the recommended procedures he or she declines. The waiver usually is part of the consent form.

Annual Assessment Updates

A risk assessment should be reviewed and, if necessary, updated at least annually. Information about family history, hormone use, biopsies, menopausal status, and smoking behavior, for example, is likely to change. Changes can be made directly on the appropriate form, initialed, and dated. If no changes have occurred, the top or bottom of the family-history and risk-factor sheet can be dated and initialed.

An annual update also provides an excellent opportunity to review significant risk factors, cancer-prevention strategies, and early-detection behaviors.

The Implications of Screening Tests

Quaid (1993) noted that, if clients are to realize the intended benefits of screening, they must understand the implications of the screening tests before they are screened and after they receive results.

After screening tests, risk may be more apparent, and nurses may need to revise screening recommendations. For example, a 50-year-old woman may have a baseline screening flexible sigmoidoscopy examination that a finds polyp. A biopsy shows hyperplasia. The woman's risk of developing colon cancer is higher than initially perceived, so the healthcare professional should tell her about her risk and ACS's guidelines, which recommend total colon examination (Byers et al., 1997).

Nursing Implications of Risk Assessment

Economic Considerations

At the clinical level, the delivery of cancer risk information takes time, and how the cost of these services are reimbursed is unclear. Sometimes the costs of genetic-risk assessment counseling are bundled with the costs of other services, such as mammography. This practice could cause healthcare and insurance administrators, clients, and the public to fail to realize the importance of risk assessment and counseling and the need for trained professionals to deliver these services.

In most cases, reimbursement for genetic-risk assessment counseling is limited. Clients may need assistance to find the means to cover the cost of the services they provide.

Practice Considerations: Identifying Potential Clients

Kramer (1999) emphasized that the process of providing a client with enough information to make an informed decision is extremely labor-intensive. Obviously, advanced practice nurses in genetics should spend their time with clients who stand the chance of benefiting most.

One approach to finding such clients is to use staff nurses as case finders, or nurses who spot clients with a likelihood of benefiting from genetic counseling. Candidates are individuals at increased risk for cancer who will benefit from a detailed risk assessment and, possibly, genetic counseling (MacDonald, 1997). Staff nurses who work with clients and get to know their families usually make effective case finders. To be an effective case finder, the nurse must understand basic cancer incidence, epidemiology, and the importance of an accurate family history.

Nurses with advanced practice degrees can perform more in-depth risk assessments, recommend cancer screening procedures, explain the risks and benefits of a particular screening examination, and, in many cases, actually perform the screening examination. Advanced practice nurses are well-suited to perform clinical breast examinations, teach breast self-examination, do rectal examinations, or complete a pelvic exam and take a Pap smear. Some advanced practice nurses with additional subspeciality training are able to perform flexible sigmoidoscopy examinations.

The Need for Future Research

Future research should evaluate the process of risk notification and the impact of this knowledge on attitudes, emotions, practices, and outcomes related to health and disease status. Vernon (1999) emphasized that most of the studies of perceived risk have been cross-sectional, making it difficult to determine whether perceived risk is a cause or an effect in relation to cancer screening. This relationship could be better understood if future longitudinal studies measured perceived risk in defined populations, with different cancer-screening histories, who have received follow-up screening and several measurements of risk perception. These studies should include controlled clinical trials to evaluate different counseling protocols. Such work would provide information about the impact and effectiveness of cancer-risk assessment and counseling.

Clearly, clinicians need more information about the roles of cognition, affective state, developmental differences, and personal values in cancer-risk communication (Maibach, 1999). Researchers also should try to determine which care providers communicate genetic risks most effectively and through what approach (Arkin, 1999). Another research goal would be to determine methods that facilitate decision making about cancer-risk management. Prospective studies are needed to determine the psychological and behavioral implications of risk information. Optimal assessments would be conducted at multiple times and include outcome variables.

More research is needed to understand why two individuals react differently to similar information regarding cancer risk. Wardle and Pope (1992) noted that little research has been done to show how people cope with information about their risk of disease. Models of coping with disease may not encompass the concept of coping with increased risk for developing a disease. In particular, the effect of cancer-risk assessment on cancer-screening behaviors merits more attention.

Currently, nurses and healthcare professionals have few options when it comes to education about communicating risk and genetic concepts. Future studies should focus on developing courses that will teach effective risk communication and the most effective way of implementing it (Visser & Bleiker, 1997; Vernon, 1999).

Conclusion

As healthcare professionals continue to search for knowledge about minimizing risk factors and improving cancer treatment, genetics will play a key role. Developments in genetic testing offer a dramatic enhancement to cancer prevention. Researchers finally opened a locked door and are beginning to understand how endogenous and exogenous sources interact to cause cancer. This theoretical knowledge is now an applied science, growing steadily and ever increasing the number of factors formerly out of one's control that they can now do something about.

References

American Cancer Society. (2001). *Cancer facts and figures, 2001.* Atlanta: Author.

American Society of Clinical Oncology. (1996). Statement of the American Society of Clinical Oncology: Genetic testing for cancer susceptibility. *Journal of Clinical Oncology, 14,* 1730–1736.

Arkin, E.B. (1999). Cancer risk communication—What we know. *Journal of the National Cancer Institute Monographs, 25,* 182–185.

Armstrong, K., Eisen, A., & Weber, B. (2000). Assessing the risk of breast cancer. *New England Journal of Medicine, 342,* 564–571.

Berry, D.A., Parmigiani, G., Sanchez, J., Schildkraut, J., & Winer, E. (1997). Probability of carrying a mutation of breast-ovarian cancer gene BRCA1 based on family history. *Journal of the National Cancer Institute, 89,* 227–238.

Bilimoria, M.M., & Morrow, M. (1995). The woman at increased risk for breast cancer: Evaluation and management strategies. *CA: A Cancer Journal for Clinicians, 45,* 263–278.

Bottorff, J.L., Ratner, P.A., Johnson, J.L., Lovato, C.Y., & Joab, S.A. (1998). Communicating cancer risk information: The challenges of uncertainty. *Client Education and Counseling, 33,* 67–81.

Brody, J.E. (1999). Communicating cancer risk in print journalism. *Journal of the National Cancer Institute Monographs, 25,* 170–172.

Byers, T., Levin, B., Rothenberger, D., Dodd, G.D., & Smith, R.A. (1997). American Cancer Society guidelines for screening and surveillance for early detection of colorectal polyps and cancer: Update 1997. *CA: A Cancer Journal for Clinicians, 47,* 154–160.

Clark, R.A. (1996). Breast cancer. In D.S. Reintgen & R.A. Clark (Eds.), *Cancer screening* (pp. 23–40). St. Louis, MO: Mosby.

Clark, R.A., & Reintgen, D.S. (1996). Principles of cancer screening. In D.S. Reintgen & R.A. Clark (Eds.), *Cancer screening* (pp. 1–20). St. Louis, MO: Mosby.

Claus, E.B., Risch, N., & Thompson, W.D. (1994). Autosomal dominant inheritance of early-onset breast cancer: Implications for risk prediction. *Cancer, 73,* 643–651.

Claus, E.B., Schildkraut, M.M., Thompson, W.D., & Risch, N. (1996). The genetic attributable risk of breast and ovarian cancer. *Cancer, 77,* 2318–2324.

Constantino, J.P., Gail, M.H., Pee, D., Anderson, S., Redmond, C.K., Benichou, J., et al. (1999). Validation studies for models projecting the risk of invasive and total breast cancer incidence. *Journal of the National Cancer Institute, 91,* 1541–1548.

Cornelisse, C.J., & Devilee, P. (1997). Facts in cancer genetics. *Client Education and Counseling, 32,* 9–17.

Couch, F.J., DeShano, M.L., Blackwood, M.A., Calzone, K., Stopfer, J., Campeau, L., et al. (1997). BRCA1 mutations in women attending clinics that evaluate the risk of breast cancer. *New England Journal of Medicine, 336,* 1409–1415.

Daly, M. (1999). NCCN practice guidelines: Genetics/familial high risk cancer screening. *Oncology, 13,* 161–184.

Emery, J., Walton, R., Murphy, M., Austoker, J., Yudkin, P., Chapman, C., et al. (2000). Computer support for interpreting family histories of breast and ovarian cancer in primary care: Comparative study with simulated cases. *BMJ, 321,* 28–32.

Fischhoff, B. (1999). Why (cancer) risk communication can be hard. *Journal of the National Cancer Institute Monographs, 25,* 7–13.

Fischhoff, B., Lichtenstein, S., Slovic, P., Derby, S.L., & Keeney, R.L. (1983). *Acceptable risk.* New York: Cambridge University Press.

Fisher, B., Costantino, J.P., Wickerham, D.C., Redmond, C.K., Kavanah, M., Cronin, W.M., et al. (1998). Tamoxifen for prevention of breast cancer: Report of the National Surgical Adjuvant Breast and Bowel Project P-1 study. *Journal of the National Cancer Institute, 90,* 1371–1388.

Florica, J.V., & Roberts, W.S. (1996). Ovarian cancer. In D.S. Reintgen & R.A. Clark (Eds.), *Cancer screening* (pp. 150–167). St. Louis, MO: Mosby.

Foltz, A. (2000). Issues in determining cancer screening recommendations: Who, what and when. *Oncology Nursing Forum, 27*(Suppl. 9), 13–18.

Frank, T.S. (1998). Hereditary risk of breast and ovarian carcinoma: The role of the oncologist. *The Oncologist, 3,* 403–412.

Frank, T.S., Manley, S.A., Olopade, O.I., Cummings, S., Garber, J.E., Bernhardt, B., et al. (1998). Sequence analysis of BRCA1 and BRCA2: Correlation of mutations with family history and ovarian cancer risk. *Journal of Clinical Oncology, 16,* 2417–2425.

Gail, M.H., Brinton, L.A., & Byar, D.P. (1989). Projecting individualized probabilities of developing breast cancer for white females who are being examined annually. *Journal of the National Cancer Institute, 81,* 1879–1886.

Gerrard, M., Gibbons, F.X., & Reis-Bergan, M. (1999). The effect of risk communication on risk perceptions: The significance of individual differences. *Journal of the National Cancer Institute Monographs, 25,* 94–100.

Hopwood, P. (1997). Psychological issues in cancer genetics: Current research and future priorities. *Client Education and Counseling, 32,* 19–31.

Huerta, E.E., & Macario, E. (1999). Communicating health risks to ethnic groups: Reaching Hispanics as a case study. *Journal of the National Cancer Institute Monographs, 25,* 23–26.

Kash, K.M., Ortega-Verdejo, K., Dabney, M.K., Holland, J.C., Miller, D.G., & Osborne, M.P. (2000). Psychosocial aspects of cancer genetics: Women at high risk for breast and ovarian cancer. *Seminars in Surgical Oncology, 18,* 333–338.

Kelly, P.T. (1991). *Understanding breast cancer risk.* Philadelphia: Temple University Press.

Kelly, P.T. (1996). Cancer risk information services: Promise and pitfalls. *The Breast Journal, 2,* 233–237.

Kelly, P.T. (1999). Will cancer risk assessment and counseling services survive genetic testing. *Acta Oncologica, 38,* 743–746.

Kelly, P.T. (2000). *Assess your true risk of breast cancer.* New York: Henry Holt & Co.

Kerber, R., & Slattery, M. (1997). Comparison of self-reported and database-linked family history of cancer data in a case-control study. *American Journal of Epidemiology, 146,* 244–248.

Kramer, B.S. (1999). Matching strength of message to strength of evidence: A discussion. *Journal of the National Cancer Institute Monographs, 25,* 85–87.

Kreuter, M.W. (1999). Dealing with competing and conflicting risks in cancer communication. *Journal of the National Cancer Institute Monographs, 25,* 27–34.

Lai, D., & Hardy, R.J. (1999). Potential gains in life expectancy or years of potential life lost: Impact of competing risks of death. *International Journal of Epidemiology, 28,* 894–898.

Leitch, M.A., Dodd, G.D., Costanza, M., Linver, M., Pressman, P., McGinnis, L., & Smith, R.A. (1997). American Cancer Society guidelines for the early detection of breast cancer: Update 1997. *CA: A Cancer Journal for Clinicians, 47,* 150–153.

Lerman, C., Rimer, B.K., & Engstrom, P.F. (1991). Cancer risk notification: Psychosocial and ethical implications. *Journal of Clinical Oncology, 9,* 1275–1282.

Leventhal, H., Kelly, K., & Leventhal, E.A. (1999). Population risk, actual risk, perceived risk, and cancer control: A discussion. *Journal of the National Cancer Institute Monographs, 25,* 81–85.

Levine, J. (1999). Risky business: Communicating scientific findings to the public. *Journal of the National Cancer Institute Monographs, 25,* 163–166.

Lipkus, I.M., & Hollands, J.G. (1999). The visual communication of risk. *Journal of the National Cancer Institute Monographs, 25,* 149–163.

Love, R.R., Evans, A.M., & Josten, D.M. (1985). The accuracy of client reports of a family history of cancer. *Journal of Chronic Disease, 38,* 2892–2893.

Love, S.M. (1989). Use of risk factors in counseling clients. *Hematology/Oncology Clinics of North America, 3,* 599–610.

Love, S.M. (1995). *Dr. Susan Love's breast book* (2nd ed.). Reading, MA: Addison-Wesley.

MacDonald, D.J. (1997). The oncology nurse's role in cancer risk assessment and counseling. *Seminars in Oncology Nursing, 13,* 123–128.

Madigan, M.P., Ziegler, R.G., Benichou, J., Byrne, C., & Hoover, R.N. (1995). Proportion of breast cancer cases in the United States explained by well-established risk factors. *Journal of the National Cancer Institute, 87,* 1681–1685.

Mahon, S.M. (1995). Using brochures to educate the public about the early detection of prostate and colorectal cancer. *Oncology Nursing Forum, 22,* 1413–1420.

Mahon, S.M. (1996). Educating women about gynecologic health using brochures. *Oncology Nursing Forum, 23,* 529–531.

Mahon, S.M. (1998). Cancer risk assessment: Conceptual considerations for clinical practice. *Oncology Nursing Forum, 25,* 1535–1547.

Mahon, S.M. (2000). Principles of cancer prevention and early detection. *Clinical Journal of Oncology Nursing, 4,* 169-176.

Mahon, S.M., & Casperson, D.S. (1991). Teaching women about mammography through use of a brochure. *Oncology Nursing Forum, 18,* 1375–1378.

Mahon, S.M., Casperson, D.S., & Wolf, J. (1994). Testicular cancer: Part 1: Screening and early detection. *Journal of Urological Nursing, 11,* 746–750.

Maibach, E. (1999). Cancer risk communication—What we need to learn. *Journal of the National Cancer Institute Monographs, 25,* 179–181.

Marcus, A.C. (1999). New directions for risk communication research: A discussion with additional suggestions. *Journal of the National Cancer Institute Monographs, 25,* 35–41.

McCall, R.B. (1988). Science and the press—Like oil and water? *American Psychologist, 43*, 87–94.

Meyerowitz, B.E., & Chaiken, S. (1987). The effect of message framing on breast self-examination attitudes, intentions, and behavior. *Journal of Personality and Social Psychology, 3*, 500–510.

Murday, V. (1994). Genetic counseling in the cancer family clinic. *European Journal of Cancer, 30*, 2012–2015.

Newell, G.R., & Vogel, V.G. (1988). Personal risk factors—What do they mean? *Cancer, 62*, 1695–1701.

Northouse, P.G., & Northouse, L.L. (1992). *Health communication strategies for health professionals* (2nd ed.). Norwalk, CT: Appleton & Lange.

Oncology Nursing Society. (1997). *Oncology Nursing Society position on cancer genetics testing and risk assessment counseling.* Retrieved September 4, 2001, from http://www.ons.org xp6ONSClinical.xml/Prevention_Detection .xml/ Genetics_Resource_Area.xmlNovember_ 1997.xmlONS_Releases_ Postion_Statements_Related_to_Cancer_Genetics.xml

Oncology Nursing Society. (2000). *Oncology Nursing Society position on the role of the oncology nurse in cancer genetic counseling.* Retrieved August 4, 2002, from http://www.ons.org/xp6/ONS/Information.xml/Journals_and_Positions .xml/Positions.xml/Role_of_the_Oncology_Nurse.xml

Press, N., Fishman, J.R., & Koenig, B.A. (2000). Collective fear, individualized risk: The social and cultural context of genetic testing for breast cancer. *Nursing Ethics, 7*, 237–249.

Quaid, K.A. (1993). Psychological and ethical considerations in screening for disease. *American Journal of Cardiology, 72*(10), 64D–67D.

Ries, L.A.G., Kosary, C.L., Hankeg, B.F., Miller, B.A., Clegg, L., & Edwards, B.K. (Eds.). (1999). *SEER cancer statistics review 1973–1996.* Bethesda MD: National Cancer Institute.

Rimer, B.K., Schildkraut, J.M., Lerman, C., Lin, T., & Audrain, J. (1996). Participation in women's breast cancer risk counseling trials. Who participates? Who declines? *Cancer, 77*, 2348–2355.

Rodgers, J.E. (1999). Introduction of section: Overarching considerations in risk communications: Romancing the message. *Journal of the National Cancer Institute Monographs, 25*, 21–22.

Rodriquez-Bigas, M.A., Boland, C.R., Hamilton, S.R., Henson, D.E., Jass, J.R., Khan, P.M., et al. (1997). A National Cancer Institute workshop on hereditary nonpolyposis colorectal cancer syndrome: Meeting highlights and Bethesda Guidelines. *Journal of the National Cancer Institute, 89*, 1758–1762.

Rohwer, J., & Wandberg, R. (1997). Evaluating cancer prevention technology with instructional strategies. *Journal of Health Education, 28*, 324–334.

Rosenberg, R.D., Hunt, W.C., Williamson, M.R., Gilliland, F.D, Wiest, P.W., Kelsey, C.A., et al. (1998). Effects of age, breast density, ethnicity, and estrogen replacement therapy on screening mammographic sensitivity and cancer stage at diagnosis: review of 183,134 screening mammograms in Albuquerque, New Mexico. *Radiology, 209*, 511–518.

Rosser, E.M., Hurst, J.A., & Chapman, C.J. (1996). Cancer families: What risks are they given and do the risks affect management? *Journal of Medical Genetics, 33*, 977–980.

Rothman, A.J., & Kiviniemi, M.T. (1999). Treating people with information: An analysis and review of approaches to communicating health risk information. *Journal of the National Cancer Institute Monographs, 25*, 44–51.

Rowan, F. (1996). The high stakes of risk communication. *Preventive Medicine, 25*(1), 24–25.

Russell, C. (1993). Hype, hysteria, and women's health risks: The role of the media. *Women's Health Institute, 3*, 191–197.

Russell, C. (1999). Living can be hazardous to your health: How the news media cover cancer risks. *Journal of the National Cancer Institute Monographs, 25*, 167–172.

Sachs, L. (1999). Knowledge of no return: Getting and giving information about genetic risk. *Acta Oncologica, 38*, 735–740.

Salovey, P., Schneider T.R., & Apanovitch, A.M. (1999). Persuasion for the purpose of cancer risk reduction: A discussion. *Journal of the National Cancer Institute Monographs, 25*, 119–122.

Schoenbach, V.J., Wagner, E.H., & Beery, W.L. (1987). Health risk appraisal: A review of evidence for effectiveness. *Health Services Research, 22*, 553–579.

Schwartz, L.M., Woloshin, S., & Welch, H.G. (1999). Risk communication in clinical practice: Putting cancer in context. *Journal of the National Cancer Institute Monographs, 25*, 124–133.

Shattuck-Eidens, D., Oliphant, A., & McClure, M. (1997). BRCA1 sequence analysis in women at high risk for susceptibility mutations. Risk factor analysis and implications for genetic testing. *JAMA, 278*, 1242–1250.

Slovik, P. (1986). Informing and educating the public about risk. *Risk Analysis, 6*, 403–415.

Smith, R.A., Mettlin, C.J., Davis, K.J., & Eyre, H. (2000). American Cancer Society guidelines for the early detection of cancer. *CA: A Cancer Journal for Clinicians 50*, 34–49.

Spiegelman, D., Colditz, G.A., Hunter, D., & Hertzmark, E. (1994). Validation of the Gail et al. model for predicting individual breast cancer risk. *Journal of the National Cancer Institute, 86,* 600–607.

Stopfer, J.E. (2000). Genetic counseling and clinical cancer genetics services. *Seminars in Surgical Oncology, 18,* 347–357.

Struewing, J.P., Hartge, P., Wacholder, S., Baker, B.S., Berlin, M., McAdams, M., et al. (1997). The risk of cancer associated with specific mutations of BRCA1 and BRCA2 among Ashkenazi Jews. *New England Journal of Medicine, 336,* 1401–1408.

Strecher, V.J., Greenwood, T., Wang, C., & Dumont, D. (1999). Interactive multimedia and risk communication. *Journal of the National Cancer Institute Monographs, 25,* 134–139.

Tischkowitz, M., Wheeler, D., France, E., Chapman, C., & Lucassen, A. (2000). *Annals of Oncology, 11,* 451–454.

University of Texas M.D. Anderson Cancer Center Cancer Prevention and Detection Programs Staff. (1988). *Cancer prevention and detection in the cancer screening clinic.* Houston, TX: University of Texas M.D. Anderson Cancer Center.

Vasen, H.F., Mecklin, J.P., Khan, M.P., & Lynch, H.T. (1991). The International Collaborative Group on Hereditary Nonpolyposis Colorectal Cancer (ICG-HNPCC). *Diseases of the Colon and Rectum, 34,* 424–425.

Vasen, H.F., Watson, P., Mecklin, J.P., & Lynch, H.T. (1999). New clinical criteria for hereditary nonpolyposis colorectal cancer (HNPCC, Lynch Syndrome) proposed by the International Collaborative Group on HNPCC. *Gastroenterology, 116,* 1453–1456.

Vernon, S.W. (1999). Risk perception and risk communication for cancer screening behaviors: A review. *Journal of the National Cancer Institute Monographs, 25,* 101–119.

Visser, A., & Bleiker, E. (1997). Introduction: Genetic education and counseling. *Client Education and Counseling, 32,* 1–7.

Vogel, V. (2000). Breast cancer prevention: A review of current evidence. *CA: A Cancer Journal for Clinicians, 50,* 156–170.

Walker, B. (1997). Cancer risk assessment. *JAMA, 89,* 21–26.

Wardle, J., & Pope, R. (1992). The psychological costs of screening for cancer. *Journal of Psychosomatic Research, 36,* 609–624.

Weinstein, N.D. (1999). What does it mean to understand a risk? Evaluating risk comprehension. *Journal of the National Cancer Institute Monographs, 25,* 15–20.

Weitzel, J.N. (1999). Genetic cancer risk assessment. Putting it all together. *Cancer, 86*(Suppl. 11), 2483–2492.

Westman, J., Hampel, H., & Bradley, T. (2000). Efficacy of a touchscreen computer based family cancer history questionnaire and subsequent cancer risk assessment. *Journal of Medical Genetics, 37,* 354–360.

White, L.N. (1986). Cancer risk assessment. *Seminars in Oncology Nursing, 2,* 184–190.

Wijnen, J.T., Vasen, H.F.A., Khan, P.M., Zwinderman, A.H., van der Klift, H., Mulder, A., et al. (1998). Clinical findings with implications for genetic testing in families with clustering of colorectal cancer. *New England Journal of Medicine, 339,* 511–518.

Wolf, A.M., Nasser, J.F., Wolf, A.M., & Schorling, J.B. (1996). The impact of informed consent on client interest in prostate-specific antigen screening. *Archives of Internal Medicine, 156,* 1333–1336.

Wolpaw, D.R. (1996). Early detection in lung cancer: Case finding and screening. *Medical Clinics of North America, 80,* 63–82.

Worthen, H.G. (1999). Inherited cancer and the primary care physician: Barriers and strategies. *Cancer, 86,* 2583–2588.

6

The Impact of Genetic Information in the Management of Cancer

Paula Trahan Rieger, RN, MSN, CS, AOCN®, FAAN

Editors' note: The terms that appear in boldface in this chapter are defined in the glossary. Glossary terms also are highlighted in Chapters 3 and 5.

Introduction

The explosion, in the past two decades, of knowledge about cancer genetics and the molecular basis of neoplasia is now changing the basic management of cancer. The hope is that these advances will ultimately translate into improved patient survival or even the prevention of cancer (Alberts, 1999; Cannistra, 1997; Sausville & Johnson, 2000). The discovery of genes that are altered during carcinogenesis provides new insights into how to determine an individual's cancer risk, provides prognostic indicators for those who develop cancer, and generates new modalities for cancer treatment.

Much of the knowledge gained in this regard has resulted from work related to the **Human Genome Project,** initiated in 1990. The ultimate goal of this project is to generate information, tools, and molecular approaches that will facilitate the understanding of both normal and abnormal gene structure and function. The first-draft sequence of the human genetic code has been completed, and scientists now estimate that humans have some 30,000–40,000 genes in their **genomes** (Sachidanandam et al., 2001; Venter et al., 2001). This juncture represents just the end of the beginning for the Human Genome Project as scientists now work to produce a finished sequence with extremely high accuracy. This will allow for ultimate determination of gene function, so that this growing knowledge will be converted into treatments than can lengthen and enrich lives. Although excitement abounds regarding the potential of these discoveries, some experts have raised concerns about the effect of recent achievements in genetics. Holtzman and Marteau (2000) cautioned that, in the rush to fit medicine with a genetic mantle, we are losing sight of other possibilities for improving public health. Differences in social structure, lifestyle, and environment, Holtzman and Marteau continued, account for much larger proportions of disease than do genetic differences.

This chapter will discuss the integration of genetic information into three major areas of cancer management: risk management and cancer prevention, diagnosis and prognosis, and treatment. As a prerequisite to understanding these advances in cancer care, oncology nurses must have a solid foundation in cell biology, genetics, and the molecular basis of cancer. (A portion of this information is provided in Chapter 3.) Specific clinical examples will illustrate current and future incorporation of this knowledge into cancer management.

Risk Management and Cancer Prevention

The goals of risk management and cancer prevention are to lessen an individual's susceptibility to cancer and to stop or reverse the multistep process of carcinogenesis (Heusinkveld, 1997; Loescher & Reid, 2000). Maximizing prevention will require identifying individuals at increased risk of cancer and understanding the risk factors associated with cancer development. The most effective cancer-prevention interventions relate to the principles of carcinogenesis (see Figure 6-1) (Loescher, 1993; Mahon, 1998).

The field of cancer epidemiology provides insights into the host factors (e.g., genetic predisposition) and the mutagenic or carcinogenic agents that make individuals susceptible to developing cancer. Cancer epidemiologists study the frequencies, patterns of distribution, and determinants of tumor occurrence in humans (Thun & Wingo, 2000). By studying people who develop cancer, epidemiologists can generate hypotheses about why certain individuals develop cancer while others do not. Causal relationships can be determined by examining both host factors and environmental factors. Identification of etiologic influences can facilitate prevention, especially for individuals at increased risk, and detection of cancer at an early stage makes cure a realistic expectation.

Risk management and cancer prevention involve identification of
- Carcinogenic agents
- Host factors that make individuals susceptible to cancer development
- Individuals at increased risk
  - Risk factors that affect populations
  - Genetic risk factors
- Inherited genes that predispose individuals to cancer
- Genes that determine response to carcinogens.

Figure 6-1. A Futuristic View of Cancer-Prevention and Screening Strategies

Cancer is a multifactorial condition in that genetic, environmental, and lifestyle factors affect its development. Cancer arises following a complex, multistep process characterized by the accumulation of multiple mutations in genes within one cell. These mutations may be spontaneous (i.e., occur as a result of aging or errors in DNA replication), carcinogen-induced, or inherited (i.e., inheritance of a mutation in a known cancer-predisposition gene). In general, two classes of mutations are important in the development of cancer: mutations that result in activation of oncogenes and mutations that result in inactivation of tumor suppressor genes. Oncogenes cause increased cell proliferation. The two types of tumor suppressor genes are caretaker genes (which maintain the integrity of the genome) and gatekeeper genes (which regulate proliferation, viability, and cell senescence). When tumor suppressor genes become mutated, caretaker and gatekeeper genes do not function properly. This figure represents a futuristic view of the cancer-prevention and screening strategies—strategies that will become realities as research improves understanding of the molecular basis of cancer development.

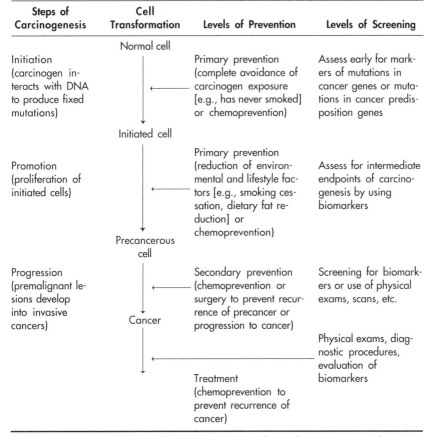

Steps of Carcinogenesis	Cell Transformation	Levels of Prevention	Levels of Screening
	Normal cell		
Initiation (carcinogen interacts with DNA to produce fixed mutations)		Primary prevention (complete avoidance of carcinogen exposure [e.g., has never smoked] or chemoprevention)	Assess early for markers of mutations in cancer genes or mutations in cancer predisposition genes
	Initiated cell		
Promotion (proliferation of initiated cells)		Primary prevention (reduction of environmental and lifestyle factors [e.g., smoking cessation, dietary fat reduction] or chemoprevention)	Assess for intermediate endpoints of carcinogenesis by using biomarkers
	Precancerous cell		
Progression (premalignant lesions develop into invasive cancers)	Cancer	Secondary prevention (chemoprevention or surgery to prevent recurrence of precancer or progression to cancer)	Screening for biomarkers or use of physical exams, scans, etc.
		Treatment (chemoprevention to prevent recurrence of cancer)	Physical exams, diagnostic procedures, evaluation of biomarkers

Note. From "Commentary: Expanding Our Horizons With an Alternative Approach to Cancer Prevention and Detection," by L.J. Loescher, 1996, *Seminars in Oncology Nursing, 9,* pp. 147–149. Copyright 1996 by W.B. Saunders. Adapted with permission.

Identification of Individuals at Increased Risk

The Genetic Basis of Cancer

Cancer results from a stepwise process of acquired genetic mutations (Cavanee & White, 1995; Gribbon & Loescher, 2000). Thus, at the level of the somatic cell, cancer is now considered a genetic disease. Several types of genetic damage seem to occur in cancer cells.

- Conversion of proto-oncogenes (genes that have a role in the regulation of normal cell growth) into oncogenes (which give cells an abnormal growth advantage)
- Inactivation of the tumor suppressor genes that normally slow or stop abnormal cell growth
- Inactivation of "mismatch-repair" genes, which are responsible for repairing errors that occur during **DNA replication;** mismatch-repair genes are the genes that mediate genetic stability
- Bypassing of genes that cause aberrant cells to die by programmed cell death (apoptosis)
- Ability to override genes that regulate cell senescence.

When one or more of the listed genetic errors occur, the end result is that cells can reproduce without restriction; invade local tissues; and, ultimately, establish distant metastases.

Of all cancers, 5%–10% occur in recognizable familial clusterings. Hereditary mutations, in conjunction with acquired mutations, play a fundamental role in the development of these cancers. The **inherited** mutations place individuals at a heightened risk for the development of cancer and have important implications for the prevention and detection of cancer. More than 50 types of cancer demonstrate a familial clustering that is indicative of inherited predisposition; such cancers include colorectal cancer, breast and ovarian cancer, melanoma, and medullary thyroid cancer (Fraser, Calzone, & Goldstein, 1997; Lindor, Greene, & the Mayo Familial Cancer Program, 1998; Ponder, 2001; Rieger, 2000). The recent discovery of genes associated with some of these hereditary cancers has translated into the ability to test for the presence of these genes in individuals. This type of testing is known as cancer-predisposition genetic testing, or predisposition testing.

Genetic Testing

Broadly defined, cancer-predisposition tests analyze, for clinical purposes, human DNA, ribonucleic acid (RNA), chromosomes, proteins, or other gene products to detect disease-related genotypes, mutations, phenotypes, or **karyotypes** (Holtzman & Watson, 1999; Task Force on Genetic Testing, 1996). The tests may help identify people at risk of developing the disease in question, identify carriers of mutated genes, establish diagnosis or prognosis, and establish genetic identity. The cost of commercial predisposition testing ranges from several hundred to several thousand dollars, depending on the tests being performed and the approach used. The waiting time for results from commercial laboratories generally is three to eight weeks.

Current technologies: A variety of techniques exist for performing commercial genetic tests; common methods include protein-truncation assays, heteroduplex analysis, versions of single-strand conformational polymorphism, and direct **DNA sequencing** of the gene of interest (see Table 6-1). Protein-truncation assays are sensitive to mutations that introduce a novel stop codon and thus produce a shortened (or truncated) version of the normal protein. Although they are relatively easy to perform, these assays miss mutations that do not shorten the protein. Further, protein-truncation assays miss cases in which messenger RNA (mRNA) becomes unstable, a condition that commonly occurs with novel stop codons or where abnormalities in the **promoter** or regulatory regions of the gene occur. Direct sequencing is the most sensitive technique and is considered the "gold standard" of genetic testing. Direct sequencing determines the sequence of both copies of the gene. Although highly accurate, the test is expensive and labor-intensive (Weber, 1996), and, generally, it assesses exons and contiguous regulatory regions only.

Emerging technologies: Newer technologies, now emerging, will provide more accurate results more quickly, test for multiple genes at once, and be less expensive. One particularly promising technology is the DNA chip (also referred to as **microarray**) (King & Sinha, 2001). DNA chips, similar in construction and concept to computer chips, are filled with dense grids of DNA probes. DNA probes have been likened to molecular tweezers in that they are able to pick out DNA sequences that are complementary to their own DNA sequence. Extracts from tumor cells are incubated with the chip. Gene fragments bind to the DNA probes that are tailored to them. A laser scans the chip, producing brilliantly colored readouts that can reveal defects in genes. Once a gene has been cloned (i.e., its DNA sequence identified), probes could be designed that pick out that gene or known alterations in the gene. A DNA chip that detects the *TP53* mutation, the most common mutation in human cancers, is on the market. Chips to detect *BRCA1* mutations are being evaluated. As

> Cancer-susceptibility tests involve analysis of
> • Human DNA
> • Human RNA
> • Chromosomes
> • Proteins or other gene products.
>
> The goal of cancer-susceptibility tests: To detect disease-related genotypes, mutations, phenotypes, and karyotypes for clinical purposes.

Table 6-1. Techniques for Identifying Mutations in Disease-Associated Genes

Technique	Description	Benefits	Limitations
Single-strand conformational polymorphism (SSCP)	A suspect fragment of DNA is expanded using polymerase chain reaction. The DNA obtained is heated to separate the complementary strands. An electric current is applied and the strand is run through a gel. The DNA is dyed so that it is visible. Normal DNA produces a reference band. Altered DNA produces a band that is higher or lower than normal.	Can detect 50%–75% of mutations, depending on the type. Technique is fast, and multiple samples can be screened quickly at a relatively low cost. Technique uses DNA, which is stable and easy to handle. Detects deletions and insertions well.	Technique lacks sensitivity and does not detect point mutations well.
Protein truncation	Protein from an unknown sample and a normal reference sample are compared on a gel similar to that described for SSCP heteroduplex analysis. The test detects a shortened protein easily because its mobility differs from that of a larger protein: Small proteins travel faster.	Detects nonsense or frameshift mutations that introduce a stop signal. The stop signal results in the production of a shortened protein.	Will not detect mutations other than nonsense and frameshift mutations. Requires the use of DNA that does not have intervening sequences (introns).
Direct sequencing	Analyzes the sequence of both copies of each gene being analyzed. This is considered the "gold standard" of testing.	Will detect all changes in the sequences being analyzed, including coding and noncoding regions of the gene. The analysis can be automated to process large numbers of specimens.	Expensive and labor-intensive. Requires skilled technicians. Misses regulatory mutations that are outside the coding region and result in absence of RNA transcribed from a gene.
Functional analysis of protein	Inserts gene into a functional assay (generally, yeast).	The analysis is gene specific.	Emerging. Requires knowledge of the function of the gene or the binding partners of the protein. Misses certain mutations.

Note. Based on information from Weber, 1996.

envisioned, DNA chip technology will be able to check for thousands of genes at once. In the future, a few cells might be placed in a gene-chip scanner and quickly analyzed to determine a person's risk of developing numerous diseases. In addition, the ability to customize cancer therapy for individual patients by "profiling" to identify all the genetic defects present and/or the ability to design gene therapy to correct defects may become a reality (Snijders, Meijer, Brakenhoff, van den Brule, & van Diest, 2000; Stipp, 1997).

Genetic profiling also is a goal of pharmacogenetics. This rapidly evolving field is identifying genetic markers that will predict an individual's therapeutic or toxic response to drugs, including chemotherapy (Krynetski & Evans, 1998).

Limitations of current means of assessment: Though several commercial tests are available to identify cancer-predisposition genes, current testing technology has limited application in the clinical setting. The traditional assessment means—evaluation of environmental and lifestyle factors (such as fat intake, smoking habits, and exposure to known carcinogens)—still play an important role in establishing an individual's risk. Even though technology is rapidly moving forward, a gap exists between the ability to identify individuals who carry an increased risk and the ability to reduce mortality and morbidity associated with increased risk.

Management of Individuals at Increased Risk

Emerging in cancer management are strategies designed to reduce the risk of developing invasive and metastatic cancers. As research reveals more about the nature of carcinogenesis, the ability to intervene at the earliest stages is rapidly becoming possible. For example, recognition that dysplastic lesions, such as oral leukoplakia, are biologically significant represents a paradigm shift that can lead to effective risk-reduction measures. In addition, study of the intrinsic biologic mechanisms that may prevent these lesions from becoming invasive and metastatic can offer insight into the design of new, effective therapeutic strategies (Chemoprevention Working Group, 1999; Sporn & Lippmann, 2000).

> Management of individuals at increased risk may include:
> • Chemoprevention (the use of agents that arrest or reverse cancer development)
> • Prophylactic surgery
> • Screening and early detection.

Chemoprevention

One new strategy is the use of pharmacologic agents that arrest or reverse the multistage process of cancer development—that is, chemoprevention (Greenwald, 1996).

Categories of chemopreventive agents: Chemoprevention agents may be classified into two basic categories: agents that prevent initiation of the carcinogenic process (blocking agents) and those that prevent further promotion or progression of lesions that have already been established (suppressing agents). In reality, the distinction between these categories is often artificial.

Major types of agents used in the chemoprevention of cancer (Greenwald, Kelloff, Burch-Whitman, & Kramer, 1995; Sporn & Lippmann, 2000; Swan & Ford, 1997) include

- Retinoids (natural and synthetic analogs of vitamin A)
- Estrogen response modifiers (e.g., tamoxifen, raloxifene)
- Deltanoids (natural and synthetic analogs of vitamin D)
- Androgen analogs (e.g., finasteride)
- Agents that alter ovulation (e.g., oral contraceptives)
- Agents that suppress cell proliferation (e.g., difluoromethylornithine)
- Nonsteroidal anti-inflammatory drugs (NSAIDs) (e.g., aspirin, ibuprofen, sulindac)
- Agents that protect cells from oxidative stress (e.g., vitamin E)
- Agents that block carcinogens from binding to DNA (e.g., oltipraz, acetylcysteine)

Applications of chemoprevention: Randomized trials have evaluated the use of chemopreventive agents in the following areas: risk reduction for solid tumors, such as breast, prostate, lung, and colorectal cancers in those at increased risk; reversal of premalignant conditions, such as cervical dysplasia, premalignant skin lesions, and oral premalignancies; and risk reduction of second primary cancers in patients who have had head or neck, lung, or bladder cancers (Singh & Lippman, 1998a, 1998b; Sporn & Lippmann, 1997; Swan & Ford, 1997). An example of how chemoprevention can be applied to high-risk populations is the use of NSAIDs for the prevention of colorectal cancer. In several large, observational epidemiologic studies, participants who elected to take NSAIDs lowered their risk of colorectal cancer. The studies were limited in that controlling for confounding variables was difficult and randomization lacking. Nevertheless, these observational and basic research studies supported the rationale for the use of NSAIDs in preventing colorectal cancer (Clapper, Chang, & Meropol, 2001; Lee, Hennekens, & Buring, 1997). The U.S. National Cancer Institute (NCI) is now sponsoring several trials using NSAIDs for the chemoprevention of adenomas in those at high risk for developing colorectal cancer owing to an inherited predisposition (familial adenomatosis polyposis [FAP] and hereditary nonpolyposis colorectal cancer [HNPCC]). The U.S. Food and Drug Administration has approved celecoxib as a means of reducing the number of colorectal polyps in patients with FAP.

The efficacy of tamoxifen in reducing a second primary breast cancer in postmenopausal women with a diagnosis of breast cancer led to its evaluation as a chemopreventive agent. The Breast Cancer Prevention Trial (BCPT), sponsored by the NCI-funded National Surgical Adjuvant Breast and Bowel Project (NSABP), evaluated the ability of tamoxifen to decrease breast cancer incidence in women at high risk for developing the disease. The trial, started in 1992, reached full accrual in 1997. Eligibility for the trial was based on risk of developing breast cancer and was determined by both family history and nongenetic risk factors, such as age at menarche, parity, and history of breast biopsies. In April 1998, preliminary results demonstrated a 45% decreased incidence of breast cancer in women taking tamoxifen versus those taking placebo (Fisher et al., 1998). In September 1998, tamoxifen citrate received regulatory approval for use in decreasing the incidence of breast cancer in high-risk women. The NSABP is conducting a follow-up to the BCPT, the Study of Tamoxifen and Raloxifene, or STAR trial. The trial will determine whether raloxifene also is effective in reducing the risk of breast cancer in women who have not had the disease and whether the drug is more beneficial than tamoxifen.

An area for future research is the design of chemoprevention trials for women who are carriers of a cancer-predisposition gene, such as *BRCA1*, which greatly increases lifetime risk of developing breast cancer. Research by King et al. (2001) showed that tamoxifen may not decrease the risk of breast cancer development in women who have mutations in *BRCA1*. Women who are carriers of *BRCA1* alterations tend to develop estrogen receptor negative tumors. In the original BCPT trial, the breast cancers that developed tended to be estrogen-receptor negative. In the King study, women who carried *BRCA2* alterations did appear to derive benefit (i.e., have a decreased risk for developing breast cancer) as a result of tamoxifen use.

Prophylactic Surgery

Given the current lack of definitive pharmacologic measures to modify cancer risk, many individuals at high risk for developing cancer consider prophylactic surgery as their only option for truly preventing cancer. In some hereditary cancer syndromes, the use of prophylactic surgery is standard practice. For example, in cases of FAP, the entire colon is removed to prevent colorectal cancer. In cases of multiple endocrine neoplasia II (MEN II), the entire thyroid is removed to prevent medullary thyroid cancer. The genes responsible for these diseases have a high (90%–100%) penetrance; thus, most individuals who inherit the abnormal gene will ultimately develop cancer. In regard to FAP, colectomy is generally performed after numerous polyps are present (Petersen

& Brensinger, 1996). In regard to MEN II, thyroidectomy is often performed following detection of a predisposing mutation in the *RET* gene, which is associated with hereditary medullary thyroid cancer (Gagel, 1997; Giarelli, 1997; Lairmore, Frisella, & Wells, 1996). The American Society of Clinical Oncology (ASCO) has recognized these two syndromes as being in a category for which predisposition testing may be considered part of the standard management of affected families. Medical management is then guided by the genetic test results (ASCO, 1997).

The use of prophylactic surgery as a risk-management measure in other hereditary cancer syndromes is more controversial, especially in the management of increased risk for breast and ovarian cancers (Houshmand, Campbell, Briggs, McFadden, & Al-Tweigeri, 2000). On one hand, the availability of predisposition testing represents a means of identifying carriers of mutations that impart a 40%–85% lifetime risk of developing breast cancer. Because of this level of predictive certainty, women who have close relatives with breast cancer often seek opinions regarding prophylactic mastectomy as a means to decrease and manage their risk (Stefanek, Helzlsouer, Wilcox, & Houn, 1995). On the other hand, the identification of genes, such as *BRCA1* and *BRCA2*, that confer a high risk of breast and ovarian cancer is a recent event, and knowledge concerning these genes continues to evolve. A major question is whether different mutations within the gene confer different levels of absolute lifetime risk for developing a cancer.

Also sounding a note of caution in regard to prophylactic mastectomy are those who find the use of an irreversible procedure to manage risk worrisome, especially when breast-preserving procedures are often used to treat women who have already developed a breast cancer (Eisen & Weber, 2001; Healy, 1997). Because the inherited mutation is present in all body cells, a cancer can still develop after a prophylactic procedure. Primary peritoneal carcinoma has been found in women who have had prophylactic oophorectomies (Piver, Jishi, Tsukada, & Nava, 1993), as has breast cancer after prophylactic mastectomy (Stefanek, 1995).

Some of the latest research may serve to resolve the controversy about prophylactic mastectomy. Hartmann et al. (1999) conducted a retrospective study of all women with a family history of breast cancer who underwent bilateral prophylactic mastectomy at the Mayo Clinic between 1960 and 1993. The women were divided into two groups, high risk and moderate risk, on the basis of family history. The researchers reported that prophylactic mastectomy was associated with a reduction in the incidence of breast cancer by at least 90% and concluded that, in women with a high risk of breast cancer on the basis of family history, prophylactic mastectomy can significantly reduce the incidence of breast cancer. (Hartmann and colleagues presented a follow-up to this study at the annual meeting of the American Association of Cancer in 2000 [Hartmann et al., 2000]). So far, Hartmann and colleagues have completed **germline** *BRCA1* or *BRCA2* analyses for 110 high-risk families. If no affected relative was available or willing to give a blood specimen, the researchers tested the unaffected proband. The team has identified 18 women who have inherited mutations in either *BRCA1* or *BRCA2*; 12 of these are known deleterious mutations, and six are mutations of uncertain significance. None of the women has developed breast cancer. They have been followed a median of 16.1 years since prophylactic mastectomy. Their median age at prophylactic mastectomy was 37.5. With no cancers in 12 carriers, the lower limit of the 95% confidence interval for risk reduction following prophylactic mastectomy is 74%; with no cancers in 18 carriers, it is 82%. The researchers concluded that bilateral prophylactic mastectomy yields a significant reduction in breast cancer risk, even in *BRCA1* or *BRCA2* mutation carriers.

Meijers-Heijboer et al. (2001) conducted a prospective study of 139 women with a pathogenic *BRCA1* or *BRCA2* mutation who were enrolled in a breast-cancer surveillance program at the Rotterdam Family Cancer Clinic. At the time of enrollment, none of the women had a personal history of breast cancer. Seventy-six of these women eventually underwent prophylactic mastectomy, and the other 63 remained under regular surveillance. The researchers did not discover any cases of breast cancer after prophylactic mastectomy after a mean follow-up of approximately 2.9 years, whereas eight breast cancers developed in women under regular surveillance after a mean follow-up of 3.0 years. Although the results demonstrate only three years of follow-up, the work of Meijers-Heijboer et al. is the first published prospective study of prophylactic mastectomy in carriers of a *BRCA1* or *BRCA2* mutation.

Rebbeck et al. (1999) evaluated the effect of bilateral prophylactic oophorectomy (BPO) on breast cancer risk reduction in 122 *BRCA1* mutation carriers from five centers in North America. They compared two groups of women: women who had undergone BPO and a matched set of women who did not but who were born at approximately the same time and were seen at the same study site as the BPO subjects. Mean follow-up time for both groups was 10 years. The researchers concluded that BPO significantly reduced the risk of developing breast cancer.

A model developed by Schrag, Kuntz, Garber, and Weeks (1997) suggested that, for young women with a *BRCA1* or *BRCA2* mutation, prophylactic mastectomy substantially increased life expectancy by 2.9 to 5.3 years. For the same group, prophylactic oophorectomy increased life expectancy by 0.3 to 1.7 years. The authors used available data about the incidence of cancer, the prognosis for women with cancer, and the efficacy of prophylactic mastectomy and oophorectomy in preventing breast and ovarian cancer to estimate the effects of these interventions on life expectancy among women with different levels of cancer risk, rather than to women who had not undergone prophylactic surgery.

The Society of Surgical Oncology (2001), in an updated position statement concerning indications for prophylactic mastectomy, recommended the following criteria for prophylactic mastectomy in women with no history of breast cancer: personal history of breast biopsy showing atypical hyperplasia or a family history of breast cancer in a first-degree relative who was premenopausal at the time of diagnosis and has had bilateral breast cancer; or dense breasts that are difficult to evaluate by mammography and/or physical examination and women who have at least one or both of the other indications. In contrast, a task force from the Cancer Genetics Studies Consortium (CGSC) concluded that, based on available data, task force members could make no recommendations at this time regarding prophylactic mastectomy for carriers of *BRCA1* and *BRCA2* mutations (Burke, Daly, et al., 1997). Like the CGSC, the National Comprehensive Cancer Network recommended offering prophylactic mastectomy as an option for women to consider (Daly, 1999).

All these studies and recommendations can help clients to make difficult decisions about prophylactic procedures. Clients also should consider, however, the limited availability of long-term outcome data as well as the impact of such procedures on body image and sexual and reproductive function (Baron & Borgen, 1997; Frost et al., 2000; Schrag et al., 1997).

Screening and Early Detection

Cancer screening means searching for cancer in persons who have no symptoms of the disease. The purpose of screening is to find cancer at the earliest stage possible. Early detection of precancerous lesions or localized—and thus manageable—cancers maximizes the ability to cure, slow the progress of disease, prevent complications, limit disability, and enhance quality of life (Frank-Stromborg, 1997).

The American Cancer Society and professional medical organizations have, based on the best available evidence, developed screening guidelines for specific cancers. These recommendations are intended to help clinicians know when to begin screening in specific populations and what types of screening measures to use. Screening criteria are generally based on age, family and personal history of cancer, and other known risk factors related to the disease in question (Eyre, Smith, & Mettlin, 2000). With the advent of predisposition testing and other technologic advances, the goal of targeting cancer screening to the populations most at risk and tailoring the measures used is becoming a reality.

Under the auspices of the National Institutes of Health National Human Genome Research Institute, a task force of the CGSC evaluated published studies of cancer risk, surveillance, and risk reduction in individuals genetically susceptible to breast, ovarian, and colon cancers. In 1994, as a result of its evaluations, the task force released screening guidelines for individuals who have mutations in *BRCA1*, *BRCA2*, or genes associated with hereditary nonpolyposis colorectal carcinoma (HNPCC) (see Tables 6-2 and 6-3). The task force established a cancer-risk management framework based on the best data available (Burke, Daly, et al., 1997; Burke, Petersen, et al., 1997).

Although effective, current screening measures for those at high risk of developing a breast or ovarian cancer have limitations. For example, mammography is less accurate in regard to younger women than to older women because young women's breasts tend to be denser than older women's breasts. Dense tissue can obscure lesions. Researchers should investigate new and existing mammography technologies to optimize them for screening high-risk women. These technologies include digital mammography (which stores images elec-

Table 6-2. Screening Recommendations for Carriers of *BRCA1* or *BRCA2* Mutations

Cancer and Screening Modality	Frequency
Breast cancer	
Breast self-exam	Monthly
Breast exam by a clinician	Annually or semiannually, beginning at age 25–35
Mammography	Annually beginning at age 25–35
Ovarian cancer	
Transvaginal sonography (with color Doppler)	Annually or semiannually, beginning at age 25–35
CA-125 level	Annually or semiannually, beginning at age 25–35
Prostate cancer[a]	
Digital rectal exam	Annually beginning at age 50
Prostate-specific antigen level	Annually beginning at age 50
Colon cancer	
Fecal occult blood test	Annually beginning at age 50
Sigmoidoscopy	Every 3–5 years, beginning at age 50

[a] Male carriers of *BRCA* only.

Note. Based on information from Burke, Daly, et al., 1997.

Table 6-3. Screening Recommendations for Carriers of Mutations for Hereditary Nonpolyposis Colorectal Cancer (*MLH1, MSH2, PMS1, PMS2*)

Cancer and Screening Modality	Frequency
Colon cancer	
Colonoscopy	Every 1–3 years, beginning at age 20–25
Endometrial cancer[a]	
Transvaginal ultrasonography	Annually beginning at age 25–35
Endometrial biopsy	Annually beginning at age 25–35

[a] No clear consensus about screening for endometrial cancer exists. Screening consists of either transvaginal ultrasonography or endometrial biopsy.

Note. Based on information from Burke, Peterson, et al., 1997.

tronically rather than on film), ultrasonography, magnetic resonance imaging with and without contrast agents, and radionuclide scanning after the injection of radionuclide-labeled substances that concentrate in breast tumors (e.g., ^{99m}Tc-sestamibi) (Eyre et al., 2000).

Transvaginal ultrasonography is effective in detecting ovarian lesions before they cause a palpable mass, and the technology is currently used to screen women at high risk for ovarian cancer. However, transvaginal ultrasonography has a significant limitation: It produces a high number of false-positive results that call for further evaluation. Furthermore, the technology may not effectively detect primary peritoneal carcinomatosis at a curable stage.

An important question applies to radiographic screening: Does the technology itself increase cancer risk? For women without a cancer-predisposing gene, the answer appears to be no. Studies have shown that, even for these women who begin having mammography screenings at age 35 and continue for 40 years, the benefit of reduced mortality resulting from screening exceeds the risk caused by radiation by more than 25 times (Feig, 1996; Mettler et al., 1996). However, for women who carry a cancer-predisposing mutation, the risk posed by radiographic screening is unknown. Recent evidence has shown that both *BRCA1* and *BRCA2* bind to *RAD51*, a protein involved in maintaining the integrity of the genome. The *RAD51* gene is involved in repairing double-stranded DNA breaks and in recombination-linked repair. Thus, disruption of the *BRCA-RAD51* pathway may result in genetic instability (Kinzler & Vogelstein, 1997; Offit, 2000). In regard to radiographic risk, interest also has focused on the *ATM* gene, which causes ataxia telangiectasia (AT). AT is an inherited autosomal-recessive condition; affected people inherit a mutated *ATM* gene from each asymptomatic parent. Characteristics of this condition are defective DNA repair and radiation hypersensitivity (Lavin & Shiloh, 1996). Are heterozygous carriers of an altered *ATM* gene (about 1% of the population) also radiation sensitive? Studies suggest that the answer is yes. Broeks et al. (2000) concluded that *ATM* heterozygotes have an approximately nine-fold increase in risk of developing breast cancer characterized by bilaterality, early age of onset, and long-term survival. A study by Swift (1994) of blood relatives of persons with AT found that exposure to a relatively modest radiation dose, such as the dose that a woman might receive from x-ray fluoroscopy of the chest and abdomen, led to an almost six-fold increase in breast cancer risk. For people with an altered *ATM* gene, who are likely to be radiation sensitive, radiographic screening may do more harm than good. Now that the *ATM* gene has been cloned, studies will hopefully elucidate the risks associated with being a carrier of an altered *ATM* gene.

Biomarkers

Imagine a test that could, long before tumors arose, detect biologic clues that signal tissue injury by specific cancer-causing agents or the impending evolution of precancerous changes. Such clues are biomarkers, biologic substances that are either produced by the tumor or released by the host in response to the tumor. Biomarkers have long been used to monitor the efficacy of treatment and to follow a patient's status after treatment (Bosl, 1995; Wu, 1999). The goal now is to use biomarkers to identify cancer predisposition.

The emerging view of cancer as a genetic disorder has made it possible to identify genetic markers that may be associated with malignant transformation. Studies designed to determine the association between a particular environmental exposure and a specific genetic alteration associated with a given tumor type are ongoing. For example, new assays based on **polymerase chain reaction (PCR)** amplification of genetic material, a sort of molecular photocopying, and sequence-specific DNA probes can be used to identify oncogene activation and/or loss of tumor suppressor genes in premalignant lesions or body fluids. Researchers have assayed cells from people with adenomatous polyps, obtained by colonic washing, and looked for mutations in the *RAS* gene. Other researchers, analyzing stool specimens, have learned that *RAS* mutations are associated with colorectal cancer. Testing for *RAS* mutations is under investigation as a method of screening for colorectal cancer. Similar studies—using sputum and bladder washings in the early detection of head or neck, lung, and bladder cancer—have promising results. (For optimal screening of high-risk populations, assays that use blood and body fluids are desirable because these substances are more readily available than tissue.) It is now becoming possible to assay for oncogene products, tumor-derived growth factors, and genetic alterations in exfoliated cells. The hope is that, in the future, it will be possible to identify individuals at risk for the development of cancer before it occurs, in contrast to current screening, which, in the majority of cases, detects cancers after they have developed (Israel, 1996; Sullivan et al., 2001).

> Tumor markers are biological
> • Substances produced by the tumor or released by the host
> • Clues that may be or are used in the prevention, screening, treatment, and surveillance of cancer.

Molecular epidemiology: An emerging field, molecular epidemiology, combines the standard tools of epidemiology (case histories, questionnaires, and exposure monitoring) with the sensitive laboratory techniques of molecular biology. The goal of molecular epidemiologists is to uncover critical precancerous events taking place inside the body and to identify measurable biologic flags that signal their occurrence. Through a series of steps, markers can be "validated" and then used to determine the need for intervention in individuals exhibiting those markers (Perera, 2000). Markers may be used to determine exposure to carcinogenic agents and resultant increased risk; for example, aflatoxin B1-DNA adducts (complexes formed when a carcinogen combines with DNA or a protein) in urine or liver tissues indicate an increased risk of hepatic cancer.

Biomarkers of susceptibility: Another growing area is the identification of individual traits that may explain why, after exposure to a known carcinogen, some individuals are more susceptible to developing cancers than are others. Carcinogens include cigarette smoke (associated with upper and lower respiratory tract cancers) and ultraviolet light (associated with skin cancers). Such research may lead to the discovery of biomarkers of inborn and acquired susceptibility to cancer. Genes that determine an individual's response to a carcinogen also fall into this category. Examples include variations in genes that encode a family of enzymes known as cytochrome p450 (*CYP* family). As a group, these enzymes detoxify a wide range of internal and external substances. Epidemiologists believe that having certain forms of the *CYP1A1* gene, which codes for an enzyme that acts on polycyclic aromatic hydrocarbons, increases a smoker's susceptibility to lung cancer. Researchers hope that advances in molecular epidemiology will allow them to refine estimates of cancer risk by considering variations in innate and acquired susceptibility within populations. In reality, however, the events leading to the development of cancer are complex, so more than one single event or characteristic probably plays a role in cancer development (Amos, Xu, & Spitz, 1999; Perera, 1996).

Monoclonal antibodies: Among the newer methods used to detect existing or recurrent disease is the use of monoclonal antibodies (Britton, 1997). Monoclonal antibodies recognize tumor-specific proteins or antigens. They also recognize smaller molecules, called ligands, which bind to large numbers of receptors expressed by tumors. Monoclonal antibodies may be labeled with a variety of isotopes (e.g., indium^{111}, technetium^{99m}), administered to patients, and identified by external scintigraphy after the isotopes have localized to the tumor. Among the antibodies that have received regulatory approval are indium (In^{111}) satumomab pendetide (OncoScint® [Cytogen, East Princeton, NJ]), for the detection of colorectal and ovarian cancer, and In^{111} capromab pendetide (ProstaScint® [Cytogen]), for the detection of prostate cancer. ProstaScint binds to prostate-specific membrane antigens, which are found in larger quantities in malignant cells than in nonmalignant tissue.

The Truquant® BR™ (Fujirebio Diagnostics, Malvern, PA) radioimmunoassay blood test kit uses the monoclonal antibody B27.29 to detect the CA27.29 antigen, which is associated with breast cancer. Clinical trials have proven the kit, which has received regulatory approval, to be a significant and independent predictor for recurrent breast cancer (Chan et al., 1997). Guidelines are beginning to emerge to help clinicians in the use of biomarkers in clinical practice. ASCO recently published an updated set of guidelines for the use of tumor marker tests in the prevention, screening, treatment, and surveillance of breast and colorectal cancers. These guidelines are intended for use in the care of patients outside of clinical trials (Bast et al., 2001).

Imaging Techniques in Multidrug Resistance

A cancer's ability to have complete drug resistance or to develop drug resistance is the major basis for treatment failure. This phenomenon is called multidrug resistance (MDR) and is thought to have multiple cellular mechanism as its causation (Larsen, Escargueil, & Skladanowski, 2000). One of the mechanisms of MDR is altered drug delivery within the cell. It is associated with the overexpression of P-glycoproteins. The P-glycoproteins were initially thought to affect the permeability of cells to drugs, but they were later found to act as pumps able to extrude drugs from cells. The P-glycoproteins belong to a class of transport proteins known as the ATP-binding cassette transporter proteins (*ATCB*). Targeting genes in the ATP-binding cassette subfamily B (formally known at *MDR* genes), such as *ABCB1* or *ABCB4*, via imaging techniques might be helpful in identifying tumors and cancers that have developed drug resistance. Imaging techniques such as electron microscopy with cellular immunolabeling (Calcabrini et al., 2000) and radiographic tagging of cellular transport substrates (Crankshaw et al., 1998; Sun, Hsieh, Tsai, Ho, & Kao, 2000) are helping to detect genes involved in MDR. These imaging techniques are elucidating the MDR mechanism and present pathways by which P-glycoprotein mediated MDR could be reversed.

Diagnosis and Prognosis
Diagnosis

An accurate, specific, and sufficiently comprehensive diagnosis helps a clinician develop an optimal plan of treatment and, when possible, estimate prognosis (Connolly, Schnitt, Wang, Dvorak, & Dvorak, 2000). Until recently, a cancer diagnosis was conclusively established based on clinical; laboratory; radiologic; and, ultimately, histologic examination of tissue (generally by a surgical pathologist). A pathologist reaches a histologic diagnosis by using light microscopy to evaluate the morphologic features of cells and tissues. Recent advances in understanding the molecular basis of cancer, and associated technologies, are affecting the way cancer is diagnosed, however. Today, diagnosis may involve molecular pathology and involve immunohistochemistry, molecular genetics, and cytogenic analysis (Sklar & Costa, 1997) (see Table 6-4).

Immunohistochemistry

An immunohistochemist uses antibodies directed toward specific antigens, mostly cytoplasmic proteins and cell-membrane receptors, to make diagnoses. Immunohistochemistry is now used routinely in clinical practice. Immunohistochemical techniques are sometimes used to achieve a primary cancer identification. They are used more often to classify tumors, especially leukemias and lymphomas, and to attain a differential diagnosis of melanoma, and epithelial or mesenchymal malignancies. Immunohistochemistry also is used to definitely diagnose morphologically similar tumors, such as pulmonary carcinomas and pleural mesothelioma, and to distinguish melanoma from poorly differentiated carcinomas. The use of monoclonal antibodies targeted toward cell-surface antigens, in conjunction with chromosomal and molecular techniques, has contributed notably to the understanding of the immunology of non-Hodgkin's lymphoma and to current classification schemes. These techniques have demonstrated that most non-Hodgkin's

Table 6-4. Technologic Advances for the Diagnosis of Cancer

Technology	Description	Current and Potential Clinical Uses
Cytogenetic analysis	Evaluates the gross morphologic features of chromosomes.	Detection of consistent, nonrandom chromosomal abnormalities (translocations, deletions). Evaluates dividing cells only.
DNA diagnostics (for specific examples, see Southern blot analysis and polymerase chain reaction)	Recognizes sequences in target DNA by using a complementary molecular probe.	Diagnosis of genetic disease. Determination of the presence of oncogenes (both dominant and recessive). Identification of infectious agents. Identification of donor origin of tissue and blood (DNA fingerprinting).
DNA sequencing	Determines the sequence of nucleotides in a stretch of chromosomal DNA. Manual: Autoradiography reads DNA fragments as bands. Automated: Laser beams cause fluorescently tagged nucleotides to emit a signal as they pass through a light beam. A computer stores and translates signals as a nucleotide sequence.	Detection of mutations that lead to disease. Used in large-scale sequencing projects (e.g., Human Genome Project).
Fluorescent in situ hybridization	Uses incubation of recombinant prepared DNA probes that are complementary to a known DNA sequence.	Analysis of a single cell for a known DNA sequence in either metaphase or interphase nuclei. Detection of chromosomal deletions, inversions, translocations, and gene amplification.
Immunohistochemistry	Directs antibodies against tissue sections on cells. Assessed by fluorescent tags in flow-cytometry suspension.	Correlation of protein antigens with cytologic features. Classification of leukemias, lymphomas, and solid tumors. Detection of the tissue origin of solid tumors.
Flow cytometry	Analyzes DNA content and protein expression.	DNA index: Ratio of tumor-cell DNA content. S-phase fraction: Proportion of cells with higher DNA content (used as a prognostic indicator of select cancers). Immunophenotyping.

(Continued on next page)

Table 6-4. Technologic Advances for the Diagnosis of Cancer *(Continued)*

Technology	Description	Current and Potential Clinical Uses
Polymerase chain reaction	Amplifies defined DNA segments.	Detection of chromosomal changes in primary diagnosis of a neoplasm. Sequence analysis of minute genetic changes in tumor samples. Detection of minimal residual disease in cancer (e.g., detection of the Philadelphia chromosome in chronic myelogenous leukemia). Detection of DNA mutations that indicate genes that may predispose a person to medical conditions (e.g., diabetes, cancer, hypertension).
Southern blot analysis	Recognizes DNA sequences in target DNA by using a complementary molecular probe.	Characterization of genetic abnormalities in select tumors. Diagnosis and follow-up of progression and remission of disease. Detection of lost or rearranged DNA sequences. Detection of DNA mutation that indicates genes that may predispose a person to medical conditions (e.g., diabetes, cancer).

Note. From "Future Projections in Biotherapy," by P.T. Rieger, 1996, *Seminars in Oncology Nursing, 12,* 163–171. Copyright 1996 by W.B. Saunders. Reprinted with permission.

lymphoma cells have normal cellular counterparts that correspond to stages of lymphocyte development. This information will be useful in designing therapeutic strategies and for estimating prognosis (Skarin & Dorfman, 1997) (see Table 6-5).

The diagnosis of cancer involves
• Histologic examination of tissue
• Molecular pathology
  - Immunohistochemistry
  - DNA content analysis
  - Molecular genetics.

Molecular Genetics

Molecular genetic methods of cancer diagnosis involve a variety of techniques to analyze nucleotide sequences to detect the presence of malignant cells in fluids and tissues obtained from patients. One such technique is the use of polymerase chain reaction (PCR). PCR amplifies short segments of DNA from

Table 6-5. Diagnostic Methods for the Study of Non-Hodgkin's Lymphomas

Diagnostic Methods	Tissue	Results	Comments
Routine histologic study	Formalin and/or B5 fixed, paraffin-embedded	Morphologic classification	Traditional
Immunoperoxidase staining	Fresh, unfixed tissue (full range of markers); fixed, embedded tissue (subset of markers)	B cell, T cell, tumor subtyping, other tissue types	Technically demanding
Flow cytometry	Fresh, unfixed tissue; peripheral blood; bone marrow	B cell, T cell	Rapid
Cytogenetic analysis	Fresh, unfixed tissue; peripheral blood; bone marrow	Chromosomal translocations and other abnormalities	Technically demanding
Molecular geologic methods (Southern blot, polymerase chain reaction)	Fresh, unfixed tissue; peripheral blood; bone marrow; fixed tissue in some cases	Gene rearrangements and deletions; subtle alterations	Technically demanding
Electron microscopy	Glutaraldehyde-fixed tissue	Ultrastructural details	Differentiates between non-Hodgkin's lymphomas and other neoplasms

Note. From "Non-Hodgkin's Lymphomas: Current Classification and Management," by A.T. Skarin and D.M. Dorfman, 1997, *CA: A Journal for Clinicians, 47,* p. 357. Copyright 1997 by Lippincott-Raven Publishers. Reprinted with permission. Additional material based on *Pathology and Genetics of Tumours of Haematopoietic and Lymphoid Tissues,* by E. Jaffe, N. Harris, H. Stein, and J. Vardiman, 2001, Lyon, France: IARC Press.

extremely small quantities of cells, providing sufficient DNA for analysis. The advantages of PCR are its sensitivity, specificity, and simplicity. Its shortcomings are oversensitivity and a proclivity toward false-positive results due to contamination. An awareness of the shortcomings of PCR amplification is critical to accurate interpretation of PCR results. When the DNA or RNA of the tumor differs from that of normal tissues, PCR-based assays can be used to analyze the cancer. Such assays are currently being evaluated for the detection of point mutations, chromosomal **translocations,** and antigen-receptor gene rearrangements in the diagnosis of lymphocytic cancers. PCR-based assays have been used to detect and diagnose minimal residual disease in patients with chronic myelogenous leukemia, through detection of the Philadelphia chromosome, t(9;22). The assays also have detected and diagnosed acute promyelocytic leukemia by finding t(15;17) chromosomal translocation.

Presently, molecular diagnostic techniques are not being used as often in the evaluation of solid tumors as they are in hematologic malignancies. This may change, however, because researchers are now studying whether mutations of the *TP53* gene can be used as markers for early relapse in certain solid tumors. Mutations of the *TP53* tumor suppressor gene are the most common known mutations in cancer. In cases of bladder cancer that exhibit a known *TP53* mutation, researchers are evaluating techniques to identify *TP53* mutations in bladder washings (Mashal & Sklar, 1995; Schlechte et al., 2000.)

Cytogenetic Analysis

Cytogenetic analysis is the evaluation of the gross morphologic characteristics of chromosomes. In oncology, cytogenetic analysis has been used most often to assess leukemias and lymphomas. Newer techniques, such as PCR-based assays (described earlier) and **fluorescence in situ hybridization (FISH)** have revolutionized the detection of genetic changes in cancer. Both techniques are applicable to small amounts of nondividing cells and can precisely identify genetic changes in tumor cells. FISH is a technique that uses fluorochrome-conjugated DNA probes to visualize specific changes on individual chromosomes in metaphase and interphase cells. The technique yields information about different chromosomal abnormalities through evaluation of the number and localization of hybridization signals (Patel, Hawkins, & Griffin, 2000; Sheer & Squire, 1996). FISH is more sensitive and specific than banding analysis (karyotyping), and FISH provides better resolution regarding chromosome aberrations and allows the screening of a larger number of cells. FISH's limitations include the low number of currently available probes and spectrally nonoverlapping fluorochromes. These limitations prevent FISH from being used to discriminate all human chromosomes simultaneously.

One of the newest techniques being evaluated, multicolor spectral karyotyping of human chromosomes (a technique sometimes referred to as SKY FISH), is designed to overcome the limitations of FISH. By means of computer separation (classification) of spectra, spectrally overlapping chromosome-specific DNA probes can be resolved, and the entire genome identified simultaneously. In essence, in SKY FISH, each chromosome fluoresces a different color by which it can be identified. Although SKY FISH is still experimental, it has tremendous potential for rapid and automatic karyotyping and for the identification of complex chromosomal aberrations (Schrock et al., 1996).

Developments in cytogenetics and molecular biology will continue to provide insight into the process of carcinogenesis. The ability to identify specific genetic abnormalities through molecular techniques represents an improvement in both the specificity and sensitivity of methods to detect tumor cells or their products. Although these new techniques are not yet fully integrated into standard practice, they will continue to be studied for their utility in cancer diagnosis, determination of tumor burden, determination of prognosis, assessment of response to therapy, and guidance in designing novel therapies (Rabbitts, 1998).

Prognosis

Phenotypic Markers

Pathologic diagnosis involves determination of tumor grade, pathologic stage, and prognosis. *Grade* pertains to a tumor's degree of differentiation; *stage*, to the degree of spread (e.g., tumor size, nodal status). Prognostic indicators are most needed in three specific situations: to identify patients who:

- Require no therapy following surgery versus those who will most benefit from adjuvant therapy, such as chemotherapy and/or radiation therapy
- Have a predicted poor outcome with conventional therapy
- Would likely benefit from special therapies.

As prognostic indicators become more refined, they may be used to ensure comparability of treatment groups and provide markers to measure the success or failure of specific therapies (Connolly et al., 2000; Donegan, 1997). In recent years, the number of tumor-specific features available for use as prognostic indicators has grown substantially. Indicators have already been integrated into practice in regard to breast cancer and bladder cancer (de Vere White & Stapp, 1998; Donegan). However, it is important to remember that the role of many of the newer prognostic indicators remains uncertain; further study is needed. Several new categories of prognostic indicators are under evaluation.

> Prognostic indicators identify patients who
> - Require no therapy following surgery.
> - Have a predicted poor outcome with conventional therapy.
> - Might benefit from special therapies.
>
> Prognostic indicators under investigation include
> - Tumor neovascularization: The number of microvessels within a tumor specimen.
> - DNA content: A proliferative index of DNA ploidy.
> - Proliferation-associated markers: Enzymes, cell-surface antigens.
> - Oncogenes and tumor suppressor genes.

Neovascularization

The degree of tumor neovascularization (angiogenesis), or veins and artery development within a tumor specimen, may have value as a prognostic indicator.

The rationale is that ingrowth of blood vessels is necessary for sustained tumor growth and metastasis. At present, microvessel assessment has limited general application and is used primarily in research settings. Researchers are evaluating the use of neovascularization as a prognostic indicator in cases of breast, head or neck, lung, and prostate cancer (Connolly et al., 2000; Donegan, 1997).

DNA Content and S-Phase Fraction

DNA **ploidy** and S-phase fraction have been studied extensively. Flow cytometry techniques with laser-stimulated DNA fluorescence make possible automated measurement of the DNA content of individual cells and the number of cells in each phase of the cell cycle (Sklar & Costa, 1997). Two types of information are derived from such analyses: the proliferative index and DNA ploidy.

Cells actively synthesizing DNA incorporate tritiated thymidine, a radioactive label. The thymidine labeling index is a direct measure of the cells in the S phase. In large multivariate analyses of patients with breast cancer, the thymidine labeling index ranked fourth (behind nodal status, tumor size, and nucleus size) as an indicator of relapse-free survival (Meyer & Province, 1994). Unfortunately, the methodology involved in assessing the thymidine labeling index is cumbersome; at present, determining S-phase fraction through flow cytometry is easier.

The degree of departure from the normal DNA content (diploid) is calculated as the DNA index (i.e., the DNA content of the predominant cell population divided by diploid DNA content). Thus, a diploid tumor has a DNA index of 1.0. In general, patients with breast cancer who have diploid tumors or tumors with a low S-phase fraction tend to have more favorable outcomes than do those with aneuploid tumors or tumors with a high S-phase fraction. However, these differences may be small, and standardization of techniques from lab to lab is difficult.

An international consensus conference in 1992 evaluated evidence for the use of DNA cytometry findings as prognostic indicators in breast cancer (Hedley et al., 1993). In general, ploidy tended not to survive as a prognostic indicator in multivariate analyses because of its correlation with more powerful prognostic indicators. S-phase fraction, however, seemed to be associated with recurrence and mortality for both node-positive and node-negative breast cancers (Donegan, 1997; Hedley et al.).

Proliferation-Associated Markers

Newer markers of proliferative activity include Ki-67, a nuclear antigen that is identified by the monoclonal antibody MIB-1. The Ki-67 labeling index is considered a marker of normal and abnormal cell proliferation (Mastronardi, Guiduccil, & Puzzilli, 2001). Enzymes, such as **proteases,** are involved in the degradation of basement membranes and have been implicated in the process of invasion and metastasis. Two such enzymes, cathepsin D and urokinase plasminogen activator, have been evaluated as prognostic indicators in breast cancer. Although further research is needed, as indicators the enzymes seem promising.

Oncogenes and Tumor Suppressor Genes

Many investigators are considering whether the products of proto-oncogenes, oncogenes, and tumor suppressor genes can be used as prognostic indicators.

Researchers have studied the overexpression of oncogenes, such as epidermal growth-factor receptor *ERBB2 (HER2/NEU)*. This oncogene affects epidermal growth factor and is a transmembrane receptor molecule. To date, studies have not strongly validated the use of *ERBB2* as a prognostic indicator. However, evidence points to a link between *ERBB2* expression and response to cyclophosphamide, doxorubicin, and fluorouracil (CAF) in cases involving patients with breast cancer who exhibit expression of both *ERBB2* and *TP53* and derive the greatest benefit from dose-intensive CAF (Clark, 1998).

The *TP53* tumor suppressor gene is a negative regulator of cell proliferation and is believed to function by blocking cells in the G_1 phase or inducing programmed death (apoptosis) of cells with DNA damage. Mutated *TP53* is the most common genetic defect found in human cancers. In breast cancer, expression of mutated *TP53* is strongly associated with other markers of high tumor-proliferation rate (e.g., poor nuclear grade, *ERBB2* protein overexpression, aneuploidy, high S-phase fraction, estrogen receptor negative status); however, it has not survived as an independent prognostic factor in multivariate analyses (see Table 6-6).

Many of these genetic markers are being evaluated in other solid tumors, such as lung cancer and soft-tissue sarcomas (Gershenson et al., 1999; Levine et al., 1997; Pastorino, Andreola, Tagliabue, Pezzella, & Sozzi, 1997).

Treatment

Current modalities of cancer treatment include surgery, radiation, chemotherapy, and biologic therapy. Surgery is often curative when tumors are detected early, and radiation and chemotherapy are effective therapies for some types of tumors. However, the cure of many common tumors, especially when diagnosed at an advanced stage, remains elusive.

New insights into the biology of cancer will affect traditional therapies and propel the development of new molecular therapies.

Molecular therapies designed to correct molecular changes in cancer cells include
• Gene-directed therapies
• Control of aberrant cellular proliferation
• Exploitation of cell death
• Inhibition of neovascularization
• Reversal of multidrug resistance.

Table 6-6. Prognostic Significance of Various Factors Relevant to Breast Cancer

Prognostic Factor	Favorable Significance	Unfavorable Significance
Axillary lymph nodes	No metastasis	Metastasis present
Number of positive axillary nodes	One to three	Four or more
IM lymph nodes	No metastasis	Metastasis present
Tumor size	Small	Large
Histologic grade	I (well differentiated)	III (poorly differentiated)
Nuclear grade	I (well differentiated)	III (poorly differentiated)
Estrogen-receptor status	≥ 10 fmol/mg protein	< 10 fmol/mg protein
Progesterone-receptor status	≥ 10 fmol/mg protein	< 10 fmol/mg protein
pS2 protein	High (≥ 11 ng/mg)	Low ($<$ ng/mg)
S-phase fraction	Low	High
Ploidy	Diploid	Aneuploid
Mitotic index	Low	High
TLI	Low	High
ERBB2 (HER2/NEU)	Absent	Present
TP53	Absent	Present
Ki-67	Low	High
PCNA/cyclin	Low	High
Cathepsin D	Low	High
uPA	Low	High

[a] The pS2 protein is an estrogen-regulated secretory protein of unknown function.

IM = internal mammary, PCNA = proliferating-cell nuclear antigen, TLI = thymidine labeling index, uPA = urokinase plasminogen activator

Note. From "Tumor-Related Prognostic Factors for Breast Cancer," by W.L. Donegan, 1997, *CA: A Cancer Journal for Clinicians, 47,* p. 40. Copyright 1997 Lippincott-Raven Publishers. Reprinted with permission.

Targeted Therapies

Advances in Molecular Biology

Advances in molecular biology may one day guide the selection of therapies for a specific cancer (Mills, Schmandt, Gershenson, & Bast, 1999). For example, individuals demonstrating one set of prognostic indicators may respond best to therapy X; others may respond best to therapy Y (Caron et al., 1996; Fisher, 1997). Molecular biology would guide therapy assignment.

Prognostic indicators also may be useful in regard to adjuvant therapy, by determining which patients will develop metastatic disease and which will not. Many patients might be spared months of chemotherapy by the ability to better determine, based on their tumor's biologic properties or the existence of micrometastases, the need for such therapy (Hellman & Weichselbaum, 1995). Additionally, genetic information about a patient's ability to metabolize chemotherapy regimes would help to optimize therapy or reduce potential toxicities (Krynetski & Evans, 1998).

Aromatase Inhibitors

Aromatase inhibitors are the standard second-line treatment for estrogen receptor positive metastatic breast cancer. Recent studies suggested that aromatase inhibitors might be more effective than tamoxifen in the treatment of both early-stage and advanced breast cancer (Goss & Strasser, 2001). Data suggested that patients with breast cancers that exhibit *HER2/NEU* overexpression show a statistically significantly improved response and survival when treated with an aromatase inhibitor instead of standard tamoxifen (Goss & Strasser).

Pharmacogenetics

Another way to maximize treatment is to use genetic profiles evolving from the new field of pharmacogenetics. The goal of chemotherapy is to produce damage and ultimately the death of tumor cells at doses that do not inflict intolerable toxicity on normal cells. The variation in response to chemotherapy is due to the tumor response as well as an individual's ability to activate or inactivate cancer drugs. Pharmacogenetics, the study of the role of genes in an individual's therapeutic or toxic response to drugs, is helping to identify genetic mutations that predispose individuals to optimal or adverse drug reactions (Roses, 2000).

All drug metabolism involves enzyme activity, controlled by gene expression, for absorption, distribution, drug-cell interaction, inactivation, and excretion. Individuals and certain populations have variations in their genes called polymorphisms, or benign mutations, that affect enzymatic activity. The variations of interest usually occur in more than 1% of a given population and effect a change in one single nucleotide, single-nucleotide polymorphisms (SNPs). A major effort—spearheaded by pharmaceutical companies, bioinformation companies, five academic centers, and a charitable trust—is under way to construct an SNP map of the human genome (International SNP Map Working Group, 1999).

Information about SNPs is providing genetic profile classifications of drug-metabolizing enzymes. Recognizing that there are multiple genes involved in any drug action, individuals are being classified according to their SNP profile. An individual who has two normal functioning drug-metabolizing enzyme alleles is classified as an efficient metabolizer (EM). EMs usually activate and inactivate a drug effectively and have a low chance for toxicity. Another individual, with a polymorphism in both alleles, who lacks the same ability to metabolize compounds, is called a poor metabolizer (PM). PMs are at higher risk for adverse drug events and require lower dosing to adjust for a prolonged drug effect (Evans & Relling, 1999).

This information is now being applied clinically in the treatment of acute lymphoblastic leukemia (ALL) with 6-mercaptopurine, a purine-based drug. Critical to the metabolism of any purine-based drug is the enzyme thiopurine S-methyl transferase (TPMT). A TPMT genetic test is now used to identify the 10% of children with ALL who have a polymorphism that makes them TPMT deficient. Their deficiency, in turn, makes them PMs of 6-mercaptopurine and at high risk for neutropenia, hepatic toxicities, and fatalities. ALL patients who are genetically tested and found to have a TPMT-deficiency polymorphism may experience a 10- to 15-fold decrease in dose and still have therapy that is tolerable and effective when compared to that of patients with normal TPMT activity who receive conventional dosing (Relling et al., 1999).

Genetics-Based Decisions About Surgery and Radiation

Cancer genetics also may guide decisions about surgery and radiation. Consider, for example, a woman diagnosed with breast cancer who is a carrier for a mutation of the *BRCA1* gene. She is at substantial risk, estimated to be up to 60%, for the development of a contralateral breast cancer in her lifetime (Shattuck-Eidens et al., 1995). In the future, instead of selecting a lumpectomy with radiation for an early tumor in such a patient, the surgeon might recommend a bilateral mastectomy because of the high risk of tumor development in the remaining ipsilateral or contralateral breast. Knowledge regarding sensitivity to radiation because of an inherited gene alteration (e.g., heterozygosity for the *ATM* gene) may affect decision making concerning the use of radiation therapy or perhaps even mammography.

Advancement of Control-Paradigm Therapies

The traditional cancer-treatment modalities—surgery, radiotherapy, and chemotherapy—are based on a nonselective "killing paradigm," in which the goal is complete elimination of cancer cells, albeit along with many normal cells. New approaches in the management of cancer are based on a new paradigm, a highly selective "control paradigm," which recognizes aberrancy in tumor cells and attempts to reassert normal regulation (Shipper, Goh, & Wang, 1995). The six control-paradigm approaches are gene-directed therapies, control of cellular proliferation, exploitation of cell death, inhibition of metastasis, inhibition of neovascularization, and reversal of multidrug resistance (Gottesman, 1994; Israel, 1996; Rieger, 1997) (see Figure 6-2).

Gene-Directed Therapies

Gene-directed therapies affect protein production at the level of the gene. Thus, gene-directed therapies affect the overproduction, underproduction, or production of mutated or altered forms of proteins crucial for normal cell function.

Anticode drugs: Comprising triplex and **antisense** agents, anticode drugs consist of synthetic short strings of nucleotides (i.e., strands of nucleic acid). These so-called oligomers or **oligonucleotides** (*oligo* means a little, or a few) have been designed to bind to selected sites on DNA (a gene) or RNA (the gene's transcript) and inhibit transcription or translation (i.e., gene expression of disease-related proteins).

The triplex approach blocks transcription. The name *triplex* derives from the oligomer, which winds around the double-stranded helix of DNA to form a triple-stranded helix. Triplex therapy has not yet entered clinical trials (Chan & Glazer, 1997; McGuffie, Pacheco, Carbone, & Catapano, 2000). Before this approach can move from concept to reality, researchers must overcome several significant constraints: Current studies are focusing on solving such problems as induction of binding between the oligonucleotide and the DNA, specificity of oligonucleotide binding to the target DNA, stability of the triplex after binding occurs, and specificity of delivery (i.e., delivery to tumor cells but not to normal cells) (Askari & McDonnell, 1996; Maher, 1996).

The name *antisense* derives from the fact that the strategy involves an oligonucleotide designed to be complementary to an RNA segment. In other words, the oligonucleotide can bind to the RNA. The sequence on the RNA transcript makes "sense" by serving as the code for production of a protein; thus, the oligonucleotide sequence designed to bind with the transcript is "antisense." The goal of antisense therapy is to inhibit the translation of RNA into protein.

Figure 6-2. Emerging Anticancer Approaches

Enhancement or refinement of current anticancer strategies
- Receptor-focused therapy
- Immunotoxins
- Radioimmunoconjugates
- Monoclonal antibodies targeted to cell-surface antigens and receptors
- Receptor antagonists (e.g., interleukin-1 receptor antagonist)

Vaccines
- Activation of normal cellular immunity to tumor-specific antigens
- Prevention of cancers with specifically defined mutations

Blocking the ability of cancer cells to resist the lethal effects of chemotherapy
- Reversal of multidrug resistance
- Expanding use of growth factors
- Reversal of blocked apoptosis

Clinical development of new agents
- New biologic proteins (e.g., new interleukins)
- Thrombopoietin
- Stem-cell factor

Alteration of host cells (gene therapy)
- Increasing antitumor activity of immune cells (addition of interleukin-2, granulocyte macrophage colony-stimulating factor, or tumor necrosis-factor gene)
- *ABCB1* gene in bone marrow stem cells
- Increasing cytokine production (insertion of cytokine gene into normal cells)

Alteration of the balance between factors stimulating cell growth and those inhibiting growth (Consider the analogy of the accelerator and brake.)
- Reduction of the activity of gene products that stimulate growth
- Restoration of factors that suppress growth

Control of the cell cycle
- Restoration of normal *TP53* function
- De-repression of apoptosis
- Blocking activity of telomerase

Interference in interactions between proteins or between proteins and DNA that are crucial to oncogene activity or factors essential for cell growth
- Alteration of signal-transduction pathways
- Drugs of low molecular weight that block the interaction of larger molecules
- Alteration of gene expression
- All-trans-retinoic acid to treat acute promyelocytic leukemia
- Antisense and triplex therapies

Interference in the process of metastasis
- Blocking invasion through the basement membrane
- Blocking tumor-cell migration or adhesion
- Blocking angiogenesis
- Blocking signal-transduction pathways (communication from cell membrane to nucleus)
- Blocking cell-surface receptors with monoclonal antibodies or small molecules
- Blocking function of mutated ras proteins

Note. From "Emerging Strategies in the Management of Cancer," by P.T. Rieger, 1997, *Oncology Nursing Forum, 24,* p. 734. Copyright 1997 by the Oncology Nursing Society. Reprinted with permission.

Although antisense therapy remains in its infancy, improvements in synthetic chemistry have led to the development of cost-efficient, large-scale oligodeoxynucleotide synthesis (Calogero, Hospers, & Mulder, 1997; Narayanan, 1997; Temsamani & Guinot, 1997). As a result, approximately a dozen companies have formed over the past 10 years to develop this technology. In the United States, researchers are testing numerous oligonucleotides in human trials involving cancer and other diseases (Crooke, 2000). The majority of these compounds remains in phase I or phase II clinical trials. Among the cancer-related genes that have been targets of antisense compounds in clinical trials are *TP53*, *BCL2*, *RAF*, *RAS*, and protein kinases. The phosphorothioate backbone common to the first generation of antisense compounds was associated with significant side effects. Inhibition of target-gene expression was modest at most, and clinical activity was primarily anecdotal. Combinations of the antisense compounds with chemotherapy and second-generation oligonucleotides are promising; and researchers hope that someday these agents will become a standard part of future cancer therapy (Yuen & Sikic, 2000).

In August 1998, the first antisense drug received regulatory approval. The U.S. Food and Drug Administration approved fomivirsen (Vitravene™, Novartis Pharmaceuticals, East Hanover, NJ) to slow the progression of cytomegalovirus retinitis in patients with acquired immunodeficiency syndrome.

Researchers are now trying to determine if other antisense agents can be effective against numerous targets: *MYC* or *MYB* oncogenes; the *BCR-ABL* fusion gene in chronic myelogenous leukemia (Kronenwett & Haas, 1998); *BCL2* overexpression, which suppresses apoptosis and heightens resistance to chemotherapy; the gene that encodes basic fibroblast growth factor, a stimulator of neovascularization; and mutated genes involved in signal transduction. The key problems researchers must overcome in regard to antisense agents involve cellular uptake and compartmentalization, specificity, and the undesired digestion of antisense oligonucleotides by extracellular and intracellular enzymes (Bennett, 1998).

STI571, imatinib mesylate (Gleevec™, Novartis Pharmaceuticals), is an exciting, rationally designed oral medication that has produced significant responses in most patients with chronic myelogenous leukemia (CML). As a signal-transduction inhibitor, STI571 selectively blocks the specific abnormality, the *BCR-ABL* fusion gene (Philadelphia chromosome), that is vital to the survival and proliferation of CML cells (Mauro, O'Dwyer, Heinrich, & Drucker, 2002).

Ribozymes: Ribozymes provide another approach to blocking translation. This approach is based on the principle that specific RNA structures have the ability to function as enzymes. These "RNA enzymes" can split RNA. The insertion of genes that code for selected ribozymes into cells could result in the elimination of unwanted RNA strands—in other words, the genes could block the manufacture of unwanted proteins. Ongoing preclinical studies in this area are targeting transcripts for the *BCR-ABL* fusion gene, the *RAS* mutant gene, and aberrant *TP53* (James & Gibson, 1998).

Molecules that suppress inappropriate transcription: Yet another approach to controlling gene expression involves molecules that suppress inappropriate transcription. Suppression occurs when the molecules bind to activator or coactivator proteins, preventing them from attaching to promoter or enhancer regions of DNA and initiating creation of inappropriate RNA transcripts. Currently, the majority of research in this area has focused on identifying and cataloging transcription factors, but researchers will soon turn to the development of treatments that act on transcription factors involved in the misexpression of specific proteins (Papavassiliou, 1998).

Gene therapy: Gene therapy involves the insertion of genetic material into a patient's cells. Thus far, only somatic-cell gene therapy is approved for use in humans. Another use of gene therapy, however, is to label cells, such as bone marrow cells. Such labeling has been used in an attempt to identify whether residual tumor cells within transplanted marrow contribute to relapse. Gene therapy also may be used to insert a

- Functioning gene into a patient's cells (such as *TP53*) to correct an error
- Gene for a biologic protein (such as tumor necrosis factor or interleukin-2), to achieve a sustained release of a therapeutic molecule close to the tumor site (that is, to achieve an effective local drug concentration)
- Gene such as the *ABCB1* gene into normal cells, such as bone marrow stem cells, as protection against the effects of chemotherapy and radiotherapy.

Researchers in clinical trials are evaluating gene therapies in patients with a variety of solid tumors (Blaese, 1997; Dranoff, 1998; Hall, Chen, & Woo, 1997; Robinson, Abernathy, & Conrad, 1996; Roth, Swisher, & Meyn, 1999). Over the last decade, researchers have conducted more than 400 phase I and phase II gene-based clinical trials that focused on the treatment of cancer and monogenic disorders. More than three thousand patients have been treated in these trials. As of December 2000, the United States Recombinant DNA Advisory Committee had reviewed over 400 gene-therapy protocols (see http://www4.od.nih.gov/oba). Researchers must overcome many barriers before achieving the hoped-for success for fully effective gene therapy. Examples of barriers include effective delivery of the gene into the appropriate host cell, selection of key genetic changes to target, and optimization of gene regulation. It is hoped that novel developments in the field of cancer gene therapy, which attempt to overcome these obstacles, will ultimately result in the widespread clinical application of gene therapy.

Control of Cellular Proliferation

Growth-signal interference: One strategy for affecting cellular proliferation is to interfere with growth-regulation signals from the cell surface to the nucleus. Such signals regulate cell-cycle progression and proliferation. One potential target for this strategy is the *RAS* oncogene. When mutated, *RAS* becomes "locked" in its active state, continually signaling the nucleus for growth. *RAS* mutations are particularly prevalent in gastrointestinal malignancies, such as colorectal and pancreatic cancers. Farnesylation is a process necessary for biologic activation of *RAS*. By post-translational farnesylation of a cysteine residue to a select site on the ras protein, the protein becomes anchored to the cytoplasmic side of the cell plasma membrane. The enzyme that recognizes and farnesylates ras is known as ras farnesyltransferase. Novel anticancer compounds are being designed to inhibit the function of *RAS* by interfering at different stages of the farnesylation process (Adjei, 2001; Qian, Sebti, & Hamilton, 1997). The goal is to render *RAS* inactive and unable to send signals for growth to the nucleus.

Researchers also are studying other molecules important in the process of signal transduction, with the goal of designing compounds to inhibit the activity of the molecules. Potential targets include inhibitors of tyrosine kinases (Klohs, Fry, & Kraker, 1997) and protein kinase C. Small molecular inhibitors of the epidermal growth factor receptor, platelet-derived growth factor receptor, fibroblast growth factor receptor, and *SRC* family of tyrosine kinases are under development. Investigators are trying to discover tyrosine kinase inhibitors with more potency and selectivity, better pharmacokinetics, and less toxicity. Some epidermal growth factor receptor tyrosine kinases are now in clinical trials or are about to enter clinical trials as potential anticancer agents. Potent and selective inhibitors, with tyrosine kinases as their target, will probably form an important new class of therapeutic agents for a variety of diseases for which current therapy is insufficient. In research literature, discussion of potent, selective inhibitors of receptors involved in neovascularization, such as fibroblast growth factor receptors, is less prevalent than discussion of tyrosine kinases. The search for tyrosine kinase inhibitors that can inhibit neovascularization is an active area of research (Klohs et al.).

One inhibitor of protein kinase C under evaluation is bryostatin 1, a macrocyclic lactone. A phase I study of patients with relapsed non-Hodgkin's lymphoma or chronic lymphocytic leukemia evaluated the maximum tolerated dose, major toxicities, and possible antitumor activity of bryostatin 1. Generalized myalgia was the dose-limiting toxicity. Eleven of 29 patients achieved stable disease for 2 to 19 months. Future studies will define the precise activity of bryostatin 1 in subsets of patients with lymphoproliferative malignancies and its efficacy in combination with other agents (Varterasian et al., 1998). Phase II studies evaluating the efficacy of bryostatin in the treatment of melanoma have been reported (Bedikian et al., 2001).

Many molecular approaches to controlling cellular proliferation involve *TP53* function. Potential therapeutic strategies include development of drugs that mimic the inhibitory effects of *TP53* protein on cell division; insertion, through gene therapy, of a functional, normal *TP53* gene into cells; or use of antisense oligomers to block expression of mutated *TP53* (Chang, Syrjanen, & Syrjanen, 1995).

Exploitation of Cell Death

At least two potential therapeutic approaches capitalize on natural mechanisms of cell death. The first involves restoring or stimulating apoptosis, by, for example, blocking *BCL2* expression with antisense oligonucleotides or introducing apoptosis inducers such as wild-type *TP53* into cells via liposomes or viral vectors (Duke, Ojcius, & Young, 1996; Lotem & Sachs, 1996; Shiff & Rigas, 1997). The second involves administering molecules that inhibit the effectiveness of telomerase. Normal human cells undergo a finite number of cell divisions and ultimately enter a nondividing state called replicative senescence. The proposed mechanism of this "molecular clock" that triggers senescence is telomere shortening. The enzyme telomerase, present in cancer cells and reproductive cells, retains the lengths of telomeres; thus, cells are able to replicate without limit (Hahn & Meyerson, 2001). The development of antitelomerase therapies is an active area of investigation. However, investigators must answer critical questions before they can apply this strategy: Which normal cells manufacture telomerase? What is its importance to those cells? Cells may have other mechanisms that compensate for the loss of telomerase, and researchers must identify these telomere-salvaging pathways, which could negate antitelomerase therapies (Burger, Bibby, & Double, 1997; Shay, 1997). Recent regulatory approval of the TRAPeze® (Intergen Company, Purchase, NY) enzyme-linked immunosorbent assay (ELISA) telomerase detection kit may facilitate these discoveries. The kit permits a rapid assay that detects telomerase activity in cell or tissue extracts (Bodnar et al., 1998; Hirose et al., 1997). Information about the product is available on the Intergen Web site at www.intergenco.com.

Inhibition of Metastasis

An important window for intervention in the treatment of cancer may be the period from a cell's hyperproliferative state to the point where the cell acquires the ability to invade and metastasize. Potential therapeutic approaches to inhibiting metastasis are many; the approaches fall into two major categories (Kohn & Liotta, 1995; Lyndon, 1995). The first involves cell-surface proteins and secreted proteins—such as adhesion receptors, degradative enzymes, and their inhibitors—and motility-stimulating cytokines. The second involves regulatory proteins and pathways inside the cell, such as the calcium-mediated signaling pathway. Examination of the structure and function of molecules involved at these regulatory "checkpoints" could lead to the development of agents that can block tumor invasion or growth.

Agents that target adhesion molecules: Adhesion molecules are proteins that control certain adhesive interactions of tumor cells. The presence or absence of adhesion molecules may contribute to three characteristics of neoplastic cells: uncontrolled growth, local invasiveness, and the ability to metastasize. One avenue for preventing metastasis is to target adhesion molecules (Frenette & Wagner, 1996; Huang, Baluna, & Vitetta, 1997). Many animal models have demonstrated the feasibility of using antiadhesion strategies to treat cancer. Antiadhesive **peptides** (protein fragments) or monoclonal antibodies targeted against adhesion molecules could be designed to interfere with the adhesion molecules that enable metastatic colonization by cancer cells. Antisense oligonucleotides also may inhibit tumor growth, and gene therapy may restore the functions of altered tumor-suppressive adhesion molecules.

Proteolytic-enzyme inhibitors: Another approach to inhibiting metastasis is to inhibit the **proteolytic enzymes** known as matrix metalloproteinases (MMPs). In general, proteolytic enzymes promote the breakdown of specific proteins. Cancer cells use MMPs to degrade extracellular structures (i.e., to invade adjacent tissues).

In tumor models, treatment with MMP inhibitors decreased tumor growth and metastatic spread. Research is currently under way to study batimastat (BB-94), the first member of this class to enter clinical trials, and marimastat (BB-2156) (Heath & Grochow, 2000; Rasmussen & McCann, 1997; Woodhouse, Chuaqui, & Liotta, 1997). Several compounds have entered phase III combination-therapy trials, but it is still too early to report any data. Ongoing research has been designed to correlate biological endpoints, such as levels of MMP and markers of angiogenesis, with clinical response. As understanding of MMPs and their inhibitors matures, their role in cancer therapeutics will be better defined.

Signal-transduction therapy: Altering communication circuits within the cell can produce a positive or negative downstream action, depending on the location and type of intervention. The goal of signal-transduction therapy is to suppress the hyperactive or aberrant signaling pathways associated with malignant proliferation and invasion (Kohn & Liotta, 1995). An example of this approach is the use of carboxyamide-triazole, an agent that inhibits calcium influx and, hence, signal transduction. Phase I and II trials with this agent are in progress (Bauer et al., 1999; Kohn et al., 1997). In a phase II trial conducted by Bauer and colleagues, involving patients with prostate cancer, 14 of 15 evaluable patients had progressive disease. In addition, researchers observed grade III toxicity (peripheral neuropathy) requiring drug discontinuation.

Inhibition of Neovascularization

A very active area of investigation is the inhibition of neovascularization. The goal of this work is to deprive tumors of their blood supply (Saphir, 1997). The breakdown of basement membrane and tissue matrix are processes integral to neovascularization, tumor invasion, and metastasis. Therefore, agents that inhibit neovascularization also may inhibit tumor invasion and metastasis, and vice versa (Woodhouse et al., 1997). Investigators are now evaluating several antineovascularization agents (Folkman, 1996; Twardowski & Gradishar, 1997). One of the first to enter trials is TNP-470 (AGM-1470), an analog of fumagillin, a naturally secreted antibiotic from the fungus *Aspergillus fumigatus*. Thus far, TNP-470 has been well tolerated; a dose-limiting toxicity has not yet been reached.

Also in early clinical trials are a number of compounds that are highly sulfated and capable of binding heparin-binding growth factors (HBGFs). The HBGF proteins—which include basic fibroblast growth factor, vascular endothelial growth factor, and pleotropin—stimulate neovascularization. Anti-HBGF compounds include suramin, pentosan polysulfate, and tecogalan (DS4152). Patients have not tolerated some of these agents as well as they have tolerated TNP-470. Suramin has been associated with adrenal gland toxicity, thrombocytopenia, lymphopenia, neuropathy, and renal dysfunction.

Other agents under development include receptor antagonists for neovascularization factors such as fibroblast growth factor; monoclonal antibodies against vascular endothelial growth factor (Integrated Symposium Features Promising Results of Targeted Therapies, 2000); exotoxin CM101, a polysaccharide that causes inflammation in new tumor-cell blood vessels (DeVore et al., 1996); platelet factor 4; and interferon-alfa (Hawkins, 1995). Endostatin, a natural antiangiogenic protein, has been produced through recombinant technology. Phase I trials to evaluate its utility in the treatment of cancer are under way (Herbst, Lee, Tran, & Abbruzzese, 2001).

Reversal of Multidrug Resistance

Another major focus of current cancer-therapy research is the reversal of multidrug resistance. Several trials have evaluated drugs such as calcium-channel blockers and cyclosporin A, which inhibit drug pumping by P-glycoprotein. These trials involved patients who were receiving chemotherapy for hematologic or solid tumors. In early studies, responses to chemotherapy varied from 0% to 70%; however, determining the precise contribution of the P-glycoprotein antagonist remains difficult. Moreover, some of the tested agents are associated with significant side effects. The side effects of the calcium-channel blocker dexverapamil, for example, include congestive heart failure, hypotension, and heart block. Newer drugs under clinical evaluation include PSC-833, an analog of cyclosporin. Researchers hope that PSC-833, which lacks the immunosuppressive properties of cyclosporin, will also prove less toxic than cyclosporin (Krishna & Mayer, 1997). However, coadministration of PSC-833 with the anticancer drugs daunorubicin, doxorubicin, and paclitaxel has resulted in the exacerbation of anticancer-drug toxicity. Perhaps PSC-833 alters the pharmacokinetics of the anticancer drugs.

Liposomal carriers may, by avoiding these adverse interactions, offer a significant advantage over nonencapsulated drugs (Sikic et al., 1997). Other agents under study include a monoclonal antibody (MRK16) against P-glycoprotein for both therapeutic and diagnostic purposes (Okochi, Iwahashi, & Tsuruo, 1997). Ultimately, only further phase II and III studies will establish the effectiveness of strategies designed to overcome multidrug resistance (Sonneveld & Wiemer, 1997).

Conclusion

Although more than one million people are diagnosed with cancer every year and more than 500,000 die of the disease, the future is bright for cancer management. Indeed, more than 60% of all patients with cancer currently survive their disease. Recently, the absolute number of patients dying from cancer has begun to decline. The war on cancer has never been more exciting nor has it moved at such a rapid pace. Oncology nurses, now more than ever, will be needed to educate patients. They will have to explain the complexities of new management strategies, design effective interventions for new, and as yet unknown, side effects that may be associated with emerging therapies; and assume new roles in the ever-expanding arena of cancer care. It is a challenge that initially feels overwhelming, especially to a nurse who currently lacks fundamental knowledge about cell biology, cancer biology, and genetics. However, the nursing profession must begin educating nurses now, so the wealth of knowledge and skills they currently possess can be applied to the future of cancer care.

The author would like to acknowledge Gordon B. Mills, MD, PhD, and Adel K. El-Naggar, MD, for their assistance and review of this chapter.

References

Adjei, A.A. (2001). Blocking oncogenic Ras signaling for cancer therapy. *Journal of the National Cancer Institute, 93*, 1062–1074.

Alberts, D. (1999). A unifying vision of cancer therapy for the 21st century. *Journal of Clinical Oncology, 17*(Suppl. 11), 13–21.

American Society of Clinical Oncology. (1997). Statement of the American Society of Clinical Oncology: Genetic testing for cancer susceptibility. *Journal of Clinical Oncology, 14*, 1730–1736.

Amos, C., Xu, W., & Spitz, M. (1999). Is there a genetic basis for lung cancer susceptibility? *Recent Results in Cancer Research, 151*, 3–12.

Askari, F.K., & McDonnell, W.M. (1996). Antisense-oligonucleotide therapy. *New England Journal of Medicine, 334*, 316–318.

Baron, R.H., & Borgen, P.I. (1997). Genetic susceptibility for breast cancer: Testing and primary prevention options. *Oncology Nursing Forum, 24*, 461–468.

Bast, R.C. Jr., Ravdin, P., Hayes, D.F., Bates, S., Fritsche, H. Jr., Jessup, J.M., Kemeny, N., et. al. (2001). 2000 update of recommendations for the use of tumor markers in breast and colorectal cancer: Clinical practice guidelines of the American Society of Clinical Oncology. *Journal of Clinical Oncology, 19*, 1865–1878.

Bauer, K.S., Figg, W.D., Hamilton, J.M., Jones, E.C., Premkumar, A., Steinberg, S.M., Dyer, V., Linehan, W.M., Pludar, J.M., & Reed, E. (1999). A pharmacokinetically guided phase II study of carboxyamido-triazole in androgen-independent prostate cancer. *Clinical Cancer Research, 5*, 2324–2329.

Bedikian, A.Y., Plager, C., Stewart, J.R., O'Brian, C.A., Herdman, S.K., Ross, M., et al. (2001). Phase II evaluation of bryostatin-1 in metastatic melanoma. *Melanoma Research, 11*, 183–188.

Bennett, C.F. (1998). Antisense oligonucleotides: Is the glass half full or half empty? *Biochemical Pharmacology, 55*, 9–19.

Blaese, R.M. (1997). Gene therapy for cancer. *Scientific American, 276*, 111–115.

Bodnar, A.G., Ouellette, M., Frolkis, M., Holt, S.E., Chiu, C.P., Morin, G.B., et al. (1998). Extension of life-span by introduction of telomerase into normal human cells. *Science, 270*, 349–352.

Bosl, G. (1995). Circulating tumor markers. In J.S. MacDonald, D.G. Haller, & R.J. Mayer (Eds.), *Manual of oncologic therapeutics* (pp. 49–54). Philadelphia: Lippincott.

Britton, K.E. (1997). Towards the goal of cancer-specific imaging and therapy. *Nuclear Medicine Communications, 18*, 992–1007.

Broeks, A., Urbanus, J.H., Floore, A.N., Dahler, E.C., Klijn, J.G., Rutgers, E.J., et al. (2000). ATM-heterozygous germline mutations contribute to breast cancer-susceptibility. *American Journal of Human Genetics, 66*, 494–500.

Burger, A.M., Bibby, M.C., & Double, J.A. (1997). Telomerase activity in normal and malignant mammalian tissues: Feasibility of telomerase as a target for cancer chemotherapy. *British Journal of Cancer, 75*, 516–522.

Burke, W., Daly, M., Garber, J., Botkin, J., Kahn, M.J., Lynch, P., et al. (1997). Recommendations for follow-up care of individuals with an inherited predisposition to cancer. II. BRCA1 and BRCA2. *JAMA, 227*, 997–1003.

Burke, W., Petersen, G., Lynch, P., Botkin, J., Daly, M., Garber, J., et al. (1997). Recommendations for follow-up care of individuals with an inherited predisposition to cancer. I. Hereditary nonpolyposis colon cancer. *JAMA, 277*, 915–917.

Calcabrini, A., Meschini, S., Stringaro, A., Cianfriglia, M., Arancia, G., & Molinari, A. (2000). Detection of P-glycoprotein in the nuclear envelope of multidrug resistant cells. *The Histochemical Journal, 32*, 599–606.

Calogero, A., Hospers, G.A., & Mulder, N.H. (1997). Synthetic oligonucleotides: Useful molecules? A review. *Pharmacy World and Science, 19*, 264–268.

Cannistra, S.A. (1997). "Cancer defeated": Not if, but when—Introducing the Biology of Neoplasia series. *Journal of Clinical Oncology, 15*, 3297–3298.

Caron, H., van Sluis, P., de Kraker, J., Bokkerink, J., Egeler, M., Laureys, G., et al. (1996). Allelic loss of chromosome 1p as a predictor of unfavorable outcome in patients with neuroblastoma. *New England Journal of Medicine, 334*, 225–230.

Cavanee, W.K., & White, R.L. (1995). The genetic basis of cancer. *Scientific American, 272*, 72–79.

Chan, D.W., Beveridge, R.A., Muss, H., Fritsche, H.A., Hortobagyi, G., Theriault, R., et al. (1997). Use of Truquant BR radioimmunoassay for early detection of breast cancer recurrence in patients with stage II and stage III disease. *Journal of Clinical Oncology, 15*, 2322–2328.

Chang, F., Syrjanen, S., & Syrjanen, K. (1995). Implications of the p53 tumor-suppressor gene in clinical oncology. *Journal of Clinical Oncology, 13*, 1009–1022.

Chemoprevention Working Group. (1999). Prevention of cancer in the next millennium: Report of the Chemoprevention Working Group to the American Association for Cancer Research. *Cancer Research, 59*, 4743–4758.

Clapper, M.L., Chang, W.C., & Meropol, N.J. (2001). Chemoprevention of colorectal cancer. *Current Opinion in Oncology, 13*, 307–313.

Clark, G.M. (1998). Should selection of adjuvant chemotherapy for patients with breast cancer be based on erbB-2 status? *Journal of the National Cancer Institute, 90*, 1320–1321.

Connolly, J.L., Schnitt, S.J., Wang, H.H., Dvorak, A.M., & Dvorak, H.F. (2000). Principles of cancer pathology. In R.C. Bast, D.W. Kufe, R.E. Pollock, R.R. Weichselbaum, J.F. Holland, & E. Frei III (Eds.), *Cancer medicine* (5th ed.) (pp. 362–383). Hamilton, Ontario: B.C. Decker.

Crankshaw, C.L., Marmion, M., Luker, G.D., Rao, V.D.J., Burleigh, B.D., Webb, E.D., & Piwnica-Worms, D. (1998). Novel technetium (III)-Q complexes for functional imaging of multidrug resistance (MDR1) P-glycoprotein. *Journal of Nuclear Medicine, 39*, 77–86.

Crooke, S.T. (2000). Potential roles of antisense technology in cancer chemotherapy. *Oncogene, 19*, 6651–6659.

Daly, M. (1999). NCCN Practice Guidelines: Genetics/familial high risk cancer screening. *Oncology, 13*, 161–184.

de Vere White, R.W., & Stapp, E. (1998). Predicting prognosis in patients with superficial bladder cancer. *Oncology, 12*, 1721–1723.

DeVore, R., Hellerqvist, C., Wakefield, G., Wamil, B., Thurman, G., Sundell, H., et al. (1996). A phase I study of the antineovascularization drug Cm-101 [Abstract 1558]. *Proceedings of the American Society of Clinical Oncology, 15*, 489.

Donegan, W.L. (1997). Tumor-related prognostic factors for breast cancer. *CA: A Cancer Journal for Clinicians, 47*, 28–51.

Dranoff, G. (1998). Cancer gene therapy: Connecting basic research with clinical inquiry. *Journal of Clinical Oncology, 16*, 2548–2556.

Duke, R.C., Ojcius, D.M., & Young, J.D. (1996). Cell suicide in health and disease. *Scientific American, 275*, 80–87.

Eisen, A., & Weber, B.L. (2001). Prophylactic mastectomy for women with BRCA1 and BRCA2 mutations—facts and controversy. *New England Journal of Medicine, 345*, 207–208.

Evans, W., & Relling, M. (1999). Pharmacogenetics: Translating functional genomics into rational therapeutics. *Science, 286*, 487–491.

Eyre, H.J., Smith, R.A., & Mettlin, C.J. (2000). Cancer screening and early detection. In R.C. Bast, D.W. Kufe, R.E. Pollock, R.R. Weichselbaum, J.F. Holland, & E. Frei III (Eds.), *Cancer medicine* (5th ed.) (pp. 362–383). Hamilton, Ontario: B.C. Decker.

Feig, S.A. (1996). Assessment of radiation risk from screening mammography. *Cancer, 77*, 818–822.

Fisher, B., Costantino, J.P., Wickerham, D.L., Redmond, C.K., Kavanah, M., Cronin, W.M., et al. (1998). Tamoxifen for prevention of breast cancer: Report of the National Surgical Adjuvant Breast and Bowel Project P-1 study. *Journal of the National Cancer Institute, 90,* 1371–1388.

Fisher, E.R. (1997). Pathobiological considerations relating to the treatment of intraductal carcinoma (ductal carcinoma in situ) of the breast. *CA: A Cancer Journal for Clinicians, 47,* 52–64.

Folkman, J. (1996). Fighting cancer by attacking its blood supply. *Scientific American, 275,* 150–154.

Frank-Stromborg, M. (1997). Cancer screening and early detection. In C. Varricchio, M. Pierce, C.L. Walker, & T.B. Ades (Eds.), *A cancer source book for nurses* (pp. 43–55). Atlanta: American Cancer Society.

Fraser, M.C., Calzone, K.A., & Goldstein, A.M. (1997). Familial cancers: Evolving challenges for nursing practice. *Oncology Nursing Updates, 4*(3), 1–18.

Frenette, P.S., & Wagner, D.D. (1996). Adhesion molecules—Part 1. *New England Journal of Medicine, 334,* 1526–1529.

Frost, M.H., Schaid, D.J., Sellers, T.A., Slezak, J.M., Arnold, P.G., Woods, J.E., et al. (2000). Long-term satisfaction and psychological and social function following bilateral prophylactic mastectomy. *JAMA, 284,* 319–324.

Gagel, R.F. (1997). Multiple endocrine neoplasia type II and familial medullary thyroid carcinoma. Impact of genetic screening on management. *Cancer Treatment and Research, 89,* 421–441.

Gershenson, D.M., Deavers, M., Diaz, S., Tortolero-Luna, G., Miller, B.E., Bast, Jr., R.C., et al. (1999). Prognostic significance of p53 expression in advanced-stage ovarian serous borderline tumors. *Clinical Cancer Research, 5,* 4053–4058.

Giarelli, E. (1997). Medullary thyroid carcinoma: One component of the inherited disorder multiple endocrine neoplasia type 2A. *Oncology Nursing Forum, 24,* 1007–1020.

Goss, P., & Strasser, K. (2001). Aromatase inhibitors in the treatment and prevention of cancer. *Journal of Clinical Oncology, 19,* 881–894.

Gottesman, M.M. (1994). Commentary, report of a meeting: Molecular basis of cancer therapy. *Journal of the National Cancer Institute, 86,* 1277–1285.

Greenwald, P. (1996). Chemoprevention of cancer. *Scientific American, 275*(3), 96–99.

Greenwald, P., Kelloff, G., Burch-Whitman, C., & Kramer, B. (1995). Chemoprevention. *CA: A Cancer Journal for Clinicians, 45,* 31–49.

Gribbon, J., & Loescher, L.J. (2000). Biology of cancer. In C.H. Yarbro, M. Hansen, M.H. Frogge, M. Goodman, & S. Groenwald (Eds.), *Cancer nursing: Principles and practice* (5th ed.) (pp. 17–34). Boston: Jones and Bartlett.

Hahn, W.C., & Meyerson, M. (2001). Telomerase activation, cellular immortalization and cancer. *Annals of Medicine, 33*, 123–129.

Hall, S.J., Chen, S.H., & Woo, S.L. (1997). The promise and reality of cancer gene therapy. *American Journal of Human Genetics, 61*, 785–789.

Hartmann, L.C., Schaid, D., Sellers, T., McDonnell, S., Woods, J., Sitta, D., et al. (2000). Bilateral prophylactic mastectomy (PM) in BRCA1/2 mutation carriers. *Proceedings of the American Association of Cancer Research, 41*, [Abstract 1417].

Hartmann, L.C., Schaid, D.J., Woods, J.E., Crotty, T.P., Myers, J.L., Arnold, P.G., Petty, P.M., Sellers, T.A., Johnson, J.L., McDonnell, S.K., Frost, M.H., & Jenkins, R.B. (1999). Efficacy of bilateral prophylactic mastectomy in women with a family history of breast cancer. *New England Journal of Medicine, 340*, 77–84.

Hawkins, M.J. (1995). Clinical trials of antiangiogenic agents. *Current Opinion in Oncology, 7*, 90–93.

Healy, B. (1997). BRCA genes—Bookmaking, fortunetelling and medical care. *New England Journal of Medicine, 366*, 1448–1450.

Heath, E.I., & Grochow, L.B. (2000). Clinical potential of matrix metalloprotease inhibitors in cancer therapy. *Drugs, 59*, 1043–1055.

Hedley, D.W., Clark, G.M., Cornelisse, C.J., Killander, D., Kute, T., & Merkel, D. (1993). Consensus review of the clinical utility of DNA cytometry in carcinoma of the breast: Report of the DNA Cytometry Consensus Conference. *Cytometry, 14*, 482–485.

Hellman, S., & Weichselbaum, R.R. (1995). Oligometastases. *Journal of Clinical Oncology, 13*, 8–10.

Herbst, R.S., Lee, A.T., Tran, H.T., & Abbruzzese, J.L. (2001). Clinical studies of angiogenesis inhibitors: the University of Texas MD Anderson Center Trial of Human Endostatin. *Current Oncology Reports, 3*, 131–140.

Heusinkveld, K.B. (1997). Cancer prevention and risk assessment. In C. Varricchio, M. Pierce, C.L. Walker, & T.B. Ades (Eds.), *A cancer source book for nurses* (pp. 35–42). Atlanta: American Cancer Society.

Hirose, M., Abe-Hashimoto, J., Ogura, K., Tahara, H., Ide, T., & Yoshimura, T. (1997). A rapid, useful and quantitative method to measure telomerase activity by hybridization protection assay connected with a telomeric repeat amplification protocol. *Journal of Cancer Research and Clinical Oncology, 123*, 337–344.

Holtzman, N.A., & Marteau, T.M. (2000). Will genetics revolutionize medicine? *New England Journal of Medicine, 343*, 141–144.

Holtzman, N.A., & Watson, M.S. (1999). Promoting safe and effective genetic testing in the United States. Final report of the Task Force on Genetic Testing. *Journal of Child and Family Nursing, 2*, 388–390.

Houshmand, S.L., Campbell, C.T., Briggs, S.E., McFadden, A.W., Al-Tweigeri, T. (2000). Prophylactic mastectomy and genetic testing: An update. *Oncology Nursing Forum*, *27*, 1537–1547.

Huang, Y.W., Baluna, R., & Vitetta, E.S. (1997). Adhesion molecules as targets for cancer therapy. *Histology and Histopathology*, *12*, 467–477.

Integrated symposium features promising results of targeted therapies. (2000). *ASCO Daily News*, *1*, 3–4.

International Human Genome Sequencing Consortium. (2001). Initial sequencing and analysis of the human genome. *Nature*, *409*, 860–921.

Kakol, J., Marth, G., Sachidanandam, R., Schmidt, S., Stein, L., Weissman, D., et al. (1999). A map of human genome sequence variation containing 1.42 million single nucleotide polymorphisms. *Nature*, *409*, 928–933.

Israel, M.A. (1996). Molecular genetics in the management of patients with cancer. In M.J. Bishop & R.A. Weinberg (Eds.), *Scientific American molecular oncology* (pp. 205–237). New York: Scientific American Inc.

James, H.A., & Gibson, I. (1998). The therapeutic potential of ribozymes. *Blood*, *91*, 371–382.

King, H., & Sinha, A. (2001). Gene expression profile analysis by DNA microassays: Promise and pitfalls. *JAMA*, *286*, 2280–2288.

King, M.C., Wieand, S., Hale, K., Lee, M., Walsh, T., Owens, K., et al. (2001). Tamoxifen and breast cancer incidence among women with inherited mutations in BRCA1 and BRCA2. National Surgical Adjuvant Breast and Bowel Project (NSABP-P1) breast cancer prevention trial. *JAMA*, *286*, 2251–2256.

Kinzler, K.M., & Vogelstein, B. (1997). Gatekeepers and caretakers. *Nature*, *386*, 761–762.

Klohs, W.D., Fry, D.W., & Kraker, A.J. (1997). Inhibitors of tyrosine kinase. *Current Opinion in Oncology*, *9*, 562–568.

Kohn, E.C., Figg, W.D., Sarosy, G.A., Bauer, K.S., Davis, P.A., Soltis, M.J., et al. (1997). Phase I trial of micronized formulation carboxyamidotriazole in patients with refractory solid tumors: Pharmacokinetics, clinical outcome, and comparison of formulations. *Journal of Clinical Oncology*, *15*, 1985–1993.

Kohn, E.C., & Liotta, L.A. (1995). Molecular insights into cancer invasion: Strategies for prevention and intervention. *Cancer Research*, *55*, 1856–1862.

Krishna, R., & Mayer, L.D. (1997). Liposomal doxorubicin circumvents PSC 833-free drug interactions, resulting in effective therapy of multidrug-resistant solid tumors. *Cancer Research*, *57*, 5246–5253.

Kronenwett, R., & Haas, R. (1998). Specific bcr-abl–directed antisense nucleic acids and ribozymes: A tool for the treatment of chronic myelogenous leukemia? *Recent Results in Cancer Research*, *144*, 127–138.

Krynetski, E., & Evans, W. (1998). Pharmacogenetics of cancer therapy: Getting personal. *American Journal of Human Genetics, 63*, 11–16.

Lairmore, T.C., Frisella, M.M., & Wells, S.A.J. (1996). Genetic testing and early thyroidectomy for inherited medullary thyroid carcinoma. *Annals of Medicine, 28*, 401–406.

Larsen, A., Escargueil, A., & Skladanowski, A., (2000). Resistance mechanisms associated with altered intracellular distribution of anticancer agents. *Pharmacology and Therapeutics, 85*, 217–229.

Lavin, M.F., & Shiloh, Y. (1996). Ataxia-telangiectasia: A multifaceted genetic disorder associated with defective signal transduction. *Current Opinion in Immunology, 8*, 459–464.

Lee, I.M., Hennekens, C.H., & Buring, J.E. (1997). Use of aspirin and other nonsteroidal anti-inflammatory drugs and the risk of cancer development. In V.T. DeVita, S. Hellman, & S.A. Rosenberg (Eds.), *Cancer: Principles and practice of oncology* (pp. 599–607). Philadelphia: Lippincott-Raven.

Levine, E.A., Holzmayer, T., Bacus, S., Mecnemer, E., Mera, R., Boninger, C., et al. (1997). Evaluation of newer prognostic markers for adult soft tissue sarcomas. *Journal of Clinical Oncology, 15*, 3249–3257.

Lindor, M.N., Greene, M.H., & the Mayo Familial Cancer Program (1998). The concise handbook of family cancer syndromes. *Journal of the National Cancer Institute, 90*, 1039–1071.

Loescher, L.J. (1993). Commentary: Expanding our horizons with an alternative approach to cancer prevention and detection. *Seminars in Oncology Nursing, 9*, 147–149.

Loescher, L.J., & Reid, M.E. (2000). Dynamics of cancer prevention. In C.H. Yarbro, M.H. Frogge, M. Goodman, & S. Groenwald (Eds.), *Cancer nursing: Principles and practice* (5th ed.) (pp. 135–149). Boston: Jones and Bartlett.

Lotem, J., & Sachs, L. (1996). Control of apoptosis in hematopoiesis and leukemia by cytokines, tumor suppressors and oncogenes. *Leukemia, 10*, 925–931.

Lyndon, J. (1995). Metastasis. Part I: Biology and prevention. *Oncology Nursing: Patient Treatment and Support, 2*, 1–13.

Maher, L.J. (1996). Prospects for the therapeutic use of antigene oligonucleotides. *Cancer Investigation, 14*, 66–82.

Mahon, S.M. (1998). Cancer risk assessment: Conceptual considerations for clinical practice. *Oncology Nursing Forum, 25*, 1535–1547.

Mashal, R., & Sklar, J.L. (1995). Polymerase chain reaction in the diagnosis and monitoring of cancer. In J.S. MacDonald, D.G. Haller, & R.J. Mayer (Eds.), *Manual of oncologic therapeutics* (pp. 55–61). Philadelphia: Lippincott.

Mastronardi, L., Guiduccil, A., & Puzzilli, F. (2001). Lack of correlation between Ki-67 labelling index and tumor size of anterior pituitary adenomas. *BMC Cancer, 1*(1), 12.

Mauro, M., O'Dwyer, M., Heinrich, M., & Drucker, B. (2002). STI571: A paradigm of new agents for cancer therapeutics. *Journal of Clinical Oncology, 20*, 325–334.

McGuffie, E.M., Pacheco, D., Carbone, G.M., & Catapano, C.V. (2000). Antigene and antiproliferative effects of a c-myc-targeting phosphorothioate triple helix-forming oligonucleotide in human leukemia cells. *Cancer Research, 60*, 3790–3799.

Meijers-Heijboer, H., van Geel, B., van Putten, W.L., Henzen-Logmans, S.C., Seynaeve, C., Menke-Pluymers, M.B., et al. (2001). Breast cancer after prophylactic bilateral mastectomy in women with a BRCA1 or BRCA2 mutation. *New England Journal of Medicine, 345*, 159–164.

Mettler, F.A., Upton, A.C., Kelsey, C.A., Ashby, R.N., Rosenberg, R.D., & Linver, M.N. (1996). Benefits versus risks from mammography. *Cancer, 77*, 903–909.

Meyer, J.S., & Province, M.A. (1994). S-phase fraction and nuclear size in long-term prognosis of patients with breast cancer. *Cancer, 74*, 2287–2299.

Mills, G.B., Schmandt, R., Gershenson, D., & Bast, R.C. (1999). Should therapy of ovarian cancer patients be individualized based on underlying genetic defects? *Clinical Cancer Research, 5*, 2286–2288.

Narayanan, R. (1997). Harnessing the power of antisense technology for combination chemotherapy. *Journal of the National Cancer Institute, 89*, 107–108.

Offit, K. (2000). Are BRCA1 and BRCA2 associated breast cancers different? *Journal of Clinical Oncology, 18*(Suppl. 21), 1045–1065.

Okochi, E., Iwahashi, T., & Tsuruo, T. (1997). Monoclonal antibodies specific for P-glycoprotein. *Leukemia, 11*, 1119–1123.

Papavassiliou, A.G. (1998). Transcription-factor–modulating agents: Precision and selectivity in drug design. *Molecular Medicine Today, 4*, 358–366.

Pastorino, U., Andreola, S., Tagliabue, E., Pezzella, F.I.M., & Sozzi, G. (1997). Immunocytochemical markers in stage I lung cancer: Relevance to prognosis. *Journal of Clinical Oncology, 15*, 2858–2865.

Patel, A.S., Hawkins, A.L., & Griffin, C.A. (2000). Cytogenetics and cancer. *Current Opinions in Oncology, 12*, 62–67.

Perera, F.P. (1996). Uncovering new clues to cancer risk. *Scientific American, 274*, 54–62.

Perera, F.P. (2000). Molecular epidemiology: On the path to prevention? *Journal of the National Cancer Institute, 92*, 602–612.

Petersen, G.M., & Brensinger, J.P. (1996). Genetic testing and counseling in familial adenomatous polyposis. *Oncology, 10*, 89–94.

Piver, M.S., Jishi, M.F., Tsukada, Y., & Nava, G. (1993). Primary peritoneal carcinoma after oophorectomy in women with a family history of ovarian cancer: A report of the Gilda Radner Familial Ovarian Cancer Registry. *Cancer, 71,* 2751–2755.

Ponder, B.A. (2001). Cancer genetics. *Nature, 411,* 336–341.

Qian, Y., Sebti, S.M., & Hamilton, A.D. (1997). Farnesyltransferase as a target for anticancer drug design. *Biopolymers, 43,* 25–41.

Rabbitts, T.H. (1998). The clinical significance of fusion oncogenes in cancer. *New England Journal of Medicine, 338,* 192–194.

Rasmussen, H.S., & McCann, P.P. (1997). Matrix metalloproteinase inhibition as a novel anticancer strategy: A review with special focus on batimastat and marimastat. *Pharmacology and Therapeutics, 75,* 69–75.

Rebbeck, T.R., Levin, A.M., Eisen, A., Snyder, C., Watson, P., Cannon-Albright, L., et al. (1999). Breast cancer risk after bilateral prophylactic oophorectomy in BRCA1 mutation carriers. *Journal of the National Cancer Institute, 91,* 1475–1479.

Relling, M., Hancock, M., Rivera, G., Sandlund, J., Ribeiro, R., Krynetski, E., et al. (1999). Mercaptopurine therapy intolerance and heterozygosity at the thiopurine S-methyltransferase gene locus. *Journal of the National Cancer Institute, 91,* 2001–2008.

Rieger, P.T. (1997). Emerging strategies in the management of cancer. *Oncology Nursing Forum, 24,* 728–737.

Rieger, P.T. (2000). Counseling for genetic risk. In C.H. Yarbro, M.H. Frogge, M. Goodman, & S. Groenwald (Eds.), *Cancer nursing: Principles and practice* (5th ed.) (pp. 189–213). Boston: Jones and Bartlett.

Robinson, K.D., Abernathy, E., & Conrad, K.J. (1996). Gene therapy of cancer. *Seminars in Oncology Nursing, 12,* 142–151.

Roses, A. (2000). Pharmacogenetics and future drug development and delivery. *Lancet, 355,* 1358–1361.

Roth, J.A., Swisher, S.G., & Meyn, R.E. (1999). p53 tumor suppressor gene therapy for cancer. *Oncology, 13*(10 Suppl. 5), 148–154.

Saphir, A. (1997). Angiogenesis: The unifying concept in cancer? *Journal of the National Cancer Institute, 89,* 1658–1659.

Sausville, E.A. & Johnson, J.I. (2000). Molecules for the millennium: how will they look? New drug discovery year 2000. *British Journal of Cancer, 83,* 1401–1404.

Schlechte, H.H., Sachs, M.D., Lenk, S.V., Brenner, S., Rudolph, B.D., & Loening, S.A. (2000). Progression in transitional cell carcinoma of the urinary bladder—Analysis of Tp53 gene mutations by temperature gradients and sequence in tumor tissues and in cellular urine sediments. *Cancer Detection and Prevention, 24*(1), 24–32.

Schrag, D., Kuntz, K.M., Garber, J.E., & Weeks, J.C. (1997). Decision analysis—Effects of prophylactic mastectomy and oophorectomy on life expectancy among women with BRCA1 and BRCA2 mutations. *New England Journal of Medicine, 336*, 1465–1471.

Schrock, E., du Manoir, S., Veldman, T., Schoell, B., Weinberg, J., Ferguson-Smith, M.A., et al. (1996). Multicolor spectral karyotyping of human chromosomes. *Science, 273*, 497.

Shattuck-Eidens, D., McClure, M., Simard, J., Labrie, F., Narod, S., Couch, F., et al. (1995). A collaborative survey of 80 mutations in the BRCA1 breast and ovarian cancer susceptibility gene. Implications for presymptomatic testing and screening. *JAMA, 273*, 535–541.

Shay, J.W. (1997). Telomerase in human development and cancer. *Journal of Cellular Physiology, 173*, 266–270.

Sheer, D., & Squire, J. (1996). Clinical applications of genetic rearrangements in cancer. *Cancer Biology, 7*, 25–32.

Shiff, S.J., & Rigas, B. (1997). Nonsteroidal anti-inflammatory drugs and colorectal cancer: Evolving concepts of their chemopreventive actions. *Gastroenterology, 113*, 1992–1998.

Shipper, H., Goh, C.R., & Wang, T.L. (1995). Shifting the cancer paradigm: Must we kill to cure? *Journal of Clinical Oncology, 13*, 801–807.

Sikic, B.I., Fisher, G.A., Lum, B.L., Halsey, J., Beketic-Oreskovic, L., & Chen, G. (1997). Modulation and prevention of multidrug resistance by inhibitors of P-glycoprotein. *Cancer Chemotherapy and Pharmacology, 40*(Suppl.), 13–19.

Singh, D.K., & Lippman, S.M. (1998a). Cancer chemoprevention—Part 1: Retinoids and carotenoids and other classic antioxidants. *Oncology, 12*, 1642–1653, 1657.

Singh, D.K., & Lippman, S.M. (1998b). Cancer chemoprevention—Part 2: Hormones, nonclassic natural agents, NSAIDs, and other agents. *Oncology, 12*, 1787–1800.

Sklar, J.L., & Costa, J.C. (1997). Principles of cancer management: Molecular pathology. In V.T. DeVita, S. Hellman, & S.A. Rosenberg (Eds.), *Cancer: Principles and practice of oncology* (pp. 259–284). Philadelphia: Lippincott-Raven.

Snijders, A.M., Meijer, G.A., Brakenhoff, R.H., van den Brule, A.J., & van Diest, P.J. (2000). Microarray techniques in pathology: Tool or toy? *Molecular Pathology, 53*, 289–294.

Society of Surgical Oncology. (2001). SSO updates statement on prophylactic mastectomy. *SSO News, 2*, 8.

Sonneveld, P., & Wiemer, E. (1997). Inhibitors of multidrug resistance. *Current Opinion in Oncology, 9*, 543–548.

Sporn, M.B., & Lippmann, S.M. (1997). Chemoprevention of cancer. In J.F. Holland, R.C. Bast, D.L. Morton, E. Frei III, D.W. Kufe, & R.R. Weichselbaum (Eds.), *Cancer medicine* (4th ed.) (pp. 495–508). Baltimore: Williams & Wilkins.

Sporn, M.B., & Lippmann, S.M. (2000). Chemoprevention of cancer. In R.C. Bast, D.W. Kufe, R.E. Pollock, R.R. Weichselbaum, J.F. Holland, & E. Frei III (Eds.), *Cancer medicine* (5th ed.) (pp. 351–361). Hamilton, Ontario: B.C. Decker.

Stefanek, M.E. (1995). Bilateral prophylactic mastectomy: Issues and concerns [Monograph]. *Journal of the National Cancer Institute, 17,* 37–42.

Stefanek, M.E., Helzlsouer, K.J., Wilcox, P.M., & Houn, F. (1995). Predictors of and satisfaction with bilateral prophylactic mastectomy. *Preventive Medicine, 24,* 412–419.

Stipp, D. (1997). Gene chip breakthrough. *Fortune, 135,* 56–73.

Sullivan, P.M., Etzioni, R., Feng, Z., Potter, J.D., Thompson, M.L., Thornquist, M., et al. (2001). Phases of biomarker development for early detection of cancer. *Journal of the National Cancer Institute, 93,* 1054–1061.

Sun, S.S., Hsieh, J.F., Tsai, S.C., Ho, Y.J., & Kao, C.H. (2000). Expression of drug resistance protein related to Tc-99m MIBI breast imaging. *Anticancer Research, 20,* 2021–2025.

Swan, D.K., & Ford, B. (1997). Chemoprevention of cancer: Review of the literature. *Oncology Nursing Forum, 24,* 719–727.

Swift, M. (1994). Ionizing radiation, breast cancer, and ataxia-telangiectasia [Editorial]. *Journal of the National Cancer Institute, 86,* 1571–1572.

Task Force on Genetic Testing. (1996). Interim principles of the task force on Genetic Testing. Retrieved August 15, 2000, from http://infonet.welch .jhu.edu/policy/genetics/intro.html

Temsamani, J., & Guinot, P. (1997). Antisense oligonucleotides: A new therapeutic approach. *Biotechnology and Applied Biochemistry, 26*(2), 65–71.

Thun, J.J., & Wingo, P.A. (2000). Cancer epidemiology. In R.C. Bast, D.W. Kufe, R.E. Pollock, R.R. Weichselbaum, J.F. Holland, & E. Frei III (Eds.), *Cancer medicine* (5th ed.) (pp. 283–297). Hamilton, Ontario: B.C. Decker.

Twardowski, P., & Gradishar, W.J. (1997). Clinical trials of antiangiogenic agents. *Current Opinion in Oncology, 9,* 584–589.

Varterasian, M.L., Mohammad, R.M., Eilender, D.S., Hulburd, K., Rodriguez, D.H., Pemberton, P.A., et al. (1998). Phase I study of bryostatin 1 in patients with relapsed non-Hodgkin's lymphoma and chronic lymphocytic leukemia. *Journal of Clinical Oncology, 16,* 56–62.

Venter, J.C., Adams, M.D., Myers, E.W., Li, P.W., Mural, R.J., Sutton, G.G., et al. (2001). The sequence of the human genome. *Science, 291,* 1304–1351.

Weber, B.L. (1996). Genetic testing for breast cancer. *Scientific American Science and Medicine, 3,* 12–21.

Woodhouse, E.C., Chuaqui, R.F., & Liotta, L.A. (1997). General mechanisms of metastasis. *Cancer, 80*(Suppl. 8), 1529–1537.

Wu, J.T. (1999). Review of circulating tumor markers: From enzyme, carcinoembryonic protein to oncogene and suppressor gene. *Annals of Clinical Laboratory Science, 29*(2), 106–111.

Yuen, A.R., & Sikic, B.I. (2000). Clinical studies of antisense therapy in cancer. *Frontiers in Bioscience, 5,* D588–D593.

7

How to Provide Genetic Counseling and Education

Karen Greco, RN, MN, ANP, APNG(c)

Genetic counseling is the process of collecting genetic information and communicating, in a supportive environment, the implications of that information to a client and his or her family. Traditionally, genetic counseling is nondirective—that is, it presents options, not imperatives—and counselors take special care to be sensitive to the emotional and psychosocial needs, culture, and healthcare beliefs of the client and his or her family. The focus is on helping the client and family to understand their potential genetic risk and options and discussing the complex issues related to genetic information. The client and family then use this information in making health-related decisions.

Genetic counseling for cancer includes providing education about the basic principles of cancer genetics, information about relevant cancer syndromes, assessment, and communication and interpretation of cancer-risk information in terminology that clients and families can understand. Counseling sessions also address the risks and benefits of cancer-predisposition testing; cancer-surveillance and risk-reduction options; implications for other family members; and ethical, emotional, and psychosocial issues related to genetic information. The oncology nurse providing genetic counseling must understand the importance of ethical issues such as confidentiality, privacy, and informed consent as he or she manages information about genetic makeup.

Genetic Counseling

Nurses have been involved in genetic counseling and education since the 1960s, when nurses began providing services to children with genetic disorders and to the children's families. Describing this nursing role, Forbes (1996) stated that genetic counseling requires the nurse to present statistical probabilities while dealing with the family's knowledge, feelings, and problems. As part of a multidisciplinary team, the nurse is involved in finding cases, taking detailed histories, obtaining medical records, constructing pedigrees, clarifying genetic information, helping the family to deal with the emotional impact of genetic information, and referring clients and their families to appropriate resources.

In a qualitative study, Patterson (1967) worked with mothers who had hereditary disease in their families. The mothers identified public health nurses as sources of help in dealing with emotional and homecare problems and in finding community resources for children affected by hereditary disease.

Cancer genetic counseling has been available for only a few years. In many respects, the role of the oncology nurse in cancer genetic counseling is similar to the role the nurse played in genetic counseling in the 1960s. According to Forsman (1994), what has changed is the information available and the population to which the information may be applied.

In a study by Bernhardt, Geller, Doksum, and Metz (2000), nurses and non-nurse genetic counselors were equally effective in providing education about genetic testing for breast cancer susceptibility.

Counseling Issues Related to Genetic Information

This section will present a brief overview of issues that are typical of and unique to genetic counseling, especially counseling pertaining to cancer.

The Uncertainty of Genetic Information

Clients often think that genetic services can provide a concrete explanation of why cancer has occurred in their families. They see genetic testing as a diagnostic tool that will give a clear answer about whether a person will develop cancer. Similarly, healthcare providers often want to use genetic assessments to make decisions about the treatment of cancer or precancerous conditions, without understanding the uncertainties associated with genetic assessment and cancer-predisposition testing. A positive cancer-predisposition test does not mean a person will develop cancer; a negative cancer-predisposition test does not mean a person is free from cancer risk. Communicating the uncertainty associated with genetic information is an essential part of genetic counseling.

Inappropriate Expectations

Many reasons impel a person to seek genetic services, and many reasons impel a provider to refer a client for genetic counseling or predisposition testing. A person diagnosed with cancer may be concerned about his or her potential risk of other cancers or the potential cancer risk of a relative or child. A provider may be searching for a basis for making cancer-surveillance and risk-reduction recommendations.

A nurse must understand what each person expects from the genetic counseling process. During the intake process, he or she must ask many questions to determine if the expectations are realistic and what services the client may need. Will the services meet the client's expectations? How does the client expect to use the information he or she will receive? What is the client's perception of his or her cancer risk? How well does the client understand genetic information?

Counselors must be aware that the referral provider and the client may not have the same expectations. The provider may want to use the cancer-risk assessment and genetic-test information to make decisions about cancer treatment or prophylactic surgery. The client, however, may not be ready to deal with the psychological and family issues related to testing or to make a decision about prophylactic surgery. Furthermore, the time in which the treatment decision must be made often is much shorter than the time needed to undergo genetic counseling and testing.

In a study by Bowen et al. (1999), women who were more worried about their cancer risk were less likely to participate in breast cancer risk counseling than were women who were less worried. Similarly, Burke et al. (2000) showed that women with a family history of breast cancer but a low likelihood of carrying a cancer-predisposing mutation tended to overestimate their personal breast cancer risk and be more likely than other women to consider themselves candidates for predisposition testing. Genetic counseling helped these women to develop more accurate views of their personal cancer risk and to worry less about developing breast cancer (Burke et al., 2000).

In studies regarding breast or ovarian cancer, the most common reasons that clients cited for wanting predisposition testing were to learn about their children's cancer risk, to have more cancer-screening tests, to take better care of themselves, to feel more reassured, and to make childbearing decisions (Lerman, Daly, Masny, & Balshem, 1994; Lerman, Seay, Balshem, & Audrain, 1995). In a series of women's focus groups, the major advantages to *BRCA1*-predisposition testing, as cited by participants, were the reduction of uncertainty and help with decisions about medical treatment, surveillance, and lifestyle changes (Tessare, Borstelmann, Regan, Rimer, & Winer, 1997).

The Needs of Family Members

Genetic information is unique in that it has implications for family members as well as for the individual undergoing testing. Healthcare professionals have a responsibility to inform clients who test positive for a cancer-predisposing gene that family members related by blood may carry the same mutation. If appropriate, encourage the client to contact family members and recommend that they receive genetic counseling and applicable healthcare services. Questions from family members about their own cancer risk and healthcare issues will arise, especially if family members attend genetic counseling sessions with the client. Addressing these questions can be challenging. Although in certain situations you may have a duty to inform a family member that a potential health risk to other family members may be present, the family member is not the client you are authorized to serve. Be aware that your institution has a duty to develop policies regarding informing family members that they could be at risk for a hereditary condition or disease if effective screening, prevention, or risk-reduction measures are available and there is clear evidence that withholding such information could result in harm to the family member (Leung, 2000).

Health practitioners have been successfully sued for not informing family members that they are at risk for a hereditary cancer syndrome for which effective screening and risk-reduction measures are available (Severin, 1999). Liability cases in regard to genetic information are just emerging, however. Raising the standard of care for individuals and families at risk for genetic susceptibility to cancer requires awareness of the legal precedents and skill development to meet the needs of family members.

When family members are educated together, time must be allocated to address the needs of each person. However, when family members attend a session to serve as support for a patient, they may ask questions about their own risk and health concerns. In this situation, recommend to the family members that they formalize the client-healthcare provider relationship. The best approach is to offer to schedule a separate appointment to address a family member's own healthcare concerns or to refer the family member to appropriate healthcare resources.

> To assess motivations for genetic testing, ascertain
> - The client's reasons for and expectations about testing
> - The referring provider's reasons for recommending testing and his or her expectations about test results
> - The client's perception of cancer risk
> - What the client intends to do with information gained from testing.

Potential Workplace and Insurance Discrimination

Many insurance companies now cover predisposition testing for cancer, but clients may be concerned about releasing the results of such tests to their insurance companies, fearing that the result will be health insurance cancellation or an insurance rate increase. The client may fear that the insurance company will discriminate against his or her relatives if tests reveal that the client carries a mutation associated with a high cancer risk. People who undergo genetic testing also may be at risk for workplace discrimination based on their genotype (Jacobs, 1998).

Clients need to be informed of potential insurance-discrimination issues, what state and federal protections exist, and the limitations of those protections.

State Laws Against Discrimination

State and federal laws that regulate the use of genetic information are intended to help protect the confidentiality of genetic information and prevent insurance and workplace discrimination. These laws vary greatly and are changing rapidly. Understanding the benefits and limitations of these laws and staying abreast of legislative changes can be a complicated undertaking. The work of Karen Rothenberg, University of Maryland Law and Healthcare Program, may be a helpful resource (Gould, Lynch, Smith, & McCarthy, 1997). For more information, visit www.genome.gov/policyethics.

Federal Legislation Against Discrimination

At least three federal initiatives affect the potential for discrimination by health insurers or employers based on genetic information. The Americans With Disabilities Act (ADA) was enacted in 1990 to protect the disabled, and it makes discrimination against an employee or potential employee, based solely on an impairment, illegal. The Equal Employment Opportunities Commission has interpreted the ADA to apply to genetic information. The result of this interpretation is that employers are prohibited from denying employment to an individual based on his or her genetic predisposition to cancer.

In regard to genetic information, the most significant federal legislation is the Health Insurance Portability and Accountability Act of 1996. A key provision of this legislation is that genetic information may not be treated as a preexisting condition in the absence of a diagnosis of the condition related to such information. Another key provision is that genetic information cannot be used to deny, cancel, or refuse to renew insurance coverage. This provision applies to an individual's eligibility for insurance under a group health plan offered by an employer. In addition, the employer may not require an individual to pay a premium that is higher than that paid by a similarly situated individual within the group based on the health status of the individual or his or her dependent (Berner, 1996). This legislation applies to health insurance only, not to disability or life insurance.

The third significant federal initiative is Executive Order No. 13145, enacted in 2000, which prohibits employment discrimination based on genetic information. The order prohibits agencies of the federal government from obtaining genetic information from employees or job applicants. The order also prohibits government agencies from using genetic information in hiring and promotion decisions. Additional federal and state legislation still is needed to prevent discrimination.

The Impact of a Cancer Diagnosis on Counseling Needs

Of people who seek genetic counseling, those who have been diagnosed with cancer often have needs different from those who have not. Individuals who have recently been diagnosed with cancer or who are referred for predisposition testing may be coping with multiple issues and may or may not be ready to undergo testing, which could lead to more psychosocial and family stressors.

Potential insurance and workplace discrimination tends to be less of an issue for a person with a cancer diagnosis than for someone who has not been diagnosed with cancer. It is not uncommon for a diagnosed person to say, "If they wanted to discriminate against me because of my breast cancer diagnosis, they could." Learning that he or she may be at risk for other cancers, because of a positive genetic test, is unlikely to increase potential insurance or workplace discrimination. The motivation for pursuing cancer-predisposition testing may be the individual's concern about his or her potential risk for other cancers or the potential cancer risk of unaffected family members.

People without a cancer diagnosis may be extremely anxious about their own cancer risk, and their level of anxiety may be unrelated to the number of relatives in the family who have been diagnosed with cancer. Many people in this situation turn out not to be in the high-risk category. In their case, risk assessment and appropriate health education may alleviate their anxiety.

Psychosocial Impact

Genetic counseling involves not only communicating genetic information, but also addressing the emotional and psychological issues associated with it. Psychological distress can impede the client's ability to receive information. For cancer-risk counseling to be effective, emotional issues must be identified and addressed (Peters, 1994). Psychological issues may include fear of cancer or medical procedures, past negative experiences with cancer, unresolved loss and sorrow, feelings of guilt about passing on a mutation to children, anxiety about learning test results, and concern about the effect of results on other family members (Botkin et al., 1996). For these reasons, it is important for clients to know how to access additional support services, such as those of a psychologist, social worker, or support groups.

The Client's Perception of Risk

The medical and psychosocial dimensions of cancer counseling are closely intertwined. How clients perceive their cancer risk often seems to depend more on their emotional responses and experiences than the actual numeric risk (Schneider, 2002).

Clients receiving cancer genetic services often have lost loved ones to cancer or may have had cancer themselves. Many families have survived multiple losses or had multiple family members diagnosed with cancer, and each of these experiences has left an emotional imprint. The words of one client, a woman whose parents were diagnosed with breast cancer and who herself had a genetic predisposition to the disease, described how her experience molded her attitude and outlook: "The agony of watching my mother die from breast cancer is like . . . a pencil mark [on] a piece of paper: It made an emotional imprint that can never be erased, and it caused me to view breast cancer as a disease that can never be survived" (Prouser, 2000).

Emotional responses to perception of cancer risk can include anger, fear of developing cancer, fear of disfigurement or death, grief, guilt, loss of control, negative body image, and a sense of isolation (Schneider, 2002).

Support for Decisions and During Waiting Times

The decision to have predisposition testing is difficult for many clients, as is waiting to receive test results. From the time blood is drawn to the receipt of results can be several weeks or longer. This waiting time can be a period of increased anxiety, isolation, and depression.

The counselor should maintain telephone contact with the client during this time and offer psychological support. A peer counselor may be helpful during this period, if one is available. Peer counselors are trained volunteers who have been through a similar experience and are willing to share their experience as a means of support.

Emotional Response to Predisposition Diagnosis

Typical reactions: Clients found to carry a genetic mutation may experience anxiety, depression, anger, feelings of vulnerability, or guilt about possibly having passed the mutation to children. Clients found not to carry a mutation may experience survivor's guilt, especially if close family members are found to carry the mutation. They also may experience regrets if they made major life decisions, such as the decision to have prophylactic surgery, prior to testing (Gellar et al., 1997).

Reactions cited in specific studies: Lerman et al. (1996) examined psychological outcomes related to *BRCA1* testing as assessed after clients had received test results. Participants who tested negative showed a lesser degree of depressive symptoms and functional impairment than did participants who tested positive and untested individuals. Mutation carriers, however, did not show increases in depression and functional impairment.

In a similar study, Croyle, Smith, Botkin, Baty, and Nash (1997) discovered that women found to carry a *BRCA1* mutation had higher levels of psychological distress than did women who tested negative. The researchers found the highest levels of test-related distress among mutation carriers with no history of cancer or cancer-related surgery.

In a study of clients with colorectal cancer who were undergoing genetic testing for hereditary colon cancer, higher depression scores were associated with being female and having less formal education and fewer sources of social contact. Increased anxiety was associated with younger age, less formal education, nonwhite race, and fewer social contacts (Vernon et al., 1997).

Assessment for Psychological Counseling

Extreme emotional responses to receiving predisposition test results are infrequent, but they do occur. In the ideal setting, a psychologist or social worker would consult with every client who undergoes predisposition testing. In clinical practice, however, this is rarely possible. Consequently, the nurse must be able to assess the client's emotional ability to handle test results.

Consider referring a client for psychological counseling if he or she
- Displays signs of excessive anxiety, depression, or stress
- Has a history or current indications of ineffective coping
- Has an ineffective social support system
- Shows distress regarding making decisions related to genetic information
- Has a history of psychiatric problems
- Shows signs of unresolved bereavement
- Is experiencing marital or family discord
- Has experienced multiple crises in a short time
- Expresses an interest in receiving psychological counseling.

Clients who need support must have available a psychologist or social worker who understands that predisposition-testing patients who have been affected by cancer have needs that are very different from those who have not.

Psychosocial assessment is an ongoing process that takes place as a part of each client contact and involves verbal, nonverbal, and written clues. Clinical judgment on the part of the nurse is involved in deciding how to interpret the information gathered and making appropriate referrals for psychosocial services.

Nursing considerations regarding the psychosocial impact of genetic information
1. Assessment of issues prior to testing may enhance receipt of information. Nursing assessment includes assessment of
   • Current stressors
   • Past cancer experiences and unresolved grief
   • Risk perception and its related impact (e.g., anxiety, symptom monitoring)
   • Past coping strategies and psychiatric history
   • Access to social and professional supports
   • The client's understanding of how genetic information will affect client and family.
2. Support during the time the client and family are waiting for results.
3. Assessment of immediate reaction to genetic-test results. This includes
   • Identifying and validating feelings
   • Assessing the impact of the results on the client and his or her perception of their impact on family members
   • Being aware of psychosocial or ethical issues that arise regarding third-party notification.
4. Knowing when to refer individuals for psychological counseling
5. Postcounseling follow-up to assess long-term impact.

Cancer-Predisposition Testing: Who Might Benefit?

Consideration of Personal Factors

When deciding whether to pursue cancer-predisposition testing, clients and family members must weigh the options, risks, and benefits in light of each person's unique situation. The decision is a very personal one, and the issues are different for each individual. For example, the cost of testing and reimbursement factors may be issues for some people. Not everyone who has a personal or family history that increases the risk of carrying a genetic mutation wants to know his or her genetic status. For some, however, the uncertainty of not knowing may cause such great anxiety that they are unable to make informed health choices. The physical risks of having a blood sample drawn for genetic assessment are minimal; the real risk is associated with the impact the test results have on the individual.

American Society of Clinical Oncology Guidelines

The American Society of Clinical Oncology (ASCO) (1996) recommended that cancer-predisposition testing be offered only when

• The patient has a strong family history of cancer or very early age of onset of disease (with a 10% or greater probability of having a mutation).
• The test can be adequately interpreted.

197

- The results will influence the medical management of the patient or family member.

For some hereditary cancer syndromes, genetic testing already is considered standard practice. In such cases, testing is offered in accordance with the requirements in the preceding list. These syndromes include multiple endocrine neoplasia (MEN II), von Hippel-Lindau disease, and familial adenomatous polyposis (FAP) (Eng, Hample, & de la Chapell, 2000).

ASCO guidelines cited hereditary breast-ovarian cancer syndrome and hereditary nonpolyposis colorectal cancer (HNPCC) as two hereditary cancer syndromes with high estimated probabilities of mutation detection in an affected family member and gave examples of when to consider predisposition genetic testing for these conditions. There is a greater than 10% probability of a *BRCA* mutation associated with breast-ovarian cancer syndrome in the situations in the list that follows.

- When more than two breast cancer cases and one or more cases of ovarian cancer are diagnosed at any age.
- If sister pairs with two of the following cancers are diagnosed before age 50: two breast cancers, two ovarian cancers, or a breast and an ovarian cancer.

The probability of mutations in *MSH2, MLH1, PMS1,* or *PMS2,* which are associated with HNPCC, is greater than 10% when both of the conditions that follow are met.

- If three individuals, one of whom is the first-degree relative of the other two, are diagnosed with colorectal carcinoma.
- If two generations are affected and one of the cases is diagnosed before age 50.

These two hereditary cancer syndromes are the ones that oncology nurses are most likely to encounter in clinical practice. For more information, refer to professional position statements and keep abreast of subsequent updates. The ASCO position statement is under revision in 2002.

Other Guidelines

Some cancer genetics programs have developed their own clinical guidelines to help to assess the appropriateness of predisposition testing for an individual. The commercial laboratories that perform the tests also may be sources of guidelines stating who might benefit from specific procedures. The examples that follow present situations in which testing may be indicated.

- If a blood relative has undergone predisposition testing and tested positive for a mutation known to be associated with increased cancer risk, the client may benefit from being tested for the same mutation.
- Any man diagnosed with breast cancer may benefit from predisposition genetic testing for *BRCA1* or *BRCA2,* because 5%–20% of men with breast

cancer test positive for *BRCA2*. *BRCA2* also is associated with an increased risk for breast and ovarian cancer in women and prostate cancer in men (Frank, 1998; Richardson, Deffenbaugh, & Frank, 2001; Shih et al., 2002).

Ethnic background also needs to be considered when deciding if testing may be appropriate. More than 2% of Ashkenazi Jews are estimated to carry *BRCA1* and *BRCA2* mutations associated with increased risk for breast, ovarian, and prostate cancers (Strewing et al., 1997).

Mutation-Specific Criteria

Eligibility criteria vary according to mutation. This chapter will not list the criteria but will instead refer to two Web sites essential for healthcare professionals who provide genetic counseling and testing services.

The first site is GeneTests (www.genetests.org), which comprises a directory of laboratories that offer cancer-predisposition testing. GeneTests—which is searchable by specific mutation, disease, or hereditary condition—is a tool for finding laboratories that offer specific tests. Also included on the site is a clinical overview of the diagnosis, management, and genetic counseling of individuals and families with specific inherited disorders.

The second site, PDQ (www.cancer.gov/cancer_information/pdq/), is the National Cancer Institute's comprehensive cancer database designed for patients, the public, and healthcare professionals. In addition to cancer treatment summaries, PDQ now offers genetic information, including a list of genetic professional resources (www.cancer.gov/search/genetics_services).

The Testing of Minors

In general, testing a minor for a specific hereditary disorder or syndrome is discouraged unless testing would result in a clear medical benefit to the child. For example, if someone in the family has tested positive for the *APC* gene, the gene associated with FAP, it is reasonable to test children as young as 10 years old, because scientists have recommended that individuals with FAP begin annual colon surveillance at age 10 (Petersen & Brensinger, 1996). Another example relates to multiple endocrine neoplasia type 2. When this condition is suspected, testing for a mutation in the *RET* gene is recommended because the risk of medullary thyroid cancer is very high and prophylactic thyroidectomy often is done in childhood (Wiesner & Snow, 2001). In other cases, test results would not benefit a child; indeed, they could harm the child if they trigger stigmatization by parents, siblings, or others. Children may be too young to understand the significance of genetic information (Dickens, Pei, & Taylor, 1996). The GeneTests Web site often includes information about whether to test minors for a specific hereditary disorder or syndrome.

Testing Minors for Adult-Onset Disorders

The genetic testing of unaffected minors for adult-onset disorders is controversial. Knowing a child's genetic status affects neither the course of an adult-onset disorder nor its treatment. The usual recommendation is not to test an unaffected minor. When the child reaches maturity, he or she can weigh the risks, benefits, and options of genetic testing and make his or her own decision about whether to pursue it (Gould et al., 1997).

Disclosing Results to Children

Disclosing or not disclosing genetic results to children has the potential for causing negative sequelae. When test results are shared, potential consequences include lowered self- esteem, inability to integrate with peers, parent-child bonding issues, and stigmatization. In situations in which results are not disclosed to children, a climate of secrecy can develop or parents may act in an overprotective manner (Fanos, 1997). The child's cognitive stage and emotional maturity must be considered in all aspects of the genetic testing process.

Considering Psychological and Psychosocial Issues That Affect Minors

The decision whether to test a child or adolescent for a particular hereditary cancer syndrome involves many psychological issues. If parents choose not to have the child undergo genetic testing, the risk is that later the child may have difficulty integrating such information into his or her self-concept. In addition, young children may not be able to understand the difference between being a carrier and being diagnosed with cancer (Fanos, 1997). Even when the medical benefit of knowing a child's or adolescent's genetic status is clear, consider the psychosocial consequences of testing and provide appropriate support to the child and the child's family.

Types of Test Results

The results of predisposition genetic tests generally fall into three major categories: true positive, true negative, and uninformative. The third category, uninformative, is further classified into two subcategories: indeterminate/inconclusive and mutation of uncertain clinical significance. To date, names for the types of test results have not been standardized. Different institutions use different terminology. The paragraphs that follow define some of the terminology used in practice.

- **True positive.** The result produced when a genetic test identifies in a client a germline mutation known to be associated with increased risk for cancer.
- **True negative.** The condition when a known deleterious germline mutation is present in a close blood relative but no mutation is identified in the client. This type of result also is called negative or negative in the presence of a known mutation.
- **Uninformative**
  - Indeterminate/inconclusive. No mutation is identified in the client, and there is no known mutation in the family. Three other terms for this type of result are *negative in the absence of a known mutation, indeterminate negative,* and *uninformative.*
  - Mutation of uncertain clinical significance. A novel mutation is found, but its association with cancer risk is unknown. Other terms for this type of result are *variant of uncertain significance, variant,* and *uncertain result.*

Before an individual is tested, he or she is educated regarding all potential test outcomes and the impact of each result. This usually is conducted in the pretest education and counseling session. If a mutation has not been identified in the family, the client needs to understand that results may be inconclusive. He or she should be able to take the information about potential results into consideration before deciding to commit the psychological energy and pay the financial cost associated with testing. In addition, knowing types of test results in advance may help the client and the nurse to identify issues related to the impact of receiving the results.

Implications of Test Results

Implications of a True Positive Result

A true positive occurs when the test result is positive for a mutation known to be associated with an increased cancer risk or the mutation is known to alter the function of the gene. Receiving a positive test result can have a tremendous emotional impact on some patients. If previously undiagnosed with cancer, they may feel as if they have been told that they have cancer. Initially, the patient may feel shock, disbelief, or anger. Some individuals report that they expected to have a positive result. However, they may have concerns about what to do now that the expectation has been confirmed. What to do about medical management and risk reduction often is of foremost concern. They also may have concerns about telling family members and how they will react. If other family members have been tested, dissimilar results may cause worry about the effect on family relationships. A person may feel guilty about the possibility of having passed a mutation to a child. Others may feel isolated from those who do not understand the feelings associated with learning one's genetic status.

Some clients, however, experience relief when they receive a positive result, because they now know why there is cancer in their families. As a result of the new information, they can make healthcare decisions about increased surveillance, chemoprevention, or prophylactic surgery. A positive result may solidify family relationships and increase support for those testing positive. Identifying cancer and mutation carrier risk for other family members can unify the family in a common cause.

Negative implications of a true positive result
- Anger, depression, fear, or hopelessness
- Guilt for potentially passing the mutation to children
- Worry over possible insurance or workplace discrimination
- Stress on family relationships
- Concern over increased healthcare costs associated with risk-reduction interventions
- Uncertainty about unproven risk-reduction options

Positive implications of a true positive result
- Having the information needed to make medical decisions
- Potential decrease in cancer risk or increase in early cancer detection because of risk-reduction strategies employed
- Reduced feelings of uncertainty or anxiety
- Motivation for positive health behaviors
- Increased support from family and friends

Implications of a True Negative Result

A true negative result occurs in cases in which one or more close blood relatives of the client have a known mutation and the client tests negative for the same mutation. In most cases, individuals receiving true negative results are relieved. Their level of anxiety and cancer worry decreases. The true negative result assures these clients that their cancer risk is not higher than average for the cancers associated with the tested-for mutation. In most cases, a client who receives a true negative result can return to the screening and surveillance levels recommended for the general population. In addition, as a result of testing, these clients have the knowledge that they have not passed the tested-for predisposition gene to offspring.

However, some clients develop a false sense of security about cancer risk related to the negative test result. A true negative result does not mean that the client will not get cancer. The client's cancer risk may still be increased by nongenetic factors, such as lifestyle factors or carcinogen exposure. In addition, the negative result applies to the tested-for mutation or mutations only—the mutation or mutations presumed to be causing cancer in the family. Some other genes associated with increased cancer risk, genes for which the client was not tested, could be present (Gould, Lynch, Smith, & McCarthy, 1997). In some situations, a client's anxiety and cancer worry may not decrease even with a negative test result. Clients may feel insecure in relinquishing heightened cancer surveillance. Furthermore, since a mutation is known to be in the family, the negative result may elicit feelings of survivor's guilt or alienation as a result of no longer sharing a cancer risk that is similar to that of other family members.

Negative implications of a true negative result
- False sense of security about cancer risk
- Surveillance and preventive behaviors may decrease because the client feels a false sense of security.
- Feelings of guilt or alienation if other family members test positive

Positive implications of a true negative result
- Reduced anxiety and cancer worry
- A more accurate description of cancer risk
- Sense of relief as a result of knowing that the tested-for mutation was not passed to offspring

Implications of an Indeterminate Result

A test result is categorized as indeterminate when no mutation is identified in the client and there is no known mutation in the family. This test result, also called negative in the absence of a known mutation, means that the finding is inconclusive because a genetic predisposition to cancer is not ruled out. This result is difficult to interpret and may indicate one of the following scenarios:

- There is no mutation in the family—that is, the cancers in the family are the result of some combination of genetic and environmental factors shared by the family.
- A mutation may exist in the family, but the client has not inherited it.
- The client may be a carrier of a cancer-predisposition gene that is different from the tested-for gene or genes.

- There may be a cancer-predisposition gene in the family—a gene for which testing is not yet available.

To reduce the chance of getting an indeterminate result, it is recommended that family members affected with cancer have testing first. If an affected family member tests negative, the result is still indeterminate or inconclusive. If a mutation is found in the affected family member, the unaffected client can then be tested for the specific mutation found in the family. In cases of indeterminate results, the client sill needs to be considered at risk. The surveillance and risk-reduction options are based on family history and other medical risk factors.

The indeterminate result may leave a client confused and uncertain about the cause of the cancers in his or her family or how to plan for risk-reduction interventions. Cancer worry, anxiety, and powerlessness may continue. Therefore, for clients who receive an indeterminate result, a clear follow-up plan is important.

Negative implications of an indeterminate result
- Disappointment with an inconclusive result
- Other family members do not have an option for testing for known mutation.
- Uncertainty related to medical decision making for cancer-risk reduction
- Confusion about the meaning of the result.

Implications of Receiving a "Mutation of Uncertain Clinical Significance" Result

A mutation of uncertain clinical significance means that the test detected a DNA change or genetic variation, but the variant's association with cancer risk is unknown. That is why this result also is called a variant of uncertain significance. This type of result can occur when a new DNA variation is found but not enough scientific information exists to determine if the variant is associated with an increased cancer risk (Frank, 1998). Mutations of uncertain clinical significance usually are missense mutations or splice-site mutations in an intron. These mutations may affect mRNA splicing. However, at the time of identification, no one knows if the variant causes a functional protein change, making it a deleterious mutation, or if the variant results in a nonfunctional change (i.e., a polymorphism) and is unrelated to cancer risk (Schneider, 2002). Some laboratories will test family members free of charge in an attempt to clarify the meaning of the variant. However, the client and family should be counseled that the process may be lengthy and that future laboratory findings may yield uncertain results.

When a patient receives "a mutation of uncertain clinical significance" test result, he or she may experience disappointment, anxiety, anger, or depression because the test result did not provide the information expected. He or she may feel confused and uncertain about how to make healthcare decisions regarding cancer surveillance and risk reduction. Similar to the options associated with the indeterminate result, the surveillance and risk-reduction options associated with a result of uncertain clinical significance are based on the family history and other medical risk factors.

Negative implications of a result of an uncertain clinical significance
- Uncertainty about the meaning of the result and the client's cancer risk
- Indecision about cancer-risk reduction interventions

Positive implication of a result of uncertain clinical significance
- Further testing of other family members may clarify the mutation associated with cancer risk.

Interpreting Test Results

A positive predisposition genetic test result does not necessarily mean that the client will get cancer, and a negative test result does not mean the client is free from cancer risk. There is no way to predict when or if an unaffected client will be diagnosed with cancer or when or if an affected client will be diagnosed with a different cancer. Predisposition genetic testing sometimes can help us to determine how high the probability is that a client may be diagnosed with a certain cancer or cancers in the future. Even correctly estimating the risk of certain cancers is complicated, however, because the cancer-risk estimates associated with certain mutations are changing as more information becomes available.

If the client received a "mutation of unknown clinical significance" test result, some labs will test the client's family members at no cost, as part of research to determine if the mutation is associated with increased cancer risk. The lab may enter information about the client into a confidential database, which allows the lab to contact the client if information about the client's mutation becomes available in the future. Myriad Genetics Inc., for example, provides extensive follow-up regarding mutations of uncertain clinical significance and maintains a confidential patient-tracking database (S. Manley, personal communication, March 4, 1998).

What to Do After Testing

Predisposition testing is usually a one-time event, but the results of testing can have a lasting impact, especially for people who test positive. Support groups are a typical means of helping people to deal with significant health issues.

Because of the confidential nature of predisposition testing, however, gathering people to help each other deal with the results of predisposition testing may be infeasible. Even if confidentiality is not a concern, the number of individuals needed for a support group may be available only in large metropolitan areas.

People without a previous cancer diagnosis who test positive may be most in need of some type of follow-up psychological support because, at the time they receive genetic test results, they are not receiving support services through a cancer program.

Healthcare providers have much to learn about the psychological and psychosocial follow-up needs of clients after predisposition testing. A focus of research to date has been surveillance needs and the risks and benefits of prophylactic surgery (Burke, Daly, et al., 1997; Burke, Petersen, et al., 1997; Hartmann et al., 1999; Rebbeck et al., 1999; Rebbeck, 2000). A systematic review of research assessing the impact of predictive genetic testing indicates that adverse psychological effects are common after notification of positive genetic test results but that these effects dissipate over time (Shaw, Abrams, & Marteau, 1999). A lack of informative studies about the types of support required and counseling provided to affect emotional outcomes limits current knowledge (Broadstock, Michie, & Marteau, 2000). Oncology nurses have a pivotal role in caring for clients who have received positive genetic test results; consequently, they need to participate in and carry out nursing research studies to learn more about the long-term healthcare needs of people at genetic risk for cancer. What is it like to live with the uncertainty associated with genetic risk for cancer? How can nurses best support these clients as they make decisions based on genetic information? What interventions are most helpful in addressing the emotional issues these clients and their families face?

Cancer Surveillance and Risk Reduction

Increased surveillance may lead to early detection of cancer. Prophylactic surgery may reduce the risk of certain cancers. The Cancer Genetics Studies Consortium, a group sponsored by the National Human Genome Research Institute, has published consensus statements addressing follow-up guidelines for people who carry a *BRCA1* or *BRCA2* alteration and for people diagnosed with hereditary nonpolyposis colon cancer (Burke, Daly, et al., 1997; Burke, Petersen, et al., 1997). The National Comprehensive Cancer Network has published similar recommendations and an accompanying algorithm (Daly, 1999).

For a discussion of cancer surveillance, prophylactic surgery, and chemo-prevention, see Chapter 6.

The Three-Component Counseling Model

Genetic counseling combines the provision of risk information with the provision of psychological and educational support (Nussbaum, McInnes, & Willard, 2001). Many of the clients who seek cancer genetic counseling may not be interested in cancer-predisposition testing. Some clients are referred for cancer-predisposition testing but, after the genetic assessment, decide against testing because they learn that it will not provide the answers they want or may not alter management or screening behaviors. Others may decide against genetic testing because of insurance discrimination, psychosocial and family concerns, or other issues.

The content of genetic counseling varies according to the needs of the client, the outcome of the cancer-risk assessment, and whether the client decides to pursue genetic testing. When genetic testing is involved, more than one genetic counseling session is needed. Many issues must be addressed in pretest and posttest counseling sessions (McKinnon et al., 1997). Accomplishing all the tasks included in each component may involve three or more sessions.

Component 1: Cancer-Risk Assessment

The purpose of the first session or sessions is risk assessment. In these sessions,

- Determine why the client is seeking risk counseling and if it will meet his or her needs.
- Obtain the client's health history.
- Document current health status, including lifestyle issues. Assess dietary, hormonal, environmental, and other cancer-risk factors.
- Obtain the client's family medical history.
- Construct a three- to four-generation pedigree; revise it as necessary in assessment sessions. Begin the process of obtaining pathology reports and other documentation.
- Assess and communicate
  - The client's risk of being diagnosed with the cancer or cancers of concern
  - The client's probability of having a cancer-predisposing mutation associated with the particular cancer or cancers in the client's family.
- Discuss the psychosocial issues associated with predisposition testing, including family impact.

- Perform a psychosocial assessment.
- Explain autosomal-dominant patterns of inheritance and the difference between germline and sporadic mutations.
- Discuss the confidentiality of genetic information.
- Provide information about the alternatives to predisposition testing, such as DNA banking or risk-management options.
- Discuss the risks and benefits of cancer-predisposition testing.
- Give the client handouts to reinforce information presented in the counseling session.

Figure 7-1 lists Web sites that contain educational materials. If the client decides to proceed with genetic testing, he or she moves on to Component 2.

Component 2: Pretest Education and Counseling

Component 2, pretest education and counseling, consists of the tasks involved in obtaining an informed consent for genetic testing and drawing the blood necessary for testing. (Informed consent is discussed in detail later in this chapter.) To accomplish these tasks,

- Answer the client's questions; address the client's concerns.
- Ensure that the client understands the potential risks and benefits of cancer-predisposition testing.
- Offer psychological support.
- Discuss
    - The type of genetic test and its cost and accuracy, how it will be performed, and potential test results
    - Specific information regarding institution policies related to the storage and release of test results
    - Who will provide medical follow-up to the client after test results have been received
    - Guidance regarding disclosure of test results to his or her healthcare providers, including suggestions about broaching the subject and the handling of the information in the medical record
    - Disclosing test results to family members and/or friends
    - The importance of notifying at-risk family members if a mutation is identified and sensitive approaches to notification.
- Invite the client to bring a companion to the results-disclosure visit.
- Review the format of the results-disclosure visit.
- Review the consent form with the client.
- Obtain written informed consent for predisposition testing.
- Have blood drawn, ensuring appropriate labeling, and send the blood to the lab.

Figure 7-1. Cancer Genetics Web Resources

American Society of Clinical Oncology (ASCO)
www.asco.org
Offers ASCO's cancer genetics curriculum slides and speakers notes, and ONCOCEP, a self-education module on cancer genetics, released November 2000. Both excellent programs are available for a fee. Select Shopping Cart to see descriptions of these and other products.

Breast Cancer in Men
http://interact.withus.com/interact/mbc
Provides information and resources concerning male breast cancer, including information about hereditary factors associated with male breast cancer.

CancerNet
http://cancernet.nci.nih.gov/prevention/genetics.shtml
Offers genetics-related pamphlets that can be downloaded. Also available for downloading are articles such as "Cancer Genetics Overview," "Elements of Cancer Genetics Risk Assessment and Counseling," and "Genetics of Colorectal Cancer."

FORCE
www.facingourrisk.org
Provides information for women at high risk for breast or ovarian cancer. In the "Ask the Experts" section, a site user can pose a question to a physician-specialist. This Web site is produced by Facing Our Risk of Cancer Empowered (FORCE).

Gail Breast Cancer Risk Assessment Program
http://bcra.nci.nih.gov/brc
Offers the Gail-model risk-assessment program online. The program calculates breast cancer risk.

GeneTests
www.genetests.org
Provides a directory of medical genetics laboratories, including laboratories that offer predisposition cancer genetic testing. The site—which is searchable by specific mutation, disease, or hereditary condition—tells which laboratories offer a particular test. It also gives a clinical overview of the diagnosis, management, and genetic counseling of individuals and families with specific inherited disorders.

National Cancer Institute Information Page
www.cancer.gov
Includes information about cancer, cancer treatment, and clinical trials. Also includes information about hereditary types of cancer, the contribution of genetics to cancer risk, and a list of professional resources in regard to genetics.

Genetic Alliance
www.geneticalliance.org
Offers information about specific diseases (including cancer) as well as support groups for people affected by genetic conditions. Genetic Alliance is an international coalition of individuals, professionals, and genetic support organizations working together to promote healthy lives for everyone affected by genetic disorders.

(Continued on next page)

Figure 7-1. Cancer Genetics Web Resources (Continued)

Genetics Education Center
www.kumc.edu/gec
Provides a variety of resources for educators, at all undergraduate levels, who are interested in teaching basic genetics.

Genetics Professionals Directory
www.cancernet.nci.nih.gov/genesrch.shtml
Comprises the National Cancer Institute database of cancer genetics service providers in the United States.

Glossary of Genetic Terms
www.nhgri.nih.gov/DIR/VIP/Glossary/pub_glossary.cgi
Provides the National Institute of Health's Glossary of Genetic Terms

International Society of Nurses in Genetics
http://nursing.creighton.edu/isong
Contains information about educational opportunities and links to other genetics-related Web sites.

Component 3: Post-Test Counseling

The purpose of component 3, post-test counseling, is to disclose the results of the predisposition test. In this component,

- Allow the client to process the information and assess his or her responses.
- Address the client's concerns.
- Discuss
  - What the test results may mean in relation to the client's own cancer risk and the risk of family members
  - Psychosocial issues
  - Family concerns.
- Review medical follow-up recommendations; present a cancer-surveillance and risk-reduction plan (see Figure 7-2).
- Inform the client of any follow-up telephone calls or letters he or she may receive after the session.
- Discuss available resources for additional information, psychological support or counseling, and follow-up.

Tips for Information Delivery

A great deal of information must be conveyed in cancer genetic counseling visits. A number of resources can help with this task.

Figure 7-2. Components of a Cancer-Surveillance and Risk-Reduction Plan

---

In regard to all common and unusual cancers for which the client may be at increased risk, ensure that the client knows
- Recommended frequency of suggested cancer-screening tests
- Recommended frequency of examinations by a healthcare provider
- Potential risks and benefits of chemoprevention and prophylactic surgery
- Information about lifestyle, dietary, and environmental factors known to increase cancer risk
- Any follow-up recommendations regarding additional clinic visits or referrals to outside programs or healthcare providers.

Note. From "Cancer Genetics Nursing Practice: Impact of the Double Helix" by K. Greco, 2000, *Oncology Nursing Forum, 27*(Suppl. 9), pp. 29–33. Copyright 2000 by the Oncology Nursing Society. Adapted with permission.

Information Packets

Many programs or clinics that provide cancer genetic services have prepared information packets that can be sent to people who inquire about services. In many cases, these packets
- Tell the client what information he or she will be expected to provide as part of the counseling process.
- Describe the type of information and services the client can expect to receive.
- Include a brochure describing the program or clinic's services.
- Provide other relevant educational brochures related to cancer-risk assessment and genetic testing.

Prospective clients receive information packets by mail after they call to ask about counseling or an appointment. The information can help them to decide if cancer-risk assessment and counseling is right for them. By answering initial questions before the session, the packet can save much time during the session.

Visual Aids

Handouts that summarize and illustrate session content are particularly helpful in the context of cancer-risk assessment and counseling, which deals with complex issues. The client can read the materials after the sessions to resolve any confusion that may develop.

Videos can be a helpful way of introducing information. See Figure 7-3 for a list of videos and other titles related to cancer genetic counseling. Interactive computer programs also are effective learning aids.

Small-Group Classes

Some programs offer small-group classes, lasting an hour or two, in which an oncology nurse or genetic counselor provides basic information about the genet-

Figure 7-3. Genetics Education Resources for Individuals and Families

Videos About Genetics and the Human Genome Project, Available Through the Oak Ridge National Laboratory Web Site
See www.ornl.gov/hgmis/education/videos.html#suppliers for a list of titles, prices, and ordering information. Titles include
Banking Our Genes
Gene Blues: Dilemmas of DNA Testing
Deadly Inheritance
The Burden of Knowledge
A Question of Genes: Inherited Risks
Patterns of Inheritance: Understanding Genetics
Heredity and Mutation

Video and Booklet From the National Cancer Institute (NCI)
See https://cissecure.nci.nih.gov/ncipubs for information about *Genetic Testing for Breast Cancer Risk: It's Your Choice,* a video and booklet for clients. Both are free of charge.

Printed Materials From NCI
See https://cissecure.nci.nih.gov/ncipubs for a list of printed educational materials that can be ordered free of charge. Titles include
Genetic Testing for Breast Cancer Risk: It's Your Choice
Understanding Gene Testing (a downloadable version is available at www.accessexcellence.org/AE/AEPC/NIH/index.html)

Online Tutorials From NCI
See http://newscenter.cancer.gov/sciencebehind for access to titles such as
Understanding Estrogen Receptors, Tamoxifen and Raloxifene
Understanding Cancer
Understanding Gene Testing

Note. Copyright © 2001 by Karen Greco, RN, MN, ANP. Reprinted with permission.

ics of cancer, hereditary and other risk factors, and risk-reduction and surveillance options. For many people, this type of setting allows them to obtain information and ask questions in a nonthreatening environment before deciding if they want to schedule an appointment. The limitations of group discussion include the possibility that the client will be embarrassed to speak in a group; the possibility that some disclosure, by the leader or client, could compromise confidentiality; and the possibility that individual needs are not met (Gellar et al., 1997).

Ethical and Legal Issues

Informed Consent

Informed consent involves more than having a client sign a consent form. It involves the interaction of healthcare providers and clients in making healthcare decisions. Informed consent is the willing acceptance of a medical intervention by a client after adequate disclosure by the healthcare provider of the nature of the intervention and its risks and benefits, as well as discussion of alternatives and their risks and benefits (Jonsen, Seigler, & Winslade, 1992).

As healthcare professionals, nurses must give clients sufficient information to enable them to make informed decisions. To do that, nurses must be sufficiently informed regarding genetics or know how to obtain the necessary information (Gellar et al., 1997). Obtaining informed consent can be viewed as an event model or a process model (Rieger & Pentz, 1999).

The Event Model of Informed Consent

In the event model, the nurse presents the client with several options from which to choose. The medical professional usually indicates what he or she thinks is in the client's best interest, and the client has the opportunity to agree or disagree. The event model documents informed consent through the completion of a written consent form that summarizes the medical intervention that has been proposed verbally by the healthcare provider. This model is limited in that it takes place in a single point in time. People seldom make complicated decisions in one sitting.

The Process Model of Informed Consent

The process model of informed consent assumes a relationship with the healthcare provider in which decision making is approached as a multistep process shared over time. Integral to informed, shared decision making is the entire education and counseling process that occurs when a client faces a complicated decision, such as whether to pursue predisposition testing. The decision must be consistent with the client's values and needs. The client must have time to reach and then rethink his or her decision (Gellar et al., 1997).

The practice of obtaining signed authorization is often equated with informed consent. The broader view of informed decision making, however, includes greater involvement of clients in clinical decision making. Braddock, Finn, Levinson, Jonsen, and Pearlman (1997) advocated a process model that included the six steps shown in Figure 7-4. This model can be used to support the client in making healthcare decisions that are informed. According to Gellar et al. (1995), the informed consent process must include both an educational component and a decision-making component. The decision-making component should explore the client's understanding, perceptions of barriers to testing, and reasons for and against testing.

Figure 7-4. Elements of Informed Decision Making

1. Discussion of the clinical issue and nature of the decision to be made
2. Discussion of the alternatives
3. Discussion of the pros (or benefits) and cons (or risks) of the alternatives
4. Discussion of the uncertainties associated with the decision
5. Assessment of client's understanding
6. Asking the client to express a preference

Note. From "How Doctors and Clients Discuss Routine Clinical Decisions," by C.H. Braddock, S. Finn, W. Levinson, A.R. Jonsen, and R.A. Pearlman, 1997, *Journal of General Internal Medicine, 12,* p. 340. Copyright 1997 by Blackwell Science. Reprinted with permission.

Braddock, Edwards, Hasenberg, Laidley, and Levinson (1999) studied informed decision making in outpatient practice. They devised a cross-sectional study in which they audiotaped 1,057 physician-patient interactions. Only 9% of the decisions reached in the taped interactions met researchers' criteria for completeness in informed decision making. Of the elements of informed decision making that the researchers did find, discussion of the nature of the intervention occurred most frequently (71%). Assessment of the patient's understanding occurred least frequently (1.5%).

Informed Consent for Predisposition Testing

In the informed decision-making model and according to Dickens et al. (1996), ensuring informed consent for predisposition testing means providing enough information about the risks associated with accepting, rejecting, or postponing predisposition testing to enable the client to decide whether to proceed with testing. This information must address the risks and benefits of genetic information as it applies to family members as well as the client. Alternatives to genetic testing, such as DNA banking and increased surveillance, also must be discussed.

According to Gellar et al. (1997) and Rieger and Pentz (1999), the process of obtaining informed consent should include discussion of the purpose of the test and the practical aspects of the testing, such as the amount of blood to be drawn; cost; time for results to become available; accuracy of the test; range of possible results; the privacy of genetic information; how results will be communicated; and who will answer questions. Clients must understand interpretation of results and what each potential result might mean. Discussion also should include psychosocial implications and the potential for insurance risk or employment discrimination. Clients need to know how their genetic information will be kept confidential and that additional testing will not be performed without informed consent. They should be aware of their options for medical follow-up.

The PARQ Method

A standard method of obtaining informed consent and documenting the medical record is to use the procedure, alternatives, risks, and questions (PARQ) method (Oregon Medical Association, 1996).

- **Procedure:** Explain the procedure.
- **Alternatives:** State the alternatives.
- **Risks:** State the risks of the procedure and the alternatives.
- **Questions:** Ask if the client wants more detailed information about the procedure, alternatives, or risks. In some states, such as Oregon, just asking the client if he or she has questions is not enough; the counselor must follow a specific procedure and document that the client has received information. Know the laws and guidelines that pertain to your state.

It is important that a professional, not support personnel, lead the discussion relating to informed consent.

The most common method of presenting information about a medical intervention is through one-on-one discussion. See Tips for Information Delivery, earlier in this chapter, for other ideas.

Documentation Regarding Informed Consent

When cancer-predisposition testing is involved, the medical record must contain documentation that shows that all components of the informed consent process were covered. Such documentation must list the specific content discussed, include an evaluation of the client's understanding of the issues, and be accompanied by appropriate signed consent forms.

Some counselors use the categories outlined in the PARQ method to structure documentation of the informed consent process. These counselor's records contain appropriate notations after each of the following statements.

- The procedure for the predisposition testing process was explained to the client.
- The alternatives to predisposition testing were discussed.
- Note the alternatives to testing discussed with the client.
- The potential risks associated with the specific predisposition test were discussed.

Document whether the client was asked about additional information needs. State the information, if any, that the client requested and whether he or she received it (Oregon Medical Association, 1996). Give the client a copy of the signed consent form that outlines potential risks.

Requests for Nondocumentation

Another problem arises when a client does not want genetic-testing information in his or her medical record because the client wants to protect him- or herself or a family member. The client may, however, want the healthcare provider to increase the frequency of physical examinations or order certain cancer-screening tests based on the genetic test results. Suppose, for example, that a client who carries a *BRCA1* mutation but has no family history of ovarian cancer asks the provider to order screening tests for ovarian cancer based on genetic information the client does not want documented. Will the provider be acting contrary to medical standards of practice by ordering screening tests in the absence of a documented medical need? Also, how can the genetic information be truly private when surveillance behavior has changed based on this information? Most risk-management strategies can be accomplished without documentation of gene status, based on family history alone. Educate and counsel clients who request nondocumentation about the risks and benefits of full disclosure versus privacy so that they can advocate for themselves.

Release of Information to a Third Party

Given the sensitivity of genetic information, clients need to know, during the informed-consent process, the specifics of how their genetic information and DNA test results will be handled. Assure clients that genetic information will not be released to any third party. Most genetic counseling programs require a specific written consent to release information about genetic predisposition. Such a consent specifies to whom genetic-test results can be released.

General Consent Versus Specific Consent to Release Information

Standard hospital or outpatient forms often contain a general release-of-information clause, which—with the client's written consent—allows the release of most medical information to the referring primary care provider or to the client's insurance company for billing purposes. Because the release of genetic information increases the risk of genetic discrimination against the client and his or her family, many genetics programs require clients to provide specific written informed consent before releasing genetic information about the client. Specific written informed consent helps ensure that program staff have a precise understanding of the client's wishes, and it helps protect the program from an unintended release of genetic information. A general release of information can apply to a broad category of information over a period of time without specifically naming the information to be released. Specific informed consent is much more precise about naming the information to be released, specifically to whom and what restrictions apply. Specific written consent is required in many states before the release of all sensitive medical information, such as information about a client's history of HIV or AIDS, mental conditions, or substance abuse. In many states, genetic information has been added to this category of sensitive information. Laws about specific written consent change frequently, so healthcare professionals need to stay up-to-date on these laws.

Release of Information to the Primary Healthcare Provider

Genetic information should not be released to the primary healthcare provider without the client's written informed consent, even if that provider referred the client for cancer-risk counseling and testing.

If the client chooses not to release cancer-predisposition test results to the healthcare provider, the provider may have a problem ordering appropriate cancer-surveillance tests for the client. When genetic information about a client or a client's family members is inaccessible to the healthcare provider, the provider is denied information necessary for client assessment (Dickens et al., 1996). It is best to discuss with clients, prior to testing, whether they intend to release the genetic test results to their healthcare providers and the potential implications of their decision.

Challenges to Confidentiality

Insurance Companies

Most insurance companies require preauthorization for genetic counseling and testing. This involves informing the insurance company why services are needed and including certain medical information about the cancer history of the client and his or her family. Many insurers will ask for a letter of medical necessity prior to approval. These letters should be concise, include the rationale for the specific genetic test and the syndrome diagnosis, and contain only the information about the client and family history that the insurer needs to make a coverage decision. Strip pedigrees of all labels that identify family members other than the insured individual. Include or offer as an addendum information from the scientific literature regarding the justification for testing, and provide references. See Shappell and Matloff (2001) and Bombard (2002) for examples of letters and medical necessity.

Unintentional Disclosures From the Medical Record

The greatest threat to confidentiality and the client's privacy may be from unintentional disclosures of genetic information from the medical records. Suppose, for example, that a pathologist dictates a report stating that the reason for prophylactic surgery was a positive genetic test. The pathologist, unintentionally, has disclosed confidential information without authorization from the client. Another example of an unintentional exposure is when genetic test results in the medical record are unintentionally copied along with other laboratory results and sent either to another healthcare provider or to an insurance company in the absence of a specific release regarding genetic information.

Record Storage

Record storage can be a legal issue in the sense that the way records are stored can affect confidentiality.

The Client's Records

In clinical practice in genetics, whether information related to genetic counseling and cancer predisposition testing should be kept separate from the regular medical record is not always clear. The decision may depend on the practice setting, how medical records currently are handled, and state and federal laws regulating the privacy of genetic information.

In some settings, material is kept separate, and administrators must decide where to keep it and how to document its existence. For example, if a client registers for an outpatient visit when receiving genetic services, one option is to put a special code into the computer to indicate the existence of a separate medical record. Medical records department staff then store these separate medical records in a locked room to which only genetics staff had access, to protect against accidental disclosure of genetic information when copying medical records.

If genetic information is kept with the regular medical record, confidentiality issues must be addressed. In a medical office where a client receives genetic counseling and predisposition testing in addition to other clinical services, maintaining a separate medical record may be difficult, and the chance of an accidental leak of information exists. Office staff must be educated regarding the highly confidential nature of genetic information. They must understand that a general consent for release of information may be inadequate, especially when the release is to a third party. They must understand the ways in which genetic information can inadvertently be released so they can avoid any releases without the client's specific written informed consent.

Secondary Records

The need to store medical records from other sources and about people other than the client creates problems for the staff of genetic counseling programs. Such records, called secondary records, should be stored in a way that ensures that they never are released to a third party, even with written informed consent. A third party must go to the original source to obtain secondary records.

Documents Usually Found in a Cancer Genetics Medical Record

The list that follows shows the information that usually is a part of a medical record in a cancer genetics facility. Most of this information usually is conveyed by means of forms. Whether all these documents are stored in the same location is a matter of institution policy.

- **Intake form:** An intake form contains basic information about the client and why he or she is requesting or being referred for genetic counseling.
- **Progress notes:** Progress notes are standard in all medical records. Because genetic counseling services often are multidisciplinary, a progress record that can be used by all team members may be the most useful.
- **Cancer risk and genetic risk assessment:** This may consist of a single assessment or multiple assessments, depending on who sees the client. Components include a summary of the medical and family history; clinical, genetic, hereditary, and nonhereditary risk factors; and psychosocial assessment.
- **Pedigree:** All charts should contain a pedigree, or diagram of the family history that employs standard symbols to represent family members, their relationships, who has been affected by cancer or other illnesses, and who is living. The pedigree must be as complete as possible and include at least three generations. The pedigree should be dated.
- **Client and family medical records:** Documentation of the client's personal and family history of cancer is important when interpreting the pedigree and assessing cancer risk. For this reason, the chart may contain a number of pathology reports and medical records, obtained from other sources, pertaining to the client or family members.
- **Copy of the summary letter:** Summary letters usually cite who was present during the assessment, the client's purpose for seeking genetic counseling, what information was exchanged, a summary of the cancer-risk assessment, and what the client decided to do as a result of genetic counseling. Consider stamping the letter "Confidential" and "Not for Redistribution." These stamps highlight the sensitivity of the information.
- **Consent forms:** The record should include all applicable consent forms, including forms that authorize predisposition testing and those that authorize the release of information to a third party. A lab may require that its own consent form for predisposition testing is completed in addition to the form required by the cancer genetics program.

- **Documentation about client education:** The record should contain documentation of the client education offered as well as the client's understanding of the information presented. Standard forms or flow sheets can be used for information that is routinely included in the education session; the counselor initials each category after it is completed. The flow sheet should allow documentation of the method used for information delivery and the method for evaluating the client's understanding. A more detailed outline of information routinely covered under each category can be part of a separate document, perhaps the institution policy about filling out the flow sheet. Because each client has unique education needs, cite exceptions to the standard of practice in the progress notes.

- **Lab and diagnostic test results:** The record should contain all documents regarding blood work, the results of cancer-screening tests used to assess risks, and cancer-predisposition testing.

- **Follow-up:** If a cancer genetics program is providing long-term follow-up, any testing related to maintenance of screening exams is necessary.

> Documentation of risk assessment and counseling includes
> - Intake form
> - Cancer risk and genetic-risk assessment
> - Family history and pedigree
> - The client's and family's medical records for cancer verification
> - Documentation of patient education
> - Consent forms
> - Summary letter regarding risk assessment, cancer-screening results, cancer-predisposition testing results, and medical management recommendations
> - Progress notes regarding patient contacts or clinical evaluation and follow-up.

Summary

Genetic information has implications for the entire family, not just the client. The predictive nature of genetic information may alter an individual's concept of his or her health, even if they are asymptomatic. Genetic information is permanent in that, with current technology, it cannot be changed. Genetic information can have long-term consequences for clients and their families. Health decisions are based on this information, and family relationships can be affected. Cancer-predisposition DNA testing does not provide definitive answers but can aid in risk management and decision making. Although a predisposition to cancer is not a diagnosis, insurance companies may discriminate and treat it as a preexisting condition. This can cause an individual to feel as if he or she had a disease or were "marked" in some way, even though they never may be diagnosed with cancer. Clients may be in the unique category of carrying a mutation but not being diagnosed with a disease, which can lead to feelings of isolation.

Handling of genetic information is regulated by both state and federal laws. Issues relating to confidentiality and informed decision making are held to a very high standard of care that oncology nurses must meet. Oncology nurses who provide genetic counseling and education must be guided by ethical principles and have the knowledge and skills to address the complex issues involved in providing genetic counseling, predisposition genetic testing, and education regarding genetic information.

References

American Society of Clinical Oncology. (1996). Statement of the American Society of Clinical Oncology: Genetic testing for cancer susceptibility. *Journal of Clinical Oncology, 14*, 1730–1736.

Berner, S. (1996). Federal protection of genetic information: Congress delivers. *Journal of Women's Health, 5*, 409–410.

Bernhardt, B.A., Geller, G., Doksum, T., & Metz, S.A. (2000). Evaluation of nurses and genetic counselors as providers of education about breast cancer susceptibility testing. *Oncology Nursing Forum, 27*, 33–39.

Bombard, A. (2002). Insurance justification letters [Letter to the editor]. *Journal of Genetic Counseling, 11*, 75.

Botkin, J., Croyle, R., Smith, K., Baty, B., Lerman, C., Goldgar, D., Ward, J., Flick, B., & Nash, J. (1996). A model protocol for evaluation of the behavioral and psychosocial effects of BRCA1 testing. *Journal of the National Cancer Institute, 88*, 872–882.

Bowen, D., McTiernan, A., Burke, W., Powers, D., Pruski, J., Durfy, S., Gralow, J., & Malone, K. (1999). Participation in breast cancer risk counseling among women with a family history. *Cancer Epidemiology, Biomarkers and Prevention, 8*, 581–585.

Braddock, C.H., Edwards, K.A., Hasenberg, N.M., Laidley, T.L., & Levinson, W. (1999). Informed decision making in outpatient practice: Time to get back to basics. *JAMA, 282*, 2313–2320.

Braddock, C.H., Finn, S., Levinson, W., Jonsen, A.R., & Pearlman, R.A. (1997). How doctors and clients discuss routine clinical decisions. *Journal of General Internal Medicine, 12*, 339–345.

Broadstock, M., Michie, S., & Marteau, T. (2000). Psychological consequences of predictive genetic testing: A systematic review. *European Journal of Human Genetics, 8*, 731–738.

Burke, W., Culver, J.O., Bowen, D., Lowry, D., Durfy, S., McTiernan, A., et al. (2000). Genetic counseling for women with an intermediate family history of breast cancer. *American Journal of Medical Genetics, 90*, 361–368.

Burke, W., Daly, M., Garber, J., Botkin, J., Kahn, M., Lynch, P., et al. (1997). Recommendations for follow-up care of individuals with an inherited predisposition to cancer: BRCA1 and BRCA2. Cancer Genetics Studies Consortium. *JAMA, 227*, 997–1003.

Burke, W., Petersen, G., Lynch, P., Botkin, J., Daly, M., Garber, J., et al. (1997). Recommendations for follow-up care of individuals with an inherited predisposition to cancer: Hereditary nonpolyposis colon cancer. Cancer Genetics Studies Consortium. *JAMA, 227*, 915–919.

Burke, W., Pinsky, L.E., & Press, N.A. (2001). Categorizing genetics tests to identify their ethical, legal, and social implications. *American Journal of Medical Genetics, 103*, 233–240.

Croyle, R., Smith, K., Botkin, J., Baty, B., & Nash, J. (1997). Psychological responses to BRCA1 mutation testing: Preliminary findings. *Health Psychology, 16*(1), 63–72.

Daly, M. (1999). NCCN Practice Guidelines: Genetics/familial high risk cancer screening. *Oncology, 13*, 161–184.

Dickens, B., Pei, N., & Taylor, K. (1996). Legal and ethical issues in genetic testing and counseling for susceptibility to breast, ovarian, and colon cancer. *Canadian Medical Association Journal, 154*, 813–818.

Eng, C., Hample, H., & de la Chapell, A. (2000). Genetic testing for cancer predisposition. *Annual Review of Medicine, 52*, 371–400.

Fanos, J. (1997). Developmental tasks of childhood and adolescence: Implications for genetic testing. *American Journal of Medical Genetics, 71*, 22–28.

Forbes, N. (1996). The nurse and genetic counseling. *Nursing Clinics of North America, 1*, 679–688.

Forsman, I. (1994). Evolution of the nursing role in genetics. *Journal of Obstetric, Gynecologic, and Neonatal Nursing, 23*, 481–486.

Frank, T. (1998). Hereditary risk of breast and ovarian carcinoma: The role of the oncologist. *The Oncologist, 3*, 403–412.

Gellar, G., Bernhardt, B.A., Helzlsouer, K., Holtzman, N.A., Stefanek, M., & Wilcox, P.M. (1995). Informed consent and BRCA1 testing. *Nature Genetics, 11*, 364.

Gellar, G., Botkin, J., Green, M., Press, N., Biesecker, B., Wilfond, B., et al. (1997). Genetic testing for susceptibility to adult-onset cancer: The process and content of informed consent. *JAMA, 227*, 1467–1474.

Gould, R., Lynch, H., Smith, R., & McCarthy, J. (1997). *Cancer and genetics:*

Answering your clients' questions. Huntington, NY: PRR, Inc.

Hartmann, L.C., Schaid, D.J., Woods, J.E., Crotty, T.P., Myers, J.L., Arnold, P.G., et al. (1999). Efficacy of bilateral prophylactic mastectomy in women with a family history of breast cancer. *New England Journal of Medicine, 340,* 77–84.

Jacobs, L.A. (1998). At-risk for cancer: Genetic discrimination in the workplace. *Oncology Nursing Forum, 25,* 475–480.

Jonsen, A., Seigler, M., & Winslade, W. (1992). *Clinical ethics.* New York: McGraw-Hill.

Lerman, C., Daly, M., Masny, A., & Balshem, A. (1994). Attitudes about genetic testing for breast-ovarian cancer susceptibility. *Journal of Clinical Oncology, 12,* 843–850.

Lerman, C., Narod, S., Schulman, K., Hughes, C., Hornez-Caminero, G., Bonney, G., et al. (1996). BRCA1 testing in families with hereditary breast-ovarian cancer. *JAMA, 275,* 1885–1892.

Lerman, C., Seay, J., Balshem, A., & Audrain, J. (1995). Interest in genetic testing among first-degree relatives of breast cancer clients. *American Journal of Medical Genetics, 57,* 385–392.

Leung, W.C. (2000). Results of genetic testing: When confidentiality conflicts with a duty to warn relatives. *BMJ, 321,* 1464–1466.

McKinnon, W.C., Baty, B.J., Bennett, R.L., Magee, M., Neufeld-Kaiser, W.A., Peters, K.F., et al. (1997). Predisposition genetic testing for late-onset disorders in adults: A position paper of the National Society of Genetic Counselors. *JAMA, 278,* 1217–1220.

Nussbaum, R., McInnes, R., & Willard, H. (2001). Thompson & Thompson genetics in medicine (6th ed.). Philadelphia: Saunders.

Oregon Medical Association. (1996). *Oregon legal handbook.* Portland, OR: Author.

Patterson, P. (1967). *An interview survey to ascertain common concerns among mothers regarding hereditary disease in their families.* Unpublished master's thesis, University of Washington, Seattle.

Peters, J. (1994). Breast cancer risk counseling. *The Genetic Resource, 8*(1), 20–25.

Petersen, G., & Brensinger, J. (1996). Genetic testing and counseling in familial adenomatous polyposis. *Oncology, 10,* 89–94.

Prouser, N. (2000). Case report: Genetic susceptibility testing for breast and ovarian cancer—A client's perspective. *Journal of Genetic Counseling, 9*(2), 153–159.

Rebbeck, T.R. (2000). Prophylactic oophorectomy in BRCA1 and BRCA2 mutation carriers. *Journal of Clinical Oncology, 18*(Suppl. 21), 100S–103S.

Rebbeck, T.R., Levin, A.M., Eisen, A., Snyder, C., Watson, P., Cannon-Albright,

L., et al. (1999). Breast cancer risk after bilateral prophylactic oophorectomy in BRCA1 mutation carriers. *Journal of the National Cancer Institute, 91*, 1475–1479.

Richardson, C., Deffenbaugh, A., & Frank, T. (2001). Genetic analysis of *BRCA1* and *BRCA2* in 100 males with breast cancer. Abstract presented at the annual meeting of the *American Journal of Human Genetics*, San Diego, CA.

Rieger, P.T., & Pentz, R.D. (1999). Genetic testing and informed consent. *Seminars in Oncology Nursing, 15*(2), 104–115.

Schneider, K. (2002). *Counseling about cancer: Strategies for genetic counseling* (2nd ed.). New York: Wiley-Liss.

Severin, M. (1999). Genetic susceptibility for specific cancers: Medical liability for the clinician. *Cancer Supplement, 86*, 2564–2569.

Shappell, H., & Matloff, E. (2001). Writing effective insurance justification letters for cancer genetic testing: A streamlined approach. *Journal of Genetic Counseling, 10*, 331–341.

Shaw, C., Abrams, K., & Marteau, T. (1999). Psychological impact of predicting individuals' risks of illness: A systematic review. *Social Science & Medicine, 49*, 1571–1598.

Shih, H., Couch, F., Nathanson, K., Blackwood, M., Rebbeck, T., Armstrong, K., et al. (2002). BRCA1 and BRCA2 mutation frequency in women evaluated in a breast cancer risk evaluation clinic. *Journal of Clinical Oncology, 20*, 994–999.

Strewing, J., Hartge, P., Wacholder, S., Baker, S., Berlin, M., McAdams, M., Timmerman, M., Brody, L., & Tucker, M. (1997). The risk of cancer associated with specific mutations of BRCA1 and BRCA2 among Ashkenazi Jews. *New England Journal of Medicine, 336*, 1401–1408.

Tessare, I., Borstelmann, N., Regan, K., Rimer, B., & Winer, E. (1997). Genetic testing for susceptibility to breast cancer: Findings from women's focus groups. *Journal of Women's Health, 6*, 317–327.

Vernon, S., Perz, C., Gritz, E., Peterson, S., Amos, C., Baile, W., & Lynch P. (1997). Correlates of psychologic distress in colorectal cancer clients undergoing genetic testing for hereditary colon cancer. *Health Psychology, 16*(1), 73–86.

Wiesner, G.L., & Snow, K. (2001). Multiple endocrine neoplasia type 2. Retrieved October 22, 2001 from http://www.geneclinics.org

8

Establishing a Cancer Genetics Clinic

Eileen Dimond, RN, MS

Introduction

Cancer-risk assessment has traditionally been part of oncology nursing practice, with the major purpose of individualizing information about personal, biologic, and environmental risk factors related to the development of cancer. Based on these risk factors, individuals receive counseling about the likelihood of developing cancer and they receive information comparing their risk to that of other groups or the general population. In addition, they receive recommendations about medical management (Mahon, 2000). With the advances in the Human Genome Project, genetic risk has been introduced as a major component in comprehensive cancer-risk assessment. The emergence of cancer genetic clinics (CGCs) nationwide has brought cancer-risk assessment to a new level. These programs are integrating information derived from the discovery of numerous inherited cancer-predisposition genes and findings in the area of chemoprevention, prophylactic surgery, and other risk-reduction strategies. Although this chapter focuses on the newer aspects of developing a CGC, the framework of comprehensive risk assessment should not be overlooked in the overall clinical plan.

Cancer Genetics Clinic Clientele

Clients who have a family history indicative of an inherited genetic cancer syndrome may seek out the services of a CGC to obtain information about cancer risk or determine if they possess an abnormal cancer gene. Inherited transmission, however, currently accounts for 5%–10%, at most, of all cancers diagnosed (Fearon, 1997). Other individuals without a family history of cancer may have a personal cancer history that raises suspicion because of early age of diagnosis, bilateral disease, or the presence of synchronous or metachronous tumors (Fraser, Calzone, & Goldstein, 1997). These patients also may seek out CGC services. Still others may turn to a CGC because they have read in the newspaper or seen a report on television about a cancer predisposition gene that raised their personal suspicion, and they simply need to speak to a knowledgeable professional regarding their cancer risk. Thus, not only *real*, but also *perceived* risk bring clients into a CGC.

Current and Future Focus of Cancer Genetics Clinics

Predisposition testing for cancer-susceptibility mutations and cancer-risk assessment are the primary foci of CGCs. As genetic research continues, future CGCs will have an increasingly broader mandate that will extend beyond just identifying the individual at risk. In the future, CGCs will initiate cancer-prevention strategies, perform improved surveillance to facilitate earlier diagnosis, administer targeted therapies designed to work in the context of a specific cancer gene mutation, and manage gene therapy and chemoprevention clinical trials (Grogan & Kirsch, 1997).

As cancer genetics enters mainstream oncologic practice, an increasing number of administrators will consider offering CGC services. This decision warrants careful consideration. Unlike other oncologic services, which typically use existing skills of practitioners currently employed in a program, a cancer genetics service requires practitioners with a unique and broad body of knowledge and expertise. When choosing to deliver services as complex as genetic counseling, testing, and risk assessment, providers must consider the time and expertise necessary for competent service delivery (Stopher, 2000).

This chapter will focus on the critical components of a CGC and points to consider when deciding whether to start a CGC.

Program Needs Assessment

The first step in determining whether an institution should establish a CCG is to evaluate the need for the services in the community. CGCs currently exist in many National Cancer Institute (NCI)-designated Comprehensive Cancer Centers across the country (Thompson et al., 1995). In light of this fact, one needs to carefully consider whether to initiate a program or to refer clients to an existing CGC in the area. Consult NCI's Web site for a searchable Cancer Genetics Services Directory, available at http://cancernet.nci.nih.gov/prevention/genetics.shtml, or contact a nearby NCI-designated Comprehensive Cancer Center.

If no programs are readily available in the area, consider performing a CGC needs assessment within the community (see Figure 8-1). A needs assessment not only provides information but also raises awareness of the clinic's potential existence and may stimulate interest in the program. The assessment should include competing programs within the community, potential programs that may be in a start-up phase, any services already provided, potential providers for the CGC, and the level of interest of local referring physicians.

Figure 8-1. Points to Consider Prior to Initiating a Cancer Genetics Clinic

---

- Are there available programs within the community?
- Has a needs assessment/feasibility study been performed?
- Will the program be integrated into existing structures or stand alone?
- What type of multidisciplinary team will plan the clinic's vision, mission, goals, and implementation?

Another decision is whether the CGC will be integrated into an existing clinic, unit, or office or will be a new program. Regardless of which approach is taken, the program should complement, not compete with, the supporting institution. Forming a multidisciplinary committee to sort out program feasibility, risks versus benefits, mission and goals, timelines, and overall vision is helpful in this endeavor (Calzone, Stopher, Blackwood, & Weber, 1997).

At the institutional level, it may be helpful to establish a steering or planning committee to garner administrative support for the program. Administrative support is essential to overall program goals, staff selection, space allocation, clinic time, and plan of operation.

Types of Cancer Genetics Programs

Research Versus Clinical Programs

Several types of CGCs currently are available. Some programs are strictly research programs, in which all client services (including genetic testing) are performed in the context of a protocol approved by an institutional review board (IRB). Other programs are clinical programs that provide services such as education, counseling, risk assessment, genetic testing, results notification, and medical management. Still other programs are a combination of the two, in which a clinical program operates in a fee-for-service mode in conjunction with a research program. Each model has advantages and disadvantages (see Table 8-1).

In a clinical program, most clients can be tested if they desire. Genetic predisposition testing may offer a black-and-white answer to some clients; more

Table 8-1. Comparison of Types of Cancer Genetics Programs

Type of Program	Advantages	Disadvantages
Clinical	• Open client access • Readily available testing	• Lack of clear guidelines for testing • Complex interpretation and analysis may be beyond the scope of the practice.
Research	• Focused care • Institutional review board-approved studies • Possibly, free service and testing	• May lack holistic approach • Clinical services may be unavailable.
Combination clinical and research	• Meets clinical needs plus avails client of research protocols • Meets client's need for information while promoting clinical advancement in the field	• Client may feel pressure to participate in a research protocol.

often, however, the result is more less clear-cut, challenging the clinician to interpret the results. The lack of clear results may raise client anxiety and leave the clinician unsure of what, if any, medical management is appropriate. Although change will be gradual, clinicians should be prepared to assess how to integrate cancer genetics into current and future practice models. Cunningham (1997) proposed for consideration a general model for setting up a breast-screening program.

Benefits of a research-based program include increased client protection because of the scrutiny of the IRB prior to client accrual and the use of informed consents. Also, once a gene mutation is identified, there may be a clinical trial for the client to pursue. For example, NCI and M.D. Anderson Cancer Center in Houston, TX, are involved in a chemoprevention study using a nonsteroidal anti-inflammatory drug for carriers of the hereditary nonpolyposis colorectal cancer (HNPCC) gene mutation (Physician Data Query, 2000). One of the drawbacks of research-based programs is that they may lack the capacity to provide any necessary treatment. For example, a program may perform a thorough family history assessment but not provide clinical physical exams. For this, the client must rely on his or her oncologist or private medical doctor, which may lead to fragmentation of care. Genetic testing may be the focus of the program while general cancer risk assessment is neglected. Follow-up surveillance may not be available within a research program, because surveillance is considered a service.

A combination clinical and research program allows for the client's clinical needs to be met while availing him or her of potential options for further care via a research protocol. For example, once a person is identified as a mutation carrier, he or she may opt to enter a clinical trial to identify new and more sensitive screening modalities or chemoprevention options. This type of program simultaneously meets the client's need for information and furthers the body of knowledge needed to move the specialty of cancer genetics forward.

Continued clinical trials in the area of cancer prevention will enable the cancer genetics community to present high-risk clients with options once they are identified as carrying a cancer predisposition gene. Indeed, cancer risk assessment/reduction strategies are being developed based on what is now known about age of disease onset and the cancer sites associated with various cancer syndromes in cancer-prone families (Tinley & Lynch, 1999). As critics argue that there is no reason for people to pursue genetic testing or risk assessment when they have no options for improving their situation once they learn of their gene mutation or high-risk status, this type of research becomes more important to the viability of CGCs.

Scope of Services

In defining what type of program to create, consider the scope of services that will be available through the clinic. Will clients be closely followed and encouraged to complete cancer surveillance procedures for early cancer diagnosis? Will they be able to access the program at will should they be diagnosed with cancer or be concerned over a physical change? Or will they be followed simply to track what happens to them physically and emotionally after they visited the CGC? Some clients may simply opt to be seen for consultation. Will the program provide education for other healthcare professionals, cancer centers, and the community? All of these options are possibilities.

Existing CGCs may have a narrow or broad disease focus in their approach. If a clinic is, for example, going to focus on only inherited breast/ovarian cancer syndromes, how will a family suspected to be at high risk for colon cancer be handled or referred? Some programs opt for disease specificity, whereas others handle all suspicious personal or family histories. The focus should be clarified prior to opening and marketing services.

Long-term client follow-up is costly, as well as time- and resource-consuming. Long-term longitudinal studies are beginning at selected Comprehensive Cancer Centers, and NCI also has begun to address the issue of needed clinical research via the formation of the Cancer Genetics Network. The network will facilitate the pooling of data generated from CGCs at NCI-designated Comprehensive Cancer Centers across the country to answer questions regarding clinical management for those at increased risk ("NCI Plans," 1996). The network may be accessed via the CancerNet Web site at http://cancernet.nci.nih.gov/prevention/genetics.shtml. Research is paramount if the necessary clinical care for this type of client is to be illuminated (Ponder, 1997).

Clinical Program Components

Various CGCs approach client care delivery differently. The following is an example of one model of flow adapted from the author's knowledge of various programs. Cancer genetics services should be viewed on a continuum. Clients often visit the clinic more than once as part of a process aimed at determining their personal cancer risk and the appropriate plan of care. Again, the emphasis on simply performing a genetic test is minimal. Providing a genetic test to determine cancer predisposition out of the context of the client's overall risk is irresponsible use of this technology (Alexander, 1997). Once the decision is made to proceed with a cancer genetics clinic, consider pilot testing the program for a few months to identify glitches before serious marketing and client appointments begin.

Initial Referral

Clients come to a CGC from a variety of sources. Physicians (e.g., oncologists, gynecologists, gastroenterologists, primary care providers, surgeons) may note a high-risk client or family history and refer the client for further assessment (Tinley & Lynch, 1999). Some clinics establish guidelines for what constitutes a "high-risk" pedigree or personal history. Clients can then be triaged based on their clinical situation (e.g., symptomatic versus not, high risk or not) and the clinic's services. Advanced practice oncology nurses are in a position to assist staff and clients with identification of those needing referral. Advanced practice nurses with a specialty in cancer genetics often function in the role of clinic coordinator and may be the first point of contact for referring practitioners. In this role, the nurse can assist in assessing the client's personal and family history and triage the referral appropriately. Usually, this initial client contact is via telephone (Dimond, Calzone, Davis, & Jenkins, 1998). Clients also may self-refer based on their personal concerns.

Initial Client Contact

Initial client contact often is used to discuss what the program has to offer and to assess the client's interest level; expectations; and perception, based on the individual's life experiences, of his or her cancer risk. (In many cases, a client's perceptions have been shaped by living in a family in which multiple cancer diagnoses and deaths have occurred.) This contact also includes a description of the CGC program, staff the client will meet, and any program requirements (e.g., number of expected visits, program questionnaires for needed family history or medical information, counseling costs). In many cases, initial contact is made by telephone, with program materials and family medical-history forms mailed to the client prior to the initial visit. If family history is collected via telephone, appropriate staffing should be considered. This may mean meeting the client's immediate need for information and deferring history taking until the initial visit with the nurse.

Risk-Assessment and Counseling Visits

Visits to a CGC vary in both quantity and duration from program to program. Space allocation will be influenced by the number and length of client visits. Whether or not education, risk assessment, and counseling are conducted at separate times contributes to determining the length of the visits. An initial risk-assessment visit may last nearly two hours if education, risk communication, and counseling are completed consecutively. The initial visit requires more time in order to ensure that clients receive the necessary information for decision making regarding genetic testing or risk reduction options, whereas a results disclosure session generally can be completed in 30–60 minutes.

Most CGC client visits can occur in an office or conference room setting, unless a physical exam is required. Consider separating unaffected CGC clients from the general oncology population when working with individuals who are anxious about their cancer risk. Clear reminders of unpleasant, past cancer family experiences will then be minimized.

Varied models exist for how clients are seen for risk assessment and possible genetic testing. Some clinics will offer the education and counseling session immediately followed by obtaining the sample for testing if the client desires it. Others require multiple visits before testing will be offered. Some CGCs will perform genetic testing after seeing the client only once. This can be considered if telephone contact has been initiated and pertinent history information has already been obtained and discussed. Education sessions may be offered in either individual or group settings. Sessions may include members of the extended family. It is recommended, however, that counseling sessions be for the client only. Figure 8-2 provides examples of visit schedules for different models. No data are available to support the use of one method over the others.

Preparation for client visits includes the creation of appropriate forms to collect information including, but not limited to, family- and medical-history forms (see Chapter 3 for examples), pathology release, medical record informa-

---

Figure 8-2. Sample Models of Cancer Genetic Clinic Visit Schedules

---

Multiple Visit Model
- **Visit One:** Risk assessment, pedigree construction, medical history review, and general education about hereditary cancer syndromes
- **Interim:** Validation of cancer diagnoses in family, if possible (via death certificate and pathology/operative reports), discussing case with multidisciplinary team to establish plan
- **Visit Two:** Physical exam (if part of the program), specific education and counseling regarding cancer of concern, informed consent, and obtaining of sample for genetic testing, if desired
- **Visit Three:** Results disclosure session and cancer management plan

Advantages:
Thorough, allows team to get familiar with client and family history, gives the client a lot of time within the program

Disadvantages:
Costly, time-consuming for the client and clinic staff, potentially paternalistic in approach (assumes that client needs this much preparation/exposure prior to decision making)

Two-Visit Model
- **Prior to Visit One:** Risk assessment, pedigree construction, medical history review, and general education about hereditary cancer syndromes can occur over telephone
- **Visit One:** Specific education and counseling regarding cancer of concern, informed consent, and obtaining sample for genetic testing, if desired
- **Visit Two:** Results disclosure session and cancer management plan

Advantages: More streamlined, less costly, and potentially more client friendly

Disadvantages: Less contact with clinic staff, client may feel rushed (although no data are available to suggest this)

One-Visit Model (Currently being studied)
- Clients will come into clinic for education, counseling, and testing and receive results over the telephone or via the mail (Jenkins & Dimond, 2001).

---

tion release, informed consents, tracking forms so coded blood samples can be appropriately monitored, telephone logs to document client conversations, and flow sheets to document the client's status at any given time in the process (see Figure 8-3). Members of the Oncology Nursing Society (ONS) Cancer Genetics Special Interest Group can be a resource for obtaining sample documents. Visit the Genetics Resource Area at ONS Online (www.ons.org) or call ONS at 412-859-6100 for more information.

Follow-Up

Each CGC has a different schema for client follow-up, depending on the mission of the program. Sending a follow-up letter to the client, which summarizes the risk-assessment visit or test-disclosure visit, is standard practice. Such

---

Figure 8-3. Sample Flow of a Client Through Cancer Genetics Clinic Services

1. Client referral
2. Initial telephone contact
3. Family/medical history assessment
4. Visit(s)
5. Follow-up

---

a letter serves as a reminder for the client and as legal documentation of the information and recommendations given. (Chapter 7 discussed required documentation in depth.) Deciding which members of the team sign follow-up letters should be done ahead of time. Generally, the nurse counselor draws up and signs the letter; the physician also may sign it.

A follow-up telephone call is recommended for a client who receives genetic test results, to assess how he or she is coping with the information and to ascertain the extent to which the client intends to comply with recommendations about medical management.

A program plan should be in place to indicate who bears the responsibility of notifying first-degree relatives of risk, after test results are known. In most settings, the CGC recommends that the client notify family members about their risk of being carriers and how cancer risk is related to being a carrier. The follow-up telephone call can determine if the client has followed through with family notification. If family members interested in being tested live far away, the follow-up call provides an opportunity for staff to help the client by providing referral resources where their relatives can obtain genetic counseling (Calzone et al., 1997; Egan, 1997).

Operational Issues

A number of operational issues need to be considered when contemplating the establishment of a CGC. These include

- Financial backing
- Capital and operating budgets
- Resources (human and physical)
- Billing mechanisms
- Information management
- Confidentiality and security of genetic data

A CGC requires resources and space to operate. Will the clinic function as part of an existing clinic, or will space be needed, and at what cost? Capital and operating budgets should be planned prior to seeking financial backing. Funds to start and run CGCs have come from a variety of sources, including grants, endowments, private monies, and insurance reimbursement. Historically, clinical genetic services have been fraught with economic concerns. Patient education and counseling are time- and labor-intensive, have not been self-supporting, and have brought indirect rather than direct economic gains to an institution (Bernhardt, Tumpson, & Pyeritz, 1992). Often, salary support occurs through department or institution funds until solid mechanisms for reimbursement are established.

Fees for Service

Fees for service may be itemized or clustered into a package fee that, for example, may cover multiple visits. CGCs may or may not produce revenue, depending on the program goals and costs. Because cancer risk assessment, education, counseling, and genetic testing involve a process, they are time-consuming, costly, and often inadequately reimbursed through third parties. Confirmation of familial cancer diagnoses via medical record collection also is a necessary but time-consuming activity. The blood test for a genetic mutation may be covered by insurance, but the accompanying assessment, counseling, and education may not be.

Billing

Billing within a CGC can be complex. The Current Procedural Terminology codes used in billing eventually come to reflect the activity of the clinic. Generic or unclear billing may lead to a false record of the clinic's activities (e.g., billing for "fibrocystic disease" for a potential *BRCA1* mutation carrier will not accurately reflect what services were provided within the clinic). Conversely, using codes that reflect a strong cancer family history may alert an insurance company to scrutinize the client's claim. Insurance laws vary from state to state; thus, seeking legal counsel may be useful to clarify billing and optimize reimbursement. The state nurse's association also can assist with regulations affecting reimbursement.

Staffing Needs

Staffing requirements vary based on the needs of a CGC. Estimates of the scope of services to be provided and the expected activity in the clinic are necessary to establish the number and type of positions needed. Ideally, the CGC staff is a multidisciplinary team. The team may include a nurse counselor, genetic counselor, physician, and support person. Access to psychosocial resources (e.g., social worker, psychologist) is important. Periodically, the staff may need to enlist the services of a lawyer or ethicist to establish genetic policies or resolve ethical issues related to genetic information.

When case volume is large, supportive staff helps conduct the initial contacts, deal with the program mailings, and coordinate appointments. Members of the risk assessment and counseling staff conduct education and counseling; evaluate pedigree data; devise and communicate risk estimates; and, at the client's request, prepare the client for genetic testing. When commercial testing is provided, staff members are responsible for obtaining insurance certification, ensuring completion of consent forms, mailing blood samples, and keeping in contact with the patient. When the client receives genetic-test results, the physician should be present and available to discuss the case, genetic diagnosis, and medical recommendations for risk management.

Physician coverage varies in current programs. Many programs are led by oncologists who have additional training in genetics. However, geneticists also play a role in many CGCs. In some settings, the nurse may interface with several physicians, referring clients for genetic services. Recognizing that many community-based hospitals do not have funds for a full complement of staff, at minimum there should be dedicated time for the nurse providing education and counseling and a physician committed to risk assessment. If a program does not have a medical doctor to champion the effort, it will not succeed.

Careful consideration of professional requirements in terms of certification, education (oncology and genetics), and licensure is warranted (see Chapter 11). Existing CGCs have established job descriptions. Such descriptions may serve as resources for people who are initiating programs. Members of the ONS Cancer Genetics Special Interest Group may be able to provide examples of position descriptions.

Data Management of Sensitive Information

Confidential and organized information management is critical in a CGC. Data management may be complex (e.g., because of large families being seen in one clinic). Tracking a client's test results, long-term surveillance follow-up, clinical course, clinical trial involvement (if applicable), and status requires a good relational database and someone who both understands and can manage the data that need to be captured. Methods for management of genetic information including pedigrees, test results, and visit notes should be determined prior to start-up. Confidentiality of information should extend to family members who are detailed in the pedigree assessment. Some programs utilize "shadow charts" to protect client confidentiality. These charts generally are program specific and are not circulated outside the CGC. The benefit of this system is containment of sensitive client and family data. The downside is lack of continuity, because a piece of client medical history is missing from the main medical record. The database used should be password coded or secured in various manners. Some programs opt to code client samples to avoid identification. However, other issues arise if these options are exercised (see Table 8-2).

Table 8-2. Confidentiality Issues for a Cancer Genetics Clinic

Method for Maintaining Confidentiality	Advantages	Disadvantages
Shadow charts	• Client's genetic information separate from medical record • Allows elaboration of details related to cancer genetics clinic visit	• Relevant client information inaccessible to general healthcare providers • Lack of continuity of documentation • Test results unavailable
Code samples	Client confidentiality	• Potential for error • Appropriate billing becomes problematic
Database	• Consolidation of client data, pedigree, and/or research information • Can be password-protected and secured for limited access • Allows rapid assessment of clinic and client statistics	• Unwanted browsing, if accessed by non-team members • May be unaffordable for some clinics

In addition to the issue of where to document a CGC visit, consideration also must be given to how follow-up to referring physicians will be handled. Consider sending the visit summary and recommendations directly to the client. He or she then may decide whether to share this information in writing or have an "off-the-record" discussion with the provider. Policies for release of genetic information should be clear to the client. Generally, no information is released from the CGC without the client's expressed, *written* consent.

Quality Assurance

Quality assurance and improvement is relevant to a CGC. Some clinics opt to send follow-up questionnaires to clients to assess client satisfaction with the clinic experience, both from a functional perspective (e.g., appointment desk service, time spent in waiting room) and an informational one (e.g., level of explanation of materials) (Collins, Halliday, Warren, & Williamson, 2000). Given the importance of the blood tests obtained through genetic testing, the CGC should establish a method for ensuring that samples are correctly labeled and results are matched with the right sample. A double-check of labeling is very reasonable, using both a colleague and the client to validate that what is written on the blood tube is accurate. If any suspicions arise regarding results, consider a repeat/confirmation test. Some labs do repeats of positive tests.

Any genetics research may be eligible for a federally granted "Certificate of Confidentiality." The certificate relieves the investigator from complying with compulsory legal demands (such as court orders and subpoenas) for information on research subjects. The certificate does not stop the voluntary disclosure of information about subjects by an investigator. NCI specifically deems IRB-approved research projects involving genetic testing for cancer predisposition as eligible for certificates. General information on these certificates is available on the National Institute of Mental Health Web site at http://www.nimh.nih.gov/research/confidentfaq.cfm or by calling 301-443-3877. The contact telephone number for information about certificates granted specifically by the National Cancer Institute is 301-402-7221.

Client Recruitment

Once a program is established, ongoing client referral is necessary for viability. Internal and external recruitment strategies are possible. Internally, the team or individuals may offer educational programs (e.g., grand rounds, clinical conferences based on a significant pedigree, in-services, tumor boards), publish an article in staff and system newsletters, and network with pathologists, gastroenterologists, gynecologists, and surgeons. Externally, the team can educate colleagues about the program's services; volunteer to speak about cancer genetics at lay gatherings, community groups, or professional meetings; advertise; create brochures to distribute to relevant community physicians and nurses; publish notices in newsletters for special interest groups within their field; or develop a Web site to promote the program (Peters, Graham, Stadler, & Sargent, 1999). Programs also can request to be listed as a cancer genetic resource on the Gene Tests and NCI Web sites (see Chapter 10).

Client Resources

Clients visiting a well-designed CGC generally receive a large volume of information. These summary documents that highlight what they heard are valuable, but providing clients with pre-visit information also may be beneficial. Collins et al. (2000) found that clients wished to receive more information before their visit so they could be better prepared. Ideas include education booklets or pamphlets about cancer risk, specific cancer susceptibility genes (e.g., *BRCA1*, *BRCA2*, HNPCC), surveillance recommendations, and available support groups. A follow-up letter summarizing the client's specific clinical situation and medical management recommendations is standard practice and recommended. Usually, a referring physician would be sent a visit summary, but because of the sensitive nature of cancer risk assessment and genetic testing, the client has control over how and what to convey to his or her private physician.

Professional Resources

Many professional organizations have published guidelines or position papers on genetic testing and the role of professionals in this arena (American Society of Clinical Oncology [ASCO], 1996; American Society of Human Genetics, Ad Hoc Committee on Breast and Ovarian Cancer Screening, 1994; National Action Plan on Breast Cancer, 1996; National Society of Genetic Counselors, 1997; ONS, 1998, 2000). The International Society of Nurses in Genetics has worked with the American Nurses Association (ANA) to have genetics identified as a valid subspecialty of nursing (Prows, 1997). In June 1998, ANA published the *Statement on the Scope and Standards of Genetics Clinical Practice* (ANA, 1998). The Human Genome Research Institute has spearheaded the formation of the National Coalition for Health Care Professional Education in Genetics (www.nchpeg.org), a coalition of healthcare professionals interested in educating colleagues in their specialties about genetics. ASCO hosted its first train-the-trainer program in cancer genetics in the summer of 1997 and subsequently published a cancer genetics training module. ONS also supports increased national conference presentations on cancer genetics. Internet resources are growing in number (see Resources, Chapter 10), as are available continuing education courses. Core curriculums in cancer genetics have been developed for nurses to guide in the design of nursing education programs (see Chapter 11) (Lea & Lawson, 2000). Resources for clients and professionals are expanding. It is incumbent upon healthcare professionals to avail themselves of this information to broaden their knowledge base as they embark on the establishment of a CGC.

Conclusion

A competently staffed, well-developed CGC provides a valuable service to clients and families who are at increased risk for cancer and to those clients simply concerned about their personal risk. A staff with a combined genetics and oncology background is ideal to effectively explain the clinical and molecular complexities of inherited cancer syndromes. Confusion and myths exist among providers regarding inherited cancer predisposition and cancer risk. Some argue this technology should be federally regulated in order to protect public health and keep it out of the hands of the misinformed (Cunningham, 1997). The National Institute of Health's Secretary's Advisory Committee on Genetic Testing is putting forth a significant effort to solicit public and professional consultation regarding oversight of genetic tests to address these concerns (see the committee's Web site at www4.od.nih.gov/oba/sacgt.htm for further information).

A CGC cannot simply be a testing site that applies the technology indiscriminately to the general population. The development of available molecular technologies is a profound breakthrough in cancer care. However, the clinical advances made possible by molecular genetics must be incorporated into clinical oncology with respect and preparation (Alexandre, 1997). All oncology practitioners must carefully consider knowing an individual's genetic makeup as "the gift of knowing" and use this information to deliver care competently. This knowledge may not always be such a gift, especially when a gap exists between "knowing" and knowing what to do with the information (Kenen, 1996). Given this reality, the importance of continued research cannot be overstated. The gap between knowledge and intervention will not close without continued research on the special population now being served in emerging CGCs across the country.

References

Alexandre, L.M. (1997). Genetic testing for cancer susceptibility: What your institution needs to know. *Oncology Issues, 12*(3), 18–22.

American Nurses Association. (1998). *Statement on the scope and standards of genetics clinical nursing practice*. Washington, DC: Author.

American Society of Clinical Oncology. (1996). Statement of the American Society of Clinical Oncology: Genetic testing for cancer susceptibility. *Journal of Clinical Oncology, 14*, 1738–1740.

American Society of Human Genetics, Ad Hoc Committee on Breast and Ovarian Cancer Screening. (1994). Statement of the American Society of Human Genetics on genetic testing for breast and ovarian cancer predisposition. *American Journal of Human Genetics, 55*, i–iv.

Bernhardt, B., Tumpson, J., & Pyeritz, R. (1992). The economics of clinical genetics services. IV. Financial impact of outpatient genetic services on an academic institution. *American Journal of Human Genetics, 50*, 84–91.

Calzone, K.A., Stopher, J., Blackwood, A., & Weber, B. (1997). Establishing a cancer risk evaluation program. *Cancer Practice, 4*, 228–233.

Collins, V., Halliday, J., Warren, R., & Williamson, R. (2000). Assessment of education and counseling offered by a familial colorectal cancer clinic. *Clinical Genetics, 57*, 48–55.

Cunningham, G.C. (1997). A public health perspective on the control of predictive screening for breast cancer. *Health Matrix, 7*(1), 31–48.

Dimond, E.P., Calzone, K.A., Davis, J., & Jenkins, J. (1998). The role of the nurse in cancer genetics. *Cancer Nursing, 21*, 57–75.

Egan, C. (1997). Models for cancer genetic risk assessment programs. *Oncology Issues, 12*(3), 14–17.

Fearon, E.R. (1997). Human cancer syndromes: Clues to the origin and nature of cancer. *Science, 278*, 1043–1050.

Fraser, M.C., Calzone, K.A., & Goldstein, A. (1997). Familial cancers: Evolving challenges for nursing practice. *Oncology Nursing Updates, 4*(3), 1–18.

Grogan, L., & Kirsch, I.R. (1997). Genetic testing for cancer risk assessment: A review. *The Oncologist, 2*, 208–222.

Jenkins, J., & Dimond, E. (2001). Methods in education for breast cancer genetics, a research study in progress at the National Cancer Institute, Bethesda, MD.

Kenen, R.H. (1996). The at-risk health status and technology: A diagnostic invitation and the "gift" of knowing. *Social Science Medicine, 11*, 1545–1553.

Lea, D., & Lawson, M. (2000). A practice-based genetics curriculum for nurse educators: An innovative approach to integrating genetics into nursing curricula. *Journal of Nursing Education, 39*, 418–421.

Mahon, S. (2000). Principles of cancer prevention and early detection. *Clinical Journal of Oncology Nursing, 4*, 169–176.

National Action Plan on Breast Cancer. (1996). Position paper on hereditary susceptibility testing for breast cancer. *Journal of Clinical Oncology, 14*, 1738–1740.

National Society of Genetic Counselors. (1997). Position paper: Predisposition genetic testing for late onset disorders in adults. *JAMA, 278*, 1217–1220.

NCI plans new consortium for new cancer genetics studies. (1996). *Cancer Letter, 22*(13), 6–7.

Oncology Nursing Society. (1998). Cancer genetic testing and risk assessment counseling. *Oncology Nursing Forum, 25*, 464.

Oncology Nursing Society. (2000). The role of the oncology nurse in cancer genetic counseling. *Oncology Nursing Forum, 27*, 1348.

Peters, J., Graham, J., Stadler, M., & Sargent, K. (1999). The components of a genetic cancer risk clinic. In G. Shaw (Ed.), *Cancer genetics for the clinician* (pp. 1–26). New York: Kluwer Academic/Plenum Publishers.

Physician Data Query. (2000). *Finding clinical trials*. Retrieved January 5, 2001, from http://cancertrials.nci.nih.gov

Ponder, B. (1997). Genetic testing for cancer risk. *Science, 278*, 1050–1054.

Prows, C.A. (1997). Update from the Professional Practice Committee. *International Society for Nurses in Genetics Newsletter, 8*(4), 3–4.

Stopher, J.E. (2000). Genetic counseling and clinical cancer genetic services. *Seminars in Surgical Oncology, 18*, 347–357.

Thompson, J.A., Weisner, G.L., Sellars, T.A., Vachon, C., Ahrens, M., Potter, J.D., et al. (1995). Genetic services for familial cancer clients: A survey of National Cancer Institute cancer centers. *Journal of the National Cancer Institute, 87*, 1446–1455.

Tinley, S., & Lynch, H. (1999). Integration of family history and medical management of clients with hereditary cancers. *Cancer, 86*(Suppl. 11), 2525–2532.

9

Handling Genetic Information Responsibly

Dale Halsey Lea, RN, MPH, APNG(c)

Introduction

Oncology nursing practice is broadening to incorporate the principles of human genetics into health improvement, health maintenance, and health restoration (International Society of Nurses in Genetics [ISONG], 1998). Genetic discoveries resulting from the Human Genome Project are paving the way for new cancer interventions and therapies. This new information requires that oncology nurses in all levels of practice consider their responsibilities in handling genetic information and the potential ethical, social, and legal implications associated with this information. Oncology nurses must, therefore, be prepared with knowledge and skills for practice in the new era of genetic health (Donaldson, 1997; Jenkins, 1997; Oncology Nursing Society, 2000a).

Using an ethical framework, nurses can assess clinical situations that present moral or ethical dilemmas. An ethical framework enables each oncology nurse to act with integrity as he or she supports and educates clients, families, and the public to deal responsibly with the complex ethical issues related to genetic interventions and services (Bove, Fry, & MacDonald, 1997; Cameron, 1996; Grady, 1998).

This chapter considers the use of ethical concepts to guide oncology nurses to apply genetic knowledge

Ethical Issues in Genetic-Related Health Care

- Privacy and confidentiality of genetic information
- Right to accept or refuse genetic interventions
- Potential insurance/employment discrimination when gene status is known
- Prenatal diagnosis of late-onset genetic conditions
- Just and fair use of genetic interventions
- Genetic susceptibility testing in children

responsibly to patient care when providing patient education, ensuring informed decision making and consent, advocating for confidentiality and privacy with regard to genetic information and test results, and helping clients and families to understand the complex issues involved in genetic detection, interventions, and therapeutics.

Ethical Considerations of Genetic Information

Genetics-related ethical issues that challenge oncology nurses in all levels of practice include privacy, confidentiality, access to and justice in health care, and informed health decisions. Although these ethical issues are not new, their application to clinical practice in genetics presents additional and unique ethical dimensions requiring nursing attention (Grady, 1998; Leavitt, 1996; Scanlon & Fibison, 1995; Wertz & Fletcher, 1989). For example, an individual client's concerns are of primary importance when the nurse is participating in a decision about whether a person should be tested for the presence of a gene for conditions such as breast cancer (Grundstein-Amado, 1992). Decisions about whether and under what conditions an institution or organization should offer a test or treatment to its clients fall into the institutional realm. At the societal level are decisions regarding whether private or public health insurance should pay for a genetic test or genetic screening of a specific population or group. Oncology nurses practicing at the basic level will be involved in ethical considerations in the individual realm, as this level of practice entails responsiveness and sensitivity to client wishes and concerns. Oncology nurses practicing at the advanced practice level will be concerned with ethical issues in the individual and institutional realms, while those practicing in advanced genetics practice settings will be responsible for participating in all three realms (see Figure 9-1).

Functioning Within an Ethical Framework

Ethical dilemmas and ethical analysis are best handled within the context of an ethical framework. An ethical framework that incorporates principle-based ethical thinking, an ethic of care, and virtue ethics can enable the nurse to arrive at thoughtful judgments that will be valuable to clients and families confronted with genetic-related health decisions (Cameron, 1996; Grady, 1998; Noddings, 1984; Scanlon & Fibison, 1995).

Principle-based ethics offers moral guidelines for nurses, which can be used to choose and to justify nursing practices. The emphasis is on the use of principles such as beneficence to help nurses to analyze and solve ethical dilemmas that may arise in clinical situations.

Figure 9-1. Oncology Nursing Practice Activities in Genetic Health Care That Support Responsible Handling of Genetic Information

---

General Oncology Nurse
• Participate as a member of the healthcare team in offering information about genetic topics and interventions.
• Maintain privacy and confidentiality of genetic information collected and recorded in the medical record.
• Ensure that clients have adequate information to make informed decisions.
• Advocate for clients to prevent discrimination.
• Support clients' healthcare decisions
• Be knowledgeable about local genetics resources for clients and for nursing professionals.

Advanced Practice Oncology Nurse
• Offer written information about genetic topics and interventions.
• Participate in client and family education by reinforcing genetic information.
• Participate in the informed-consent process by ensuring that clients have adequate and accurate information.
• Maintain privacy and confidentiality of genetic information collected and recorded in the medical record.
• Advocate, through education and participation with the healthcare team, against discrimination resulting from genetic evaluations.
• Help clients to understand the complex issues involved in genetic interventions.
• Be knowledgeable about local and national genetics resources for clients and nursing professionals.
• Work within institutions and support equal access to genetic health care.

Advanced Practice Oncology Nurse With a Subspecialty in Genetics
• Participate with genetics/oncology healthcare team in offering and discussing information about genetic topics and interventions.
• Participate in the informed-consent process by outlining to clients the risks, benefits, and limitations of genetic evaluations and testing.
• Support and maintain privacy and confidentiality of genetic information collected, recorded, and reported in the medical record.
• Discuss with clients the relevance and importance of sharing genetic information with family members at risk.
• Advocate, through education of clients and other oncology nurses, for equal access to and payment for genetic health services and for nondiscrimination resulting from genetic evaluations.
• Help clients and families to assimilate new genetic information.
• Be knowledgeable and educate other oncology nurses about local, regional, and national resources for clients and nursing professionals.
• Participate in social policy development with regard to genetic health care.

Note. Based on information from Oncology Nursing Society, 2000b.

An ethic of care is founded on the understanding that all clients are unique, that relationships and their value are central in moral deliberations, and that peoples' emotions and character traits have a role in moral decision making. When carrying out nursing practice based on an ethic of care, nurses make every effort to understand what the individuals involved with the ethical dilemma feel and then act intuitively on their behalf to help to arrive at a resolution (Noddings, 1984).

Virtue ethics is based on the belief that virtue is what guides and empowers people to be good and to attain harmony within them. Nurses, whose practice is based upon virtue ethics, are focused on achieving knowledge and a desire to develop excellent character by being a good person. This focus allows them to face moral and ethical dilemmas from a central belief that they will behave in a virtuous manner out of an innate desire to do so.

> **Ethical Principles Used to Resolve an Ethical Dilemma**
>
> * Respect for persons
> * Ethic of care
> * Respect for client autonomy
> * Beneficence
> * Nonmaleficence
> * Virtue ethics

Principles Involved in Ethical Decision Making

Ethics is a branch of moral philosophy that focuses on values related to human conduct and teaches individuals how to choose what is good or right and why. Ethics requires that healthcare professionals use an analytical approach and previous experiences to respond to questions such as: Is the person performing the act meeting his or her duties and obligations? Are the motives of the person virtuous? (Beauchamp & Childress, 1994). Bioethics refers to the application of ethical theory and concepts to biomedical practice and research. Ethical dilemmas are problems or situations in which there is a clash of competing rights, values, or goods. Ethical analysis is then required to clarify and perhaps solve moral problems (Beauchamp & Childress; Scanlon & Fibison, 1995).

Ethical theories and principles can guide healthcare professionals in analyzing and finding solutions to bioethical problems. Ethical theories organize and justify ethical analysis in different ways, depending upon the nature of the theory. Ethical principles, on the other hand, are general statements that provide reasons for a choice of actions and serve as guides to analyzing and resolving conflicting ethical choices. Ethical principles help to guide healthcare professionals in acting appropriately in a given situation while allowing for interpretation in clinical judgment in specific cases.

Respect for persons is the ethical foundation that directs all of nursing care. Four ethical principles, founded on respect for persons, generally are accepted as being central guides to bioethical decision making: respect for autonomy, nonmaleficence, beneficence, and justice (Beauchamp & Childress,

1994). Additional principles that are important for nursing consideration when providing genetic-related health care are confidentiality, privacy, and equity. These concepts also offer guidance to nurses when engaged in ethical analyses of relevant questions relating to genetic health care (American Nurses Association [ANA], 2001; Andrews, Fullarton, Holtzman, & Motulsky, 2001) (see Figure 9-2).

Figure 9-2. Important Ethical Principles That Guide the Nurse in Ethical Analysis

---

Respect for Persons—The obligation to respect the capacities and differences in human beings and to act in accordance with this obligation

Respect for Autonomy—The most important principle to consider in resolving an ethical dilemma: the freedom to choose; an obligation to respect the self-determined (autonomous) choices and actions of individuals. Moral decision making requires individuals who are able to judge circumstances independently, make choices based on actions freely chosen, and who are not constrained in their reasoning process.

Beneficence—The obligation to maximize benefits, minimize risks, and to promote the welfare of others; the focus of the practitioner is on positive benefits and doing good.

Nonmaleficence—The obligation to never do harm to clients, either intentionally or unintentionally

Confidentiality—The obligation to protect and not disclose personal information provided to the nurse in confidence by another

Privacy—The right to have control over one's own body, thoughts, and actions

Equity—The obligation to be fair in the distribution of social goods such as health care or in respect for people's rights; the right to be treated equally regardless of race, sex, socioeconomic status, etc.

Veracity (truthfulness)—The obligation to provide truthful information and not to intentionally deceive or mislead individuals.

Note. Based on information from Grady, 1998; Scanlon & Fibison, 1995.

Moral reasoning is the thought process that occurs when one recognizes an ethical dilemma and reacts to it. It is the decision-making process through which a healthcare professional chooses among his or her values and principles to come to a decision as to the appropriate response or behavior to an ethical dilemma (Cassells

Examples of Personal Biases That Interfere With Client Autonomy

- Genetic diseases are caused by "bad genes" and should be eliminated.
- People who have genetic conditions are "different."
- All clients at high risk for inherited genetic conditions are obligated to have testing to find out their status.
- Parents should make the decision to have their children tested for susceptibility to late-onset genetic disorders.

& Gaul, 1998; Ketefian, 1989). Figure 9-3 outlines steps that can be used to identify, analyze, and evaluate ethical conflicts, issues, and uncertainties. This framework is based upon the nurse's knowledge of ethical principles, concepts, and ethical decision making.

Recognition of Personal Biases and How Values Affect Others' Decisions

The first step in providing genetic information and in supporting clients' decisions is to recognize one's own values and how they influence the communication of genetic information (Fine, 1993). Although it may not be possible to

---

Figure 9-3. Ethical Assessment Framework (EAF) for Clinical Practice

Assessment
1. Identify the concern/issue that may be an ethical problem: uneasiness, uncertainties, and/or conflicts.
2. Gather relevant facts about the problem(s):
   Medical data: Objective and subjective data.
   Contextual data: Circumstances, people involved, institutional policies, state and federal laws.
3. Determine if the problem is an ethical dilemma.
4. Propose actions or options to assist in resolving the ethical dilemma.
5. Apply methods of ethical justification to each action or option to assist in resolving the dilemma: consequentialism (consequences), deontology (duty), principalism (principles), care (relationships), casuistry (cases), virtue (character).
6. Identify and clarify values, rights, and duties of client, self, and significant persons associated with the dilemma.
7. Apply relevant guidelines from nursing and professional codes of ethics.
8. Identify and use relevant interdisciplinary resources: Ethics Committee, consultants, administrators, clergy, ethicists, lawyers, colleagues, literature, etc.
9. Prioritize the identified actions or options to assist in resolving the dilemma.

Plan of Action
10. Select an ethically justified action or option from those identified.

Implementation
11. Act upon or support the action or option selected.

Evaluation
12. Evaluate the selected action or option taken: Short- and long-term outcomes.

Note. Framework: ASEAS Instrument (including EAF) © 1990 Judith M. Cassells, RN, DNSc, Mary C. Silva, RN, PhD; revised: EAF/11 Steps in Nursing Process, Cassells, J.M., Johnson, E., & Littlejohn, J., 1996; revised: EAF/12 Steps With Definitions, Cassells, J.M., & Gaul, A.L. 1998. Reprinted with permission from Cassells & Gaul, 1998; Cassells, Gaul, Lea, Calzone, & Jenkins, 1999; Cassells & Redman, 1989; Cassells, Silva, & Chop, 1990.

---

completely hide one's own values and beliefs, nurses, in providing genetic information, need to be able to maintain sufficient self-awareness to minimize the perception of favoring one decision or intervention over another. This includes discussing genetic information and interventions in a balanced manner; it implies that nurses providing genetic information offer all of the information that a client needs to make an informed health decision; assist the client in considering available health options and potential consequences of each, within the context of the client's experiences and circumstances; and support the decision that the client ultimately makes. For example, the oncology nurse who believes that all clients who have a significant risk for breast cancer should have predisposition testing brings this belief to the interactions with clients. If he or she is not aware of how this belief may influence the provision of information, the belief may be translated as a value judgment to clients who choose not to have the testing, and they may feel unsupported in their choice.

Consider the difference between these two nurses' approaches to describing *BRCA1* gene susceptibility testing to a client and family at increased risk. Nurse A: "This testing has its risks, though. Even if you get a negative result, you can feel guilty, and that would be hard for you since your other family members tested positive. If I were you, I would think twice before you decide to have it." Nurse B: "Making a decision to have or not to have genetic testing may take time and consideration of a number of issues, and I am here to help you discuss this process. What kinds of questions or thoughts have you had so far?" The first nurse makes assumptions, uses value-laden words such as "risk" and "guilty," interjects her own opinion, and gives advice (i.e., "I would think twice"). The second nurse opens discussion by making it clear to the client that decision making is a personal process and focuses the discussion on the client. This approach offers the client an opportunity to consider his or her thoughts and options with the knowledge that the nurse is present to support the client's personal decision.

Nurses need to maintain awareness of their personal values and beliefs and to remain objective in clinical situations where there is not a clear advantage to one option over another. Examples of this situation include decisions related to genetic testing for breast cancer and other late-onset conditions, prenatal diagnosis of cancer or other conditions, and gene therapy. In situations for which interventions are clearly beneficial, such as familial adenomatous polyposis, however, nurses can be directive in offering recommendations. In either of these situations, it is essential that nurses achieve sufficient awareness of their own values and biases so that they can allow open and supportive communication with clients and families who are making difficult genetic-related decisions.

Facilitating Autonomous Decision Making

The decision to participate in any genetic intervention should be the client's own, made after consideration of the risks and benefits and of his or her values and beliefs. This incorporates the principle of respect for autonomy of the individual and acknowledges that people have a right to make personal decisions about their own beliefs and property. This principle requires that nurses who are involved in a client's decision to undergo a particular genetic intervention provide sufficient information about the benefits, risks, and possible outcomes that allow that client to make an informed, independent, and voluntary decision about whether to participate. When nurses provide adequate information in the appropriate educational and cultural context, they allow the client to make free, unpressured decisions about the intervention and demonstrate respect for the client's autonomy. Nurses should ensure that the client has received adequate counseling and provided fully informed consent (Rieger & Pentz, 1999). Figure 9-4 outlines the central issues included in the informed-consent process.

The ability to participate with autonomy in decision making requires that the client be competent (see Figure 9-5). The client's ability to make an autonomous decision may be inhibited by a number of factors, as well (see Figure 9-6). The number of healthcare team

Promoting Beneficence and Avoiding Nonmaleficence

- Evaluate self and motives in genetic-related health care.
- Promote respect for clients and their health decisions.
- Support clients on the basis of what is "good" for the client according to his/her beliefs, values, and decisions.
- Maximize benefits of genetic interventions being considered.

Figure 9-4. Central Issues Discussed During the Informed-Consent Process

- Purpose of the genetic intervention
- Reason for offering the intervention
- Type and nature of genetic condition being tested for or treated
- Accuracy of genetic intervention
- Benefits of participating
- Associated risks, including unexpected results
- Acknowledgment of the right to refuse the intervention
- Other available therapeutic options
- Available treatment and intervention options
- Further decision making that may be needed upon receipt of genetic information
- Consent to use genetic information for further research purposes
- Availability of additional counseling and support services

Note. Based on information from Andrews et al., 1994; Bove et al., 1997; Lea, Jenkins, & Francomano, 1998; Scanlon & Fibison, 1995.

Figure 9-5. Client Competencies Needed to Make an Informed Health Decision

---

The client needs to have the ability to
- Understand information
- Consider options
- Evaluate potential risks and benefits of a genetic test/intervention
- Communicate health choices.

Note. Based on information from Lea, Jenkins, & Francomano, 1998; Scanlon & Fibison, 1995.

Figure 9-6. Factors That May Influence Informed Decision Making

---

- Hearing or language deficits
- Intellectual disabilities
- Effects of medications
- Cultural and family beliefs and practices
- Who and how many healthcare providers are providing genetic information
- The setting where informed consent is being obtained
- Whether the client is alone or with family/friends
- Presence of concurrent illness/health problems
- Insurance policy restrictions

Note. Based on information from Bove et al., 1997.

---

members who provide the information, the time allowed for communication of the information and for reflection, whether the client is alone or accompanied by family or friends, and the presence of concurrent illness or health problems all can influence the client's ability to make an autonomous decision (Bove et al., 1997).

Principles of Beneficence and Nonmaleficence

Beneficence and nonmaleficence are two fundamental and interconnected principles of nursing ethics that are based upon respect for persons and serve to guide nurses in providing patient care. *Beneficence* refers to the nurse's obligation to promote good and maximize the benefits of whatever intervention is being considered. *Nonmaleficence* is based on the obligation to do no harm—that is, to minimize risks (Scanlon & Fibison, 1995).

To promote good and minimize risks in genetics-related health care, nurses must be knowledgeable about the risks, benefits, and consequences of genetic interventions and be able to support and discuss these fully with clients to ensure that they make informed health decisions. The oncology nurse who is aware of the various facets of genetic testing and interventions for breast cancer, for example, and who articulates these to the client in a manner that helps the client to further his or her interests, acts with beneficence and nonmaleficence. The nurse who, on the other hand, recommends a particular course of action to the client that does not support the client's wishes or actions is behaving in a manner that may end up harming the client in the long run.

> **Ethnocultural Beliefs That May Influence Clients' Perceptions of Genetic Health Care**
>
> • Health is the absence of clinical symptoms.
> • Health and disease are determined by the will of God.
> • Needles take away valuable body fluids and should be avoided.
> • The spiritual leader makes all decisions about health care in a community.
> • Genes are a part of God's mystery and should not be known.

Recognition of Ethnocultural Differences

Clients' family and ethnic backgrounds and the associated cultural and social influences may have an impact on their perceptions of genetic information and interventions, including how they accept information and explanations about the genetic basis of cancer, prevention, and therapeutic intervention options. Furthermore, as Lea, Calzone, and Masny (2002) reported,

An important question facing our society is to what extent, if any, genetic traits, conditions, or predispositions should provide a basis for determining access to certain societal good, such as insurance and employment. A potential exists for genetic screening and testing to promote or increase discrimination. . . . Concern has been raised that genetic technology only will be available to the affluent. The potential also exists for private companies to use a person's genetic information for lucrative purposes. Concern regarding stigmatization of groups is pertinent when genetic testing reveals alterations that are more prevalent in minority ethnic populations. For example, specific gene mutations in *BRCA1* and *BRCA2* genes have been identified in [Ashkenazic] Jewish populations. As another example, ethical issues of potential discrimination have been raised with drug development that uses research into variations in particular ethnic or racial groups. (pp. 22–23)

Practices specific to certain ethnic groups' beliefs and aspirations surrounding health and reproduction may have an impact on the client's or family's approach to genetic health care and decision making. In some cultures, for example, the cause of a genetic condition may be attributed to magic or divine intervention. Having an understanding of these kinds of cultural influences on a client's perceptions of health and illness helps in providing education about the implications of genetics (Fisher, 1996; Lea & Tinley, 1998).

Clients' past family experiences also influence their reception and understanding of genetic information, decision making, and adaptation to their current situation. Family members may have very different reactions to a diagnosis of genetic-based cancer in the family. Likewise, individual reactions to the prospect of genetic interventions such as genetic susceptibility testing may differ among family members, depending upon whether the family has been newly identified as carrying a susceptibility gene or has been followed for the condition over years (Lea et al., 1998). A person who has grown up with a sibling who has neurofibromatosis, for example, brings all of those experiences to a prenatal counseling session. As another example, a young woman whose mother died from breast cancer at the same age as the young woman is now may view predisposition testing for hereditary breast cancer with a greater sense of urgency than a woman whose mother has survived breast cancer for 10 years and currently is healthy (Lea & Tinley, 1998).

Nurses can incorporate awareness of the impact of ethnocultural and family background when inquiring about the family's genetic history. Given the opportunity, many clients are willing to discuss their experiences and beliefs as a member of a family with a genetic disorder (Lea & Tinley, 1998). Knowledge of this information helps nurses to provide culturally sensitive and appropriate genetic information. Including family, cultural, and religious community leaders in genetic-related health decisions can help to improve the communication of genetic health information and may lessen social, ethnic, and familial barriers (Lea et al., 1998).

Privacy and Confidentiality: Nursing Responsibilities

- Obtain written consent from all clients to release genetic information to any party, including family.
- Advocate for clients to obtain information, before testing or treatment, regarding the use of stored DNA samples.
- Encourage clients to make decisions about sharing appropriate genetic information with family and relatives.

Privacy and Confidentiality

Privacy and confidentiality with regard to genetic information are significant issues for nursing consideration. Privacy, as defined in ANA's *Code for Nurses* (2001), is the right of the individual to be left alone and free of unwanted intrusions. Privacy relating to genetic information refers to the individual's right to have control over personal information. The client is considered to have ownership of the information and to have ultimate authority over its disclosure. Informed consent must be obtained from the client prior to the disclosure of information to others, including family members, and information gathered for one purpose should not be used for another purpose without additional informed consent from the client (Scanlon & Fibison, 1995).

Nurses have a central role in maintaining client privacy, and this is especially true with regard to genetic information. Oncology nurses at all levels of practice are involved in obtaining family history information and participating in physical examinations, which often provide genetic information about clients and families, which is recorded in the client's medical record. Nurses are entrusted with genetic information that most clients consider to be very private. Oncology nurses have an obligation to promote the integrity, accuracy, and confidential use of the genetic information that they collect and record. According to the ANA's *Code for Nurses* (2001), the nurse is obligated to safeguard the client's right to privacy by judiciously protecting information of a confidential nature. Confidentiality is defined as the obligation of one person to another to keep information in confidence (Scanlon & Fibison, 1995). Nurses have a duty to uphold confidentiality of client information by protecting the client's control over personal information.

Genetic information about a client, like other medical information, is handled as confidential and should not be shared with others without the client's consent. Genetic information, however, has unique characteristics that distinguish it from other medical information. Genetic information, for example, can give information about future health risks. Clients who have undergone genetic susceptibility testing for cancer may face difficulties maintaining privacy of this personal medical information about their future health when questioned by an insurance company or prospective employer. Nurses can protect the client's desire for privacy of such information by ensuring that the client always gives written consent to release sensitive material about genetic test results and other genetic data to any third party.

Another consideration is that genetic tests may produce unexpected results, such as revealing nonpaternity of a child. Such potential consequences should be discussed with families participating in family studies during the informed-consent process prior to testing.

Genetic information also may reveal information about other family members' risk. For example, a client who has a confirmed diagnosis of a gene mutation that puts him or her at higher risk for breast cancer may feel pressure from family members to share this information with family but not wish to do so. This may present a moral dilemma for the nurse who supports client confidentiality and yet wishes to support and promote the health of other family members at risk. In this situation, the duty of confidentiality needs to be explored with the healthcare team, including medical ethicists, to protect innocent family members from harm.

Oncology nurses should encourage and support clients in making decisions about sharing appropriate genetic information with relatives, explaining that by sharing this personal information, the client demonstrates respect and caring for others and allows the family members to potentially improve their health outcomes and avoid harm (Grady, 1998; Scanlon & Fibison, 1995).

Client Advocacy

Client advocacy is a longstanding nursing ethic that, like autonomy, beneficence, and nonmaleficence, is founded upon the principle of justice. In the advocate role, oncology nurses support the client's right to be given accurate genetic information, to have access to genetic interventions and treatments, and to fair use of genetic information. At the most basic level, this means that nurses are knowledgeable about genetic resources and make sure that clients have access to the most up-to-date genetic information and interventions.

Oncology nurses can help clients to locate genetics services so that they can receive appropriate genetic interventions, including genetic testing. This may require that the nurse advocate for the client and family by working with the client's insurance company to ensure medical reimbursement, or if the client and family are without financial support, to help them to obtain alternative resources. Advocacy on the part of oncology nurses practicing as genetics nurse specialists includes participation in developing and promoting social policies that support equal access to genetic information and services.

Advocating for nondiscrimination is another important nursing function. Genetic information has the potential to lead to discrimination by others, including healthcare providers. The *Code for Nurses* stipulates that the nurse will provide care with respect for human dignity and the uniqueness of the client. Nursing care is unrestricted by consideration of social or economic status, personal attributes, or the nature of the health problem. Nursing care is delivered without prejudicial behavior (ANA, 2001). When advocating for nondiscrimination, all healthcare professionals need to be aware of their own values, beliefs, and biases, as previously discussed. The professional who is aware of his or her own biases will be less likely to act upon these biases in dealing with clients. Recognition of the continuous need for values clarification is an ongoing challenge for all oncology nurses that will help them to successfully advocate against discriminatory behavior toward clients and families with genetic concerns (Scanlon & Fibison, 1995).

Identifying Potentially Discriminatory Situations

Oncology nurses, as advocates, can help clients to recognize situations in which discrimination might occur. For example, clients should be informed in advance of participating in genetic evaluation, testing, or treatment that an insurance company may deny reimbursement or coverage in the future. This knowledge has led some clients and families to pay for genetic interventions on their own, outside of their insurance company, so that they will not be denied coverage in the future. If needed, the nurse, in collaboration with the healthcare team, can engage in dialogue with insurance companies to advocate for appropriate coverage and can guide a family through an insurance appeal process. Oncology nurses also may advocate for clients by clarifying the nature of an inherited cancer syndrome to a school or community nurse in an effort to make sure that these healthcare professionals have sufficient knowledge about the nature of the condition to develop appropriate health plans (Scanlon & Fibison, 1995).

Education as Advocacy

Educating clients, organizations, and the public about the application of molecular genetics to health care is a major way for all oncology nurses to advocate for equal and just use of genetic information. Because genetics is a relatively new field, healthcare professionals need to educate themselves about the ethical and genetic health issues and the potential for inequity in access to and unjust use of genetic information and technologies. Professionals who are well versed in these and other issues related to genetic health care can educate, or provide for the education of, clients, the public, and those working for organizations or institutions who may be engaged in making genetic-related healthcare decisions (Donaldson, 1997; Scanlon & Fibison, 1995).

Emerging Ethical Issues for Nurses

- Fair use of genetic interventions
- Equal access to genetic health care
- Potential for misuse of genetic information (e.g., eugenics, cloning of humans)
- Need for social policies to prevent insurance/employment and other discrimination against those with or at risk for genetic conditions
- Potential for fragmented care of individuals and families with genetic conditions

Emerging Ethical Issues for Oncology Nurses

Ethical issues facing oncology nurses are increasing as the applications of genetic technologies expand. The technology to provide in utero prenatal diagnosis of hereditary predisposition to a specific cancer syndrome is available. A parent who has familial adenomatous polyposis may consider prenatal testing for this condition in the unborn child so that the parent has the options of receiving early information for interventions or pregnancy termination when the fetus tests positive for the same condition.

Cancer Predisposition Testing in Children

Genetic testing of children for cancer susceptibility is another pressing ethical issue that healthcare providers face today. Children are involved as informed or uninformed observers of their parents' or family's participation in predisposition testing and potentially as being tested themselves. Their involvement raises questions about communication of complex, abstract medical information to children and also about the ethics of having parents make decisions about such testing before the child has reached adulthood. Making a decision as a parent to have a child tested may eliminate that child's right as an adult not to have testing (Garber & Patenaude, 1995; Patenaude, 1996).

Stem Cell Research

The promise of stem cell research, for science and advances in health care, is creating excitement. However, the application of human stem cells to develop new therapies is creating controversy. Sources of human pluripotent stem cells include early-stage embryos created in excess of clinical need in an in vitro fertilization clinic or nonliving fetuses from terminated pregnancies. Many people do not support this type of research because of the need for destruction of an embryo. The National Institutes of Health has developed guidelines to direct such research in an ethically responsible manner (see www.nih.gov/news/stemcell/index.htm).

Human Cloning

The issue of cloning humans to create the "perfect" person or to eliminate certain genetic traits that are considered undesirable is another emerging ethical issue for nursing consideration. Oncology nurses will need to maintain a current knowledge base regarding these important ethical issues to be able to responsibly respond to personal, client, and family questions.

Maintaining a Current Knowledge Base in Genetic Developments

The need for oncology nurses to participate in ongoing education in genetics in the clinical setting, professional schools, the community, and social policy realms cannot be overemphasized. All nurses must be knowledgeable about where and how to access relevant genetic information so that they can promote competent nursing practice within the framework of genetic advances (Jenkins, 1997; Scanlon & Fibison, 1995).

National Resources

The Human Genome Project has set aside approximately 5% of its budget for the Ethical, Legal, and Social Implications (ELSI) Program of the National Human Genome Research Institute. The goal of this project is to identify and clarify the initial responses to the emerging issues raised by the Human Genome Project research. The ELSI Program supports research projects, conferences, working groups, fellowships, and other initiatives that focus on such issues as privacy and confidentiality, nursing education and preparation, insurance and employment discrimination, quality control of genetic testing procedures, and public education. Oncology nurses can obtain valuable information about the Human Genome Project and its initiatives for themselves and for clients via the Internet. This will enable them to become active participants in discussions of the ethical, legal, and social considerations and to influence the provision of quality genetic health care (Lea, Williams, & Tinley, 1994).

Other national agencies such as the National Cancer Institute (NCI) and the National Institute for Nursing Research (NINR) have participated in planning educational programs and providing resources for nurses to continue to broaden their scope of practice in genetics. Both NCI and NINR, for example, provided financial support for a task force meeting to develop nursing curricula in genetics. Recommendations from this task force are being implemented, in part, through the National Coalition for Health Professional Education in Genetics, a national coalition developed by several federal agencies, professional and private organizations, consumers, and industry to develop a coordinated and systematic genetic educational effort. Ethical issues and decision making are two important components of these educational endeavors for nurses. Through these efforts, new ways to integrate genetic information and ethical decision making into clinical nursing practice are being de-

Educational Opportunities in Genetics for Oncology Nurses

- Programs developed through the Ethical, Legal, and Social Implications Program
- National Coalition for Health Professional Education in Genetics
- International Society of Nurses in Genetics
- American Academy of Nurses Genhealth—an electronic discussion group for health professionals in genetics
- Oncology Nursing Society Cancer Genetics Special Interest Group

veloped that will have an impact on oncology nursing practice in genetics (Collins, 1997; Jenkins, 1997).

Professional Societies

Several key professional genetics and nursing societies can serve as educational and professional resources to oncology nurses when facing difficult ethical dilemmas. Societies such as ISONG, a recognized group of nursing experts in genetics, has assumed responsibility for and offers opportunities to nurses for genetics education. Through ISONG's Web site, oncology nurses can take advantage of opportunities to have dialogue with genetics nurse specialists and gain access to a genetics nursing literature database. The Oncology Nursing Society has collaborated with the ISONG in a number of educational activities to enhance educational goals and opportunities for oncology nurses. Other genetics professional societies that may offer valuable information and educational opportunities to oncology nurses are the American Society of Human Genetics and the National Society of Genetic Counselors.

Client and Public Resources

Knowing how and when to access current genetics information will help oncology nurses to responsibly address the increasing demand from clients for genetic information. Clients and the public are anxious to receive correct and appropriate genetic information. Oncology nurses should be aware of how to locate genetic information and resources that may be useful to answer their clients' questions and concerns. Support groups for clients with genetic conditions are one important resource. These can be identified through a number of voluntary and national organizations (see Figure 9-7).

Figure 9-7. Genetics and Ethics Information Resources for Nurses on the Internet

The Dartmouth Ethics Institute: www.dartmouth.edu/artsci/ethics-inst

Clinical Genetics on the Web (Gene Care Link): www.jbpub.com/clinical-genetics/index.cfm

International Society of Nurses in Genetics: http://nursing.creighton.edu/isong

National Information Resource on Ethics & Human Genetics at the National Reference Center for Bioethics Literature, Kennedy Institute of Ethics, Georgetown University: www.georgetown.edu/research/nrcbl/nirehg.htm

National Human Genome Research Institute: www.genome.gov

ONS Online: www.ons.org

Conclusion

The nursing profession faces the challenge of assuring the public that nurses are competent in understanding and using genetic information. Oncology nurses can develop new skills and roles that will enable them to significantly influence the quality of genetic health care they provide to clients, families, and communities. They can develop or enhance skills in bioethical decision making that are founded upon ethical principles, an ethic of care that focuses on the support of human growth and self-actualization and on virtue, which guides and supports their ability to do good and to be in harmony with life. This foundation supports the application of genetic knowledge to daily nursing practice and enhances oncology nurses' abilities to translate this new knowledge in an ongoing way into support of clients, families, and communities.

References

American Nurses Association. (2001). *Code for nurses with interpretive statements.* Kansas City, MO: Author.

Andrews, L.B., Fullarton, J.E., Holtzman, N.A., & Motulsky, A. (Eds.). (1994). *Assessing genetic risks.* Washington, DC: National Academy Press.

Beauchamp, T.L., & Childress, J.F. (1994). *Principles of biomedical ethics.* New York: Oxford University Press.

Bove, C.M., Fry, S.T., & MacDonald, D.J. (1997). Presymptomatic and predisposition genetic testing: Ethical and social considerations. *Seminars in Oncology Nursing, 12,* 135–140.

Cameron, M.E. (1996). An ethical perspective: Virtue ethics for nurses and health care. *Journal of Nursing Law, 3*(4), 26–39.

Cassells, J.M., & Gaul, A.L. (1998, January). An ethical assessment framework for nursing practice. *The Maryland Nurse,* pp. 9–11.

Cassells, J.M., Gaul, A.L., Lea, D.H., Calzone, K., & Jenkins, J. (1999). An ethical assessment framework: Oncology nurses evaluate usefulness for clinical practice. *Cancer Genetics Special Interest Group Newsletter, 3*(2), 4–8.

Cassells, J.M., & Redman, B.K. (1989). Preparing students to be moral agents in clinical nursing practice: Report of a national survey. *Nursing Clinics of North America, 24,* 463–473.

Cassells, J.M., Silva, M.C., & Chop, R.C. (1990). Administrative strategies to support staff nurses as moral agents in clinical practice. *Nursing Connection, 3*(4), 31–37.

Collins, F. (1997). Preparing health professionals for the genetic revolution. *JAMA, 278,* 1285–1286.

Donaldson, S.K. (1997). The genetic social revolution and the professional status of nursing. *Nursing Outlook, 45*, 278–279.

Fine, B. (1993). The evolution of nondirectiveness in genetic counseling and implications of the Human Genome Project. In D. Bartels, B. Leroy, & D. Caplan (Eds.), *Prescribing our future: Ethical challenges in genetic counseling* (pp. 101–117). New York: Aldine de Gruyter.

Fisher, N.L. (1996). *Cultural and ethnic diversity: A guide for genetics professionals.* Baltimore: Johns Hopkins University Press.

Garber, J.E., & Patenaude, A. (1995). Ethical, social and counseling issues in hereditary cancer susceptibility. *Cancer Surveys, 25*, 381–397.

Grady, C. (1998). Ethics, genetics, and nursing practice. In D.H. Lea, J. Jenkins, & C. Francomano (Eds.), *Genetics in clinical practice: New directions for nursing and health care* (pp. 225–256). Boston: Jones and Bartlett.

Grundstein-Amado, R. (1992). Differences in ethical decision-making processes among nurses and doctors. *Journal of Advanced Nursing, 17*, 129–137.

International Society of Nurses in Genetics. (1998). *Statement on the scope and standards of genetics clinical nursing practice.* Washington, DC: American Nurses Publishing.

Jenkins, J. (1997). Educational issues related to cancer genetics. *Seminars in Oncology Nursing, 13*, 141–144.

Ketefian, S. (1989). Moral reasoning and ethical practice in nursing practice. *Nursing Clinics of North America, 24*, 509–521.

Lea, D.H., Calzone, K., & Masny, A. (2002). *Genetics and cancer care: A guide for oncology nurses—An innovative teaching and learning module for integrating genetics into oncology nursing practice.* Pittsburgh: Oncology Nursing Society.

Lea, D.H., Jenkins, J., & Francomano, C. (1998). *Genetics in clinical practice: New directions for nursing and health care.* Boston: Jones and Bartlett.

Lea, D.H., & Tinley, S. (1998). Genetics in the OR: Implications for nursing practice. *AORN: The Official Journal of the Association of Operating Room Nurses, 67*, 1175–1191.

Lea, D.H., Williams J., & Tinley, S. (1994). Nursing and genetic health care. *Journal of Genetic Counseling, 3*, 113–124.

Leavitt, F.J. (1996). Educating nurses for their future role in bioethics. *Nursing Ethics, 3*(1), 39–52.

Noddings, N. (1984). *Caring: A feminist approach to ethics and moral education.* Berkeley, CA: University of California Press.

Oncology Nursing Society. (2000a). The role of the oncology nurse in cancer genetic counseling. *Oncology Nursing Forum, 27*, 1348.

Oncology Nursing Society. (2000b). Cancer predisposition genetic testing and risk assessment counseling. *Oncology Nursing Forum, 27*, 1349.

Patenaude, A.F. (1996). The genetic testing of children for cancer susceptibility: Ethical, legal and social issues. *Behavioral Sciences and the Law, 14,* 393–410.

Rieger, P.T., & Pentz, R.D. (1999). Genetic testing and informed consent. *Seminars in Oncology Nursing, 15*(2), 104–115.

Scanlon, C., & Fibison, W. (1995). Managing genetic information: Implications for nursing practice. Washington, DC: American Nurses Association.

Wertz, D., & Fletcher, J. (Eds.). (1989). *Ethics and human genetics: A cross-cultural perspective.* New York: Springer-Verlag.

10

How to Identify Appropriate Referrals and Current Resources

Elizabeth Glaser, RN, MSN

Introduction

What is the role of nursing in the rapidly advancing field of genetics? Regardless of their specialty area, how do nurses gain the basic knowledge needed to understand the implications of this burgeoning amount of information? Patients traditionally have looked to nurses to interpret the sometimes complex medical data with which they are faced. In their role as patient advocate, nurses frequently serve as resources for education, referral, and emotional support. To continue this function, nurses must take the initiative to enhance their own basic genetics knowledge, identify resources for patients, clients, and their families, and develop novel ways of incorporating new technologies into comprehensive nursing care.

Web sites published by reputable organizations (see Table 10-1) are valuable resources for nurses who want to enhance their knowledge of genetics. This chapter will cite relevant Internet addresses throughout the text.

Resources for Networking and Genetics Information

Oncology Nursing Society

One of the most accessible resources for nurses seeking to enhance their understanding of cancer genetics is often the most overlooked: their own colleagues.

The Oncology Nursing Society (ONS), the largest professional membership oncology association in the world, is at the forefront in setting the highest

Table 10-1. Web Resources for Cancer Genetics Information

Professional Organization	Web Site
American Academy of Nursing (AAN)	www.nursingworld.org/aan/index.htm
American Board of Medical Genetics (ABMG)	www.abmg.org
American College of Medical Genetics (ACMG)	www.faseb.org/genetics/acmg/index.html
American Nurses Association (ANA)	www.nursingworld.org
American Society of Clinical Oncology (ASCO)	www.asco.org
American Society of Human Genetics (ASHG)	www.ashg.org/genetics/ashg/ashgmenu.htm
International Society of Nurses in Genetics (ISONG)	www.nursing.creighton.edu/isong
National Coalition for Health Professional Education in Genetics (NCHPEG)	www.nchpeg.org
National Society of Genetic Counselors, Inc. (NSGC)	www.nsgc.org
Oncology Nursing Society (ONS)	www.ons.org
Other Sites	
Cancer Genetics Network (CGN)	http://epi.grants.cancer.gov/CGN
CancerNet (links to CANCERLIT)	www.cancernet.nci.nih.gov
GeneTests	www.genetests.org
Genetic Alliance	www.geneticalliance.org
Genetics Resources on the Web (GROW)	www.nih.gov/sigs/bioethics/grow.html
National Cancer Institute (NCI)	www.cancer.gov
National Human Genome Research Institute (NHGRI) (links to Ethical, Legal, Social Issues [ELSI] Program)	www.genome.gov
National Institute for Nursing Research (NINR)	www.nih.gov/ninr
Online Mendelian Inheritance in Man	www.ncbi.nlm.nih.gov/omim
Thomas—U.S. Congress on the Internet	http://thomas.loc.gov

standards of patient care. Through its annual Congress and Institutes of Learning, it strives to present oncology nurses with not only the most current medical information but also with guidelines to translate the data into improvements in the clinical setting. ONS is working to ensure that oncology nurses, with their established knowledge surrounding the treatment and supportive care of patients with cancer, assume a vital role in the emerging specialty of cancer genetics. ONS chapters provide an opportunity for networking within communities, and many sponsor continuing education sessions on cancer genetics.

In 1998, ONS published two positions related to genetics: "Cancer Genetic Testing and Risk Assessment Counseling" and "The Role of the Oncology Nurse in Cancer Genetic Counseling." Both papers were revised in August 2000 (ONS, 2000a, 2000b). The first of these papers stresses the need for obtaining informed consent and the importance of pre- and post-test counseling by individuals trained not only in the technical aspects of cancer genetics but also in the complex psychosocial, ethical, and legal issues surrounding genetic testing. ONS advocates research in all areas of cancer genetics, development of educational resources, and regulation of laboratories performing genetic testing.

In delineating the oncology nurse's role in cancer genetics, ONS asserts that oncology nurses are ideally prepared to assume expanded roles in cancer genetics and genetic-risk assessment and counseling. In clarifying the nurse's role, ONS outlines three levels of practice: the general oncology nurse; the advanced practice oncology nurse, basic level; and the advanced practice oncology nurse with specialty training in genetics (see Chapter 2 for a detailed description of these levels of practice). For nurses at both general and advanced levels, the society recommends a foundation in genetics knowledge provided by nursing school curricula, continuing education, and specialized cancer genetics programs.

The ONS Cancer Genetics Special Interest Group (SIG) was founded in 1997 to provide a forum for networking, exchange of information, and discussion of implications for clinical practice. In addition, the SIG encourages research in the areas of cancer genetics and cancer risk counseling; supports basic and continuing education in the field; advances the establishment of nursing practice guidelines; and serves as a liaison with other groups, such as the International Society of Nurses in Genetics (ISONG) and the National Society of Genetic Counselors (NSGC). The Cancer Genetics SIG has been instrumental in planning educational sessions at ONS meetings. The SIG's newsletter keeps members informed of new research in the field, activities of other members, legislative developments, and journal articles of interest.

In addition to these avenues for networking, ONS Online (www.ons.org) provides easy access to the latest developments in oncology nursing. It details upcoming conferences and continuing education programs and provides information on ONS chapters and SIGs. The site's News section summarizes breaking news from the cancer and general medical communities. It also lists employment opportunities and updates healthcare legislation. Major cancer centers are described and algorithms for disease management are discussed within the Clinical Practice section. The research section features discussion forums, resources, and information on grants available to oncology nurses.

The ONS Online Library contains the full text of its position papers, as well as articles from the *Clinical Journal of Oncology Nursing*, *Oncology Nursing Forum*, *Oncology Nursing Updates*, and the *Journal of the National Cancer Insti-*

tute. Search capabilities for these publications are available, as well as links to other clinical journals. Discussion forums are accessible throughout the Web site, enabling ONS Online users to confer with colleagues from around the world on an array of issues. ONS Online also has introduced a section to assist members in understanding clinical genetics and its impact on oncology nursing. The Genetics Resource Area can be accessed through the Clinical Practice—Prevention/Detection section. This area features a bibliography of genetics articles in the *Oncology Nursing Forum* and a moderated discussion forum on genetic issues. The full text of the booklet *Understanding Gene Testing*, published by the Department of Health and Human Services, also is included.

International Society of Nurses in Genetics

ISONG is a professional association for nurses working in all areas of genetics. Its purpose is to improve the quality of genetic services provided to patients by enhancing the scientific and professional growth of nurses as they incorporate genetic theory into clinical practice, research, and education. ISONG has been active in defining the scope and standards of genetic nursing practice (ISONG, 1998). These standards have been approved by the American Nurses Association (ANA) and were published in June 1998. ISONG also is active in developing standards for credentialing in genetics. As the representative organization for nurses working in all areas of genetics, ISONG encourages networking among members, genetics education for all nurses, and nursing research into human genetics. With the impact of genetic discoveries on the practice of oncology, many oncology nurses have joined the ranks of ISONG members, and the organization is actively involved in developing educational programs and guidelines for this emerging subspecialty. ISONG's annual conference, held in conjunction with the meeting of the American Society of Human Genetics (ASHG), offers presentations on a variety of genetic topics, including cancer genetics. The organization maintains a listserv that provides members with an excellent means of communicating with colleagues and sharing new developments online. The ISONG Web site (http://nursing .creighton.edu/isong) provides nurses with resources to integrate developments in human genetics into practice, education, and research activities. The site lists educational programs, employment positions, and links to sites for many other genetic and nursing organizations. One of these sites, the University of Kansas Medical Center Information for Genetic Professionals, is particularly comprehensive, introducing the user to a multitude of genetic resources.

American Academy of Nursing

The American Academy of Nursing published *The Genetics Revolution: Implications for Nursing*, a monograph that reviewed basic genetics and explored the impact of genetics on disease prevention and diagnosis (Lashley, 1997). This publication discussed ethical and public health policy implications and the need for nurses to assume research, advisory, and clinical roles in the area of genetics.

American Nurses Association

ANA is another organization that is examining the nurse's responsibility in genetic health. Its publication *Managing Genetic Information: Implications for Nursing Practice* reviews recent genetic discoveries and provides guidelines for nursing practice, including consideration of the ethical, legal, and social issues involved in obtaining informed consent (Scanlon & Fibison, 1995). These recommendations are based on findings of an ANA-conducted national survey, funded by the Ethical, Legal and Social Implications (ELSI) Branch of the National Human Genome Research Institute (NHGRI). This study was initiated to evaluate the management of genetic information by nurses and to establish professional and ethical standards for utilizing this theory in providing comprehensive patient care.

In conjunction with the American Medical Association (AMA) and NHGRI, ANA has formed the National Coalition for Health Professional Education in Genetics (NCHPEG). Its members consist of representatives from approximately 100 groups—including private industry, government, consumers, and managed care organizations—in addition to genetics professionals. This coalition aims to give primary healthcare providers the knowledge, skills, and resources they need to integrate the latest genetic knowledge and technologies into quality healthcare delivery. NCHPEG plans to develop the tools and resources necessary to assist these professionals in incorporating genetics into each discipline's knowledge base.

To provide guidance for establishing such training, NCHPEG recently published its "Recommendations of Core Competencies in Genetics Essential for All Health Professionals." (Jenkins et al., 2001), This document outlines the minimum knowledge, skills, and attitudes required for healthcare professionals to integrate genetic issues and concerns into their respective practices. These guidelines are available on the NCHPEG Web site (www.nchpeg.org).

National Society of Genetic Counselors

Although communication within the nursing profession is important, nurses also must maintain a relationship with other disciplines involved in cancer genetics. NSGC, a group of professionals specially trained in providing education and counseling to patients with all types of genetic disease, is actively involved in conducting research, establishing patient-care guidelines, and educating its members regarding cancer genetics. Approximately 70% of genetic counselors are board-certified by the American Board of Genetic Counseling (ABGC) or by the American Board of Medical Genetics (ABMG). Certification requirements include a graduate degree in genetic counseling; clinical experience in an ABGC-approved site; a log book of 50 supervised cases; and successful completion of both general and specialty certification exams, which are prepared and administered by ABGC. NSGC's Annual Education Conference (AEC) offers cancer genetics information via practice-based symposia, sponsored speakers, workshops, presented papers, and posters. Nurses may attend the AEC as associate members of NSGC or as nonmembers. The conference schedule is available through the NSGC Web site (www.nsgc.org). Nurses can be full members of NSGC if they have a master's or higher level degree, have undergone a broad range of clinical genetics training, and can cite genetic counseling as their primary responsibility.

Physician Groups

Physician groups that are involved in genetics include the American Society of Clinical Oncology (ASCO), the American College of Medical Genetics (ACMG), and ABMG. Information about ASCO's curriculum guidelines for cancer genetic and cancer predisposition testing is available on its Web site (www.asco.org) in the Guidelines section. ASCO also has published a policy paper on predisposition genetic testing, outlining recommendations on cancer risk counseling, indications for testing, informed consent, and management after testing.

ASCO is active in curriculum development for cancer genetics education and offers a genetics course prior to or during its annual spring meeting. In order to promote standards for clinical competence and excellence in patient care, ASCO supported credentialing in Familial Cancer Risk Assessment and Management (FCRAM) through the Institute for Clinical Evaluation (ICE). Unfortunately, ICE is no longer offering the FCRAM exam. Advanced practice nurses, physicians, genetic counselors, and other healthcare providers who work in clinical cancer genetics were eligible to take the competency exam. Additional information is available on the ICE Web site (www.icemed.org).

The goal of ACMG is the maintenance of high standards in education, practice, and research. Fellows of ACMG must possess a medical degree or a doctorate. Certified genetic counselors may join as associate members, and other individuals with an interest in medical genetics may join as affiliate members. ACMG is involved in professional and public education and works to increase access to medical genetic services. In 1999, it published its clinical guidelines for breast and ovarian cancer genetic risk assessment; counseling; and testing, including a recommended testing protocol.

ABMG is the credentialing group for MDs and PhDs in medical genetics. This agency accredits training programs in the field of human genetics and prepares the certifying exam.

Another genetics professional group, the ASHG, aims to unite investigators from the many research areas of human genetics. Its membership includes researchers, clinicians, laboratory personnel, genetic counselors, and nurses. ASHG's annual meeting serves as a forum for research findings and education about genetics. The group assumes an active role in establishing policy regarding standards for genetic research and testing; its numerous policy papers are available on its Web site (www.faseb.org/genetics/ashg/ashgmenu.htm).

Human Genetic Resources

Genetics Resources on the Web

Genetics Resources on the Web (GROW) (www.nih.gov/sigs/bioethics/ grow.html) is an umbrella organization that currently provides a network for collaboration and the communication of Web-based human genetics information (Guttmacher & Collins, 2000). Members of GROW's organizations share concerns about the availability of quality genetic information for both professionals and the public. In the future, GROW will address the possibility of providing a search engine for genetics information; develop criteria for member organizations; and, as a quality assurance measure, review the content of Web sites that publish information about genetics.

Online Mendelian Inheritance in Man

Online Mendelian Inheritance in Man (OMIM) (www.ncbi.nlm.nih.gov/ omim) is a Web site that provides a database of information about human genes and genetic disorders. The OMIM database contains text, references, and clinical synopses of genetic disorders.

Sources of Patient Referrals

In their role as patient advocates, nurses frequently serve as referral sources. As cancer genetics moves from the research to the clinical setting, it is essential that nurses know what resources are available for genetic counseling and testing. Several sites on the World Wide Web provide access to information on patient referral.

National Cancer Institute, National Institutes of Health

A list of professionals specializing in cancer genetics is available through the National Cancer Institute's (NCI's) CancerNet™ (http://cancernet .nci.nih.gov). This site enables users to search by geographic location, cancer type (e.g., breast, colon, endocrine), or specific genetic condition (e.g., ataxia telangiectasia). The directory lists names and qualifications of the providers, as well as telephone numbers and e-mail and mailing addresses. Also provided are directions regarding how to register as a qualified provider of cancer genetics information.

The Cancer Information Service (CIS), sponsored by NCI, provides information on facilities that offer genetic testing and counseling. CIS is a resource for up-to-date, accurate information for patients and families, healthcare professionals, and the general public. The service can be reached toll-free in the United States from 9 am to 4:30 pm Monday through Friday at 800-4CANCER (22-6237). In addition, hearing-impaired individuals can access TTY services by calling the toll-free number 800-332-8615.

To spearhead a national effort in cancer genetics clinical research, NCI has established a Cancer Genetics Network (CGN), a group of eight U.S. medical research centers. This network encourages collaborative efforts in studying the genetic basis of cancer susceptibility, establishing ways to integrate new findings into clinical practice, and clarifying the associated psychosocial, ethical, legal, and public health issues. Its goal is to use the knowledge obtained from studying individuals with inherited susceptibility to cancer to improve screening, diagnosis, treatment, and prevention of the disease. By working together, the centers hope to perform research that would not be possible in a single institution because of insufficient numbers. Information about ongoing studies and whom to contact is on the CGN Web site (http://epi.grants.cancer.gov/ CGN). Several National Institutes of Health (NIH) studies offer genetic testing as part of their protocols. Nurses seeking information about eligibility criteria for participation in such a study may call the protocol resource office toll-free at 800-411-1222.

National Society of Genetic Counselors

The NSGC Web site (www.nsgc.org) includes a provider list, accessible by clicking the Resource Link button on the home page. This information is categorized according to state and identifies which genetic specialty is available (e.g., cancer genetics, prenatal genetics). The list is updated regularly but may not provide a complete list of genetic counselors involved in cancer genetics, particularly those at university medical centers or other hospitals.

GeneTests

Genetic testing is now performed in commercial and research laboratories across the United States. GeneTests, a service funded by the National Library of Medicine of the NIH and the Maternal and Child Health Bureau of the Health Resources and Services Administration, provides a list of clinical and research labs that conduct testing for inherited disorders. It also sponsors a genetics clinics directory and introductory information about genetic counseling and testing. The section of the site called GeneClinics offers disease-specific data, including information about diagnosis, management, and counseling.

Genetic Alliance

The Genetic Alliance (formerly the Alliance of Genetic Support Groups) is a nonprofit organization dedicated to helping individuals and families with genetic disorders. It serves as a resource for consumers and professionals seeking genetic support groups and genetic services. It provides a toll-free helpline (800-336-GENE [4363]), as well as a comprehensive Web site (www.geneticalliance.org). This site contains a listing of established support groups that is searchable by genetic condition, services offered, or organization name. Recent editions of the alliance newsletter, *Alert*, are available online; links to many educational resources, including Cancer Risk Assessment and Counseling, also are provided.

Genetic and Rare Diseases Information Center

The Genetic and Rare Diseases Information Center (www.nhgri.nih.gov/Info_Center) is the result of collaboration involving the Genetic Alliance, the NIH Office of Rare Diseases, and the NHGRI. Communication specialists at the center answer questions about genetic and rare diseases; the questions come from the general public, healthcare professionals, and biomedical researchers. For information, call the center's toll-free number (888-205-2311) or e-mail gardinfo@nih.gov.

Resources for Continuing Education

The rapidly changing nature of genetic information makes quality continuing education essential for all professionals in the field. A group of nurses and genetic counselors with expertise in cancer genetics has published a series of programmed instructional models in the journal *Cancer Nursing*. These six articles cover the Human Genome Project, basic concepts of genes and inheritance, cancer genetics, genetic testing, the application of genetics to clinical oncology, and the role of nursing in this developing specialty area (Biesecker, 1997; Dimond, Calzone, Davis, & Jenkins, 1998; Dimond, Peters, & Jenkins, 1997; Middelton, Peters, & Helmbold, 1997; Peters, Dimond, & Jenkins, 1997; Peters & Hadley, 1997). This series of papers, which presents an excellent foundation on which to build further genetics expertise, is presently being revised (Middelton & Peters, 2001; Peters, Menaker, Wilson, & Hadley, 2001).

The previously described professional groups sponsor ongoing education in genetics through their annual meetings and updated Web pages. ISONG presents genetics educational sessions prior to the start of its annual fall meeting. Additional organizations also offer short courses in cancer genetics; some are highlighted in the following sections.

Fox Chase Cancer Center

Fox Chase Cancer Center in Philadelphia presents a three-day educational program, Familial Cancer Risk Counseling: A Basic Education Program for Nurses, once each year. This program covers the basics of cancer genetics and familial cancer; familial cancer risk factors; risk-counseling strategies; and the ethical, legal, and social issues associated with genetic risk assessment. Additional information, including upcoming course dates, is available at www.fccc.edu/nursing/nursingeducation.html or by calling the Department of Nursing Continuing Education at 215-728-3522. Additionally, Fox Chase offers an annual course for advanced practice nurses interested in learning about the competencies required for integration of genetics into clinical, education, research, and consultative roles.

Cincinnati Children's Hospital Medical Center

Nursing faculty who are interested in obtaining new knowledge about human genetics and incorporating this knowledge into nursing school curricula may take advantage of the Genetics Program for Nursing Faculty, conducted at Cincinnati Children's Hospital Medical Center. Information about this program is available on the hospital's Web site at www.cincinnatichildrens.org/education/Gpnf/about. The hospital also offers the Genetics Summer Institute for faculty interested in knowing more about the laboratory components of genetics in conjunction with clinical applications of genetic information. Further information is available from the Web site at www.cincinnatichildrens.org/education/gpnf/genetics.

The National Institute of Nursing Research

Each summer the National Institute of Nursing Research offers an intensive two-month training program that provides a foundation in genetics for use in clinical practice, education, and research. The Summer Genetics Institute is designed for nursing faculty, graduate students, and advanced practice nurses. For more information, see www.nih.gov/ninr/index.html.

The City of Hope National Medical Center

The City of Hope National Medical Center, in Duarte, CA (near Los Angeles), offers an interdisciplinary cancer genetics fellowship program. The training focuses on cancer genetics and cancer prevention and control research. For master's nurse fellows, the fellowship is a one-year program; for doctoral fellows, a two-year program. The fellowship provides didactic training in oncology, cancer genetics, and research methodology; closely mentored clinical training; and the opportunity to complete a research project.

For advance practice nurses, the City of Hope offers a 10-day intensive course in cancer-risk assessment. This course focuses on epidemiology, genetics, and oncology principles relevant to clinical genetics practice.

For information about the fellowship and course, telephone Deborah MacDonald at 626-256-8662 or e-mail her at dmacdonald@coh.org.

Resources for Information Regarding Genetics and Health Policy

With new discoveries in genetics taking place almost daily, staying abreast of vital information has become increasingly difficult. Many books and journals are outdated almost as soon as they are published. The World Wide Web, with its ability to be updated almost instantaneously, is an invaluable source of cancer genetics material. In addition to the Web sites of the previously mentioned professional organizations, many other sites offer extensive information about the science of genetics, cancer genetics specifically, and health policy regarding genetics (see Table 10-1).

National Cancer Institute

NCI's Web site (www.cancer.gov) is an excellent starting point. As a resource for both healthcare professionals and patients, it presents information on all types of cancer, training and funding opportunities, and the latest scientific developments. One of its largest components is CancerNet, which contains in-depth information on genetic testing and treatment. The CancerNet section called Genetics, Causes, Risk Factors, Prevention offers a comprehensive guide to cancer genetics. Within this section, the General Information area presents a cancer genetics overview and guidelines for risk assessment and counseling; a directory of cancer genetics professionals lists experts according to type of cancer, geographic location, and name. CancerNet also details information on clinical trials, presents abstracts of cancer genetics policy papers, and alerts the user to a variety of other resources.

CANCERLIT, accessible through CancerNet, is a bibliographic database of cancer literature with more than 1.3 million citations and abstracts from more than 4,000 different sources—including biomedical journals, proceedings, books, reports, and doctoral theses—from 1963 to the present. Although the site does not provide the full text of articles, it supplies authors, sources, abstracts (when available), and other basic information. It is updated monthly. Also included are predesigned searches of articles specific to cancer genetics and familial cancer syndromes.

National Human Genome Research Institute

NHGRI's Web site (www.genome.gov) is another comprehensive source of information. NHGRI was established in 1989 to head the Human Genome Project. In its efforts to map the genetic code of the entire human genome, this project applies genome technologies to find human disease genes and develop DNA-based diagnostics and therapeutics. The ELSI branch of NHGRI supports research to anticipate and resolve ethical, legal, and social issues arising from genetic research. The group also fosters public education and discussion of these issues. In addition to scientific genetic data, the NHGRI Web site features information about the Human Genome Project, public policy and grants, off-site resources, and intramural research. Its keyword-search program provides data on virtually any genetic topic.

Three short videos provide an alternative medium for delivering cancer genetic education. Two documentary videos are available online at the NHGRI Web site (www.genome.gov/Pages/Hyperion/educationkit/index.html): *The Human Genome Project—Exploring Our Molecular Selves* and *The Secret of Our*

Lives. These videos discuss the Human Genome Project and its effect on our future.

In 1997, the Hereditary Susceptibility Working Group of the now-disbanded National Action Plan on Breast Cancer produced a 14-minute video, *Genetic Testing for Breast Cancer Risk: It's Your Choice.* This presentation was designed for healthcare professionals to offer to patients as one part of an education and counseling process for informed decision making. It gives an overview of the risks and benefits of genetic testing for breast cancer susceptibility, with interviews of patients and families who have faced this choice. Copies of the video, with its accompanying brochure and fact sheet, are available free of charge by calling 800-4CANCER (22-6237) and placing a request with the Publications Division.

Genetics Legislation

Nurses need to be aware of current legislative developments regarding genetic testing. Presently, the U.S. Congress is considering laws to prohibit insurance and employment discrimination based on genetic information. Some states already have passed similar legislation, and other states have bills pending. National advocacy groups, such as the National Breast Cancer Coalition, are active in supporting this legislative agenda and informing healthcare professionals of legal developments. A Congress-sponsored Web site (www.thomas.com) provides a keyword search and the full text of proposed bills, as well as bill summary and status. The Policy, Education and Outreach Branch of the NHGRI's Office of Policy Coordination actively monitors federal legislation related to genetics. The NHGRI Web site features updated information on congressional testimony and activity (www.genome.gov/PolicyEthics).

Because cancer genetics is a new field with an abundance of emerging data and opinions, it is essential that guidelines concerning the use of this information be established. NCI's Statement on Genetic Testing for Cancer Risk outlines factors that must be considered in offering cancer predisposition testing. Other groups—such as ASHG, ASCO, ACMG, and NSGC—also have issued policy statements on genetic testing and have included the full text of these positions on their Web sites (see Figure 10-1). The Cancer Genetic Studies Consortium, a committee of ELSI that supports and fosters research on the psychosocial issues involved in genetic testing, has published position papers on surveillance recommendations for carriers of gene mutations associated with breast and colon cancer (Burke, Daly, et al., 1997; Burke, Petersen, et al., 1997).

Figure 10-1. Policy Papers

American College of Medical Genetics. (1999). *Genetic susceptibility to breast and ovarian cancer: Assessment, counseling and testing guidelines.* Retrieved August 30, 2001 from the World Wide Web: http://www.health.state.ny.us/nysdoh/cancer/obcancer/contents.htm

American Society of Human Genetics. (1991). ASHG Human Genome Committee report. The Human Genome Project: Implications for human genetics. *American Journal of Human Genetics, 49,* 687–691.

American Society of Human Genetics. (1996). ASHG report. Statement on informed consent for genetic research. *American Journal of Human Genetics, 59,* 471–474.

American Society of Human Genetics/American College of Medical Genetics. (1995). Points to consider: Ethical, legal, and psychosocial implications of genetic testing in children and adolescents. (1995). *American Journal of Human Genetics, 57,* 1233–1241.

National Action Plan on Breast Cancer. (1996, March). *Position paper: Hereditary susceptibility testing for breast cancer.* Retrieved August 30, 2001, from http:www.4woman.gov/napbc/napbc/hspospap.htm

National Advisory Council for Human Genome Research. (1994). Statement on use of DNA testing for presymptomatic identification of cancer risk. *JAMA, 271,* 785.

Oncology Nursing Society. (2000a). Cancer predisposition genetic testing and risk assessment counseling. *Oncology Nursing Forum, 27,* 1349.

Oncology Nursing Society. (2000b). The role of the oncology nurse in cancer genetic counseling. *Oncology Nursing Forum, 27,* 1348.

Statement of the American Society of Clinical Oncology. (1996). Genetic testing for cancer susceptibility. *Journal of Clinical Oncology, 14,* 1730–1736.

Statement of the American Society of Human Genetics on genetic testing for breast and ovarian cancer predisposition. (1994). *American Journal of Human Genetics, 55,* i–iv.

Statement on use of DNA testing for presymptomatic identification of cancer risk. (1994). *JAMA, 271,* 785.

Research Opportunities

Compared to the rapid progress of scientific discoveries in genetics, integration of these findings with the behavioral sciences is progressing slowly. For nurses to assume a significant role in the new arena of cancer genetics, they must conduct research regarding the clinical application of laboratory science. The field of genetics offers a variety of opportunities for nursing research, from biological studies to behavioral investigations (Sigmon, Grady, & Amende, 1997). Of particular importance is the establishment of appropriate models for the education and counseling of patients and families and evaluation of the psychosocial effects of genetic testing. ELSI funds and manages research grants and educational projects at institutions throughout the United States. Detailed information on specific programs and grant application instructions are available on the NHGRI Web site (www.genome.gov). This site features a section under Grants titled Linking Nursing and Genetic Research, which describes the many research topics relevant to nursing as outlined at a 1996 National Institute of Nursing Research (NINR) workshop: "Opportunities in Genetic Research." In collaboration with NINR, ELSI also provides long- and short-term support for individual postdoctoral and senior fellowships to scientists seeking training that will enable them to investigate the clinical implications of human genetic research. Information about the research objectives and application procedures for these programs is also available on the NINR Web site (www.nih.gov/ninr).

ISONG also provides online information about nursing research in genetics and links to Qualitative Research Methods, a site specializing in data analysis consultation.

Summary

The ongoing expansion of genetic information presents new challenges for oncology nurses. Understanding the advances in genetics and their impact on cancer prevention, diagnosis, and treatment is vital to providing comprehensive patient education and care. Nursing professional groups are an excellent resource to aid nurses in processing the growing volume of complex information. Professional organizations of other specialties complement this resource and enhance communication within this multidisciplinary field.

Because of their prominent role in patient care, nurses must familiarize themselves with the increasingly significant impact of genetics in oncology; they must possess a comprehensive knowledge of genetics and understand how to access pertinent information. It is particularly important that nurses recognize those individuals who need a referral to a cancer genetics program and acquaint themselves with available resources.

References

Biesecker, B.B. (1997). Genetic testing for cancer predisposition. *Cancer Nursing, 20,* 285–299.

Burke, W., Daly, M., Garber, J., Botkin, J., Kahn, M.J., Lynch, P., et al. (1997). Consensus statement: Recommendations for follow-up care of individuals with an inherited predisposition to cancer: II. BRCA1 and BRCA2. *JAMA, 277,* 997–1003.

Burke, W., Petersen, G., Lynch, P., Botkin, J., Daly, M., Garber, J., Kahn, M.J., McTiernan, A., Offit, K., Thomson, E., & Varricchio, C. (1997). Consensus statement: Recommendations for follow-up care of individuals with an inherited predisposition to cancer: I. Hereditary nonpolyposis colon cancer. *JAMA, 277,* 915–919.

Dimond, E., Calzone, K., Davis, J., & Jenkins, J. (1998). The role of the nurse in cancer genetics. *Cancer Nursing, 21,* 57–74.

Dimond, E., Peters, J., & Jenkins, J. (1997). The genetic basis of cancer. *Cancer Nursing, 20,* 213–225.

Guttmacher, A., & Collins, F. (2000). Genetics resources on the Web (GROW). *Genetics in Medicine, 2,* 296–299.

International Society of Nurses in Genetics. (1998). *Statement on the scope and standards of genetics clinical nursing practice.* Washington, DC: American Nurses Publishing.

Jenkins, J., Blitzer, M., Boehm, K., Feetham, S., Getting, B., Johnson, A., et al., for the Core Competency Working Group of the National Coalition for Health Professional Education in Genetics (NCHPEG). (2001). Recommendations of core competencies in genetics essential for all health professionals. *Genetics in Medicine. 3*(2), 155–158.

Lashley, F. (Ed.). (1997). *The genetics revolution: Implications for nursing.* Washington, DC: American Academy of Nursing.

Middelton, L.A., & Peters, K.F. (2001). Genes and inheritance. *Cancer Nursing, 24,* 357–370.

Middelton, L.A., Peters, K.F., & Helmbold, E.A. (1997). Genes and inheritance. *Cancer Nursing, 20,* 129–150.

Oncology Nursing Society. (2000a). Cancer predisposition genetic testing and risk assessment counseling. *Oncology Nursing Forum, 27,* 1349.

Oncology Nursing Society. (2000b). The role of the oncology nurse in cancer genetic counseling. *Oncology Nursing Forum, 27,* 1348.

Peters, J., Dimond, E., & Jenkins, J. (1997). Clinical applications of genetic technologies to cancer care. *Cancer Nursing, 20,* 359–376.

Peters, J., & Hadley, D. (1997). The Human Genome Project. *Cancer Nursing, 20,* 62–74.

Peters, K., Menaker, T., Wilson, P., & Hadley, D. (2001). The Human Genome Project: An update. *Cancer Nursing, 24,* 287–293.

Scanlon, C., & Fibison, W. (1995). *Managing genetic information: Implications for nursing practice.* Washington, DC: American Nurses Association.

Sigmon, H.D., Grady, P.A., & Amende, L.M. (1997). The National Institute of Nursing Research explores opportunities in genetics research. *Nursing Outlook, 45,* 215–219.

11

Ensuring Competence: Nursing Credentialing in Cancer Genetics

Amy Strauss Tranin, ARNP, MS, AOCN®, Credentialed in Familial
Cancer Risk Assessment and Management

Introduction

Genetics is playing an increasingly important role in the practice of oncology. Comprehension of the genetic basis of cancer continues to grow with each new molecular discovery. Because genetics provides a basis for understanding the fundamental biologic makeup of human beings, understanding genetics naturally leads to a better understanding of health and disease processes (Jorde, Carey, Bamshad, & White, 1999). Incorporated into practice, this enhanced knowledge may lead to the actual prevention of disease and more effective disease diagnosis and treatment. As such, genetics is becoming central to the delivery of health care.

It seems obvious that nurses, particularly oncology nurses, must possess at least a basic knowledge of genetics. However, the majority of nurses at all levels of educational preparation have had minimal instruction in genetics. In a study by Scanlon and Fibison (1995) of 1,000 nurses from a variety of practice settings and with varied educational preparation, only 14% of the respondents reported completing a course in genetics. Nine percent of the respondents did not take a genetics course until reaching the graduate level. However, 37% of the respondents reported that genetics was adequately covered in other courses at the basic degree level. Even with some formal education, 68% of the nurses perceived themselves as not too knowledgeable or not at all knowledgeable in genetics, though they did tend to perceive themselves as fairly knowledgeable in the areas of counseling, family dynamics, and human growth and development.

The number of continuing education opportunities in cancer genetics for oncology nurses has increased in the last five years. On the national level, the

Oncology Nursing Society (ONS) has offered either instructional sessions or workshops about cancer genetics at every annual meeting since 1994. However, these two-hour programs are available to a small number of nurses, compared to the number of oncology nurses in practice; are not comprehensive in scope (because of time constraints); and attract only self-motivated learners. Nurses who do not yet recognize the impact of the Genetics Revolution on cancer practice may not choose to attend these continuing education programs, especially when there are competing choices. It is precisely these nurses who may need the information the most.

In a position on the role of the oncology nurse in cancer genetic counseling, ONS (2000) stated that oncology nurses possess the skills to and are well suited to assume expanded roles in cancer genetics and genetic counseling. The position specifies that appropriate education and experience are prerequisites to providing comprehensive care in the area of cancer genetics and meeting the needs of the increased number of individuals requiring cancer genetic risk counseling. The position did not define the necessary educational and practice requirements, however.

Significant questions remain unanswered regarding the expanding role in cancer genetics for all oncology nurses. How are nurses motivated to learn something that basic training did not emphasize, is not perceived to be relevant to current practice, and is scientifically challenging? Because most nurses have not had formal training in human genetics, how can a nurse practicing at the advanced level in cancer genetics demonstrate competence in the field of genetics? How can the public and other professionals feel confident in the oncology nurse's knowledge and expertise in this emerging field?

One method of ensuring specialty knowledge is through credentialing. This chapter will explore issues related to the credentialing of oncology nurses as it relates to cancer genetics practice. The discussion will be limited to licensure and certification. Methods of ensuring continued competence will be summarized briefly; it is beyond the scope of this chapter to fully explore the strengths and weaknesses of different competency-assessment methods and of test development and administration. The chapter will end with strategic suggestions for the future.

The Significance of Credentialing to Clinical Practice

Credentialing by private or government agencies is the primary mechanism of documenting the professional competence of healthcare practitioners. Credentials identify qualified professionals. In the past, the principal method of ensuring competent performance was requiring graduation from an accredited training program and subsequent time-unlimited state licensure (Kassirer, 1997). Currently, time-limited board certification also provides evidence of specialized knowledge in a certain area.

Credentialing publicly attests to the achievement of specific qualitative and/ or quantitative characteristics (Murphy & Story, 1998). The Pew Health Professions Commission Taskforce on Health Care Workforce Regulation (Finocchio, Dower, McMahon, Gragnola, & the Taskforce on Health Care Workforce Regulation, 1995) reported that the public is calling for improved accountability through disclosure of health-practitioner information so that consumers can make informed choices about their caregivers. A common marketing strategy for many healthcare provider organizations, including insurance companies and hospitals, is to tout their board-certified physicians in an attempt to attract and retain customers in a competitive market (Kassirer, 1997). In keeping with the purpose and proper use of credentials, efforts to ensure that credentials are a valid representation of clinical expertise are essential.

The following section(s) will describe the characteristics and differences between the two separate and distinct forms of credentialing used to measure knowledge in nursing practice: nursing licensure and nursing certification. Both certification and licensure exams incorporate similar principles in assessing knowledge ("Reengineering a Mature Credentialing Program," 1994). These exams are designed to meet three overall standards:

- Validity: The test should measure important job-related skills.
- Reliability: The test should yield consistent results.
- Legal defensibility: The test should be fair to all candidates and provide equal opportunity to all who are eligible.

Nursing Licensure

A nursing license, conferred by a state regulatory body, is mandatory for any person who practices nursing. A board of directors governs nursing practice in each state and territory in the United States. The state boards license individuals, define a scope of practice, identify standards of practice, and limit the use of the title *licensed nurse*. The primary obligation of the regulatory boards is the protection of public health, welfare, and safety (Murphy, 1996). Inherent in that obligation is meeting the public's expectation that licensed clinicians have met the educational and professional qualifications for practice and that they practice competently and safely.

State boards are responsible for ensuring the competence of the practitioners they regulate. Boards carry out that responsibility by determining and enforcing standards of competence that are discernible, objective, and related to abilities necessary for the job of nursing. The process of ensuring competence consists of establishing the mechanisms to reduce the risk of harm to public health, welfare, and safety.

Unfortunately, standards established by the various state boards are inconsistent (Monsen et al., 2000). Inconsistency in licensure requirements creates problems in nursing practice—problems related to job mobility, titling, practice standards, consumer protection, and state compliance with federal reimbursement mandates (American Nurses Association, 1992). To further complicate the matter, some state boards of medicine or pharmacy regulate nursing practice.

Nursing Certification

Nursing certification is a voluntary process by which a nongovernment agency or association validates, based upon predetermined standards, a candidate's qualifications and knowledge of nursing practice in a defined functional or clinical area (Murphy & Story, 1998). Certification programs are usually peer-reviewed programs, reflecting the standards and scope of practice of the nursing specialty and providing the validity, reliability, and integrity of the process. Nursing certification assures employers, payors, and the public that an individual has mastered a body of knowledge in a particular specialty.

The principal advantage of certification is that it provides an additional measure, beyond licensure, of professional qualifications. Nursing certification validates and standardizes the qualifications and competencies of the nurse in a specialized practice area. Essential to providing quality nursing care is refined knowledge, skills related to job responsibilities, and the ability to integrate enhanced knowledge and skills into practice. Successfully meeting eligibility criteria for certification and passing a certification exam provides evidence of enhanced knowledge in a specialty area, thereby implying competence in that area.

Nurses usually seek certification to advance their careers, achieve professional recognition, and gain personal satisfaction. Certification is a tangible acknowledgment of professional achievement in nursing. Certification also can give a nurse a competitive edge when seeking new employment.

Measures of Competence

The pace of technological and scientific development is accelerating faster than ever before. Because of this accelerated pace, the volume of information that a practitioner needs to know accumulates continuously. Among the greatest challenges that healthcare professionals face are attaining, maintaining, and advancing professional competence in a rapidly evolving healthcare environment. Currently, integration of genetic information into nursing licensing and certification examinations is limited (Lea, Jenkins, & Monsen, 1999).

Credentialing organizations determine and enforce continued competency requirements, often adhering to professional standards for measuring continued competence. Time-limited certification and recertification are an obligation of an accountable profession (Glassock et al., 1991). Nursing credentialing organizations, such as the Oncology Nursing Certification Corporation (ONCC), offer certifications and recertifications, valid for a limited number of years, to foster and measure continued competence. Valid, reliable, and objective testing helps determine whether a nurse can use a knowledge base to make appropriate clinical decisions (Murphy, 1996).

The purpose of the American Board of Nursing Specialties (ABNS) is to set and maintain standards of professional specialty nursing certification and to increase the consumer's awareness of the meaning and value of specialty nursing certification. ABNS recognizes a nursing certification organization if the organization's certification process meets the standards ABNS has established. ONCC meets ABNS standards and became an ABNS member in 1994. ONCC also meets the standards established by the National Commission on Certifying Agencies. The American Nursing Credentialing Center also is an ABNS member.

The method viewed as most effective in ensuring the continued competence of healthcare professionals is performance-based assessment—not a multiple-choice examination. Performance-based examinations are, however, prohibitively expensive for most candidates and credentialing agencies. Credentialing organizations must determine continued competence requirements that are administratively feasible and cost-effective and that can be equitably applied. The majority of certification and licensing agencies regarding health care require certified professionals to accrue continuing education credits or pass retests to demonstrate continued competence.

Competitive examinations have value in measuring knowledge. Although nurses need a significant amount of knowledge to practice competently, knowledge is no guarantee of competence in practice. Knowledge is only part of the measure of competence. In fact, in some situations and for some individuals, the amount of factual knowledge and the ability to apply it to patient care may not correlate. Multiple-choice examinations cannot assess motivation, adaptability, manual dexterity, work habits, response to criticism, or the ability to handle stress in the workplace (McCartney, 1997; Volpintesta, 1997). Written tests cannot assess a clinician's character, compassion, or dedication to the philosophy and ideals of nursing. Multiple-choice examinations also fail to test for honesty, perseverance, or the ability to work with others—all important qualities for a nurse. Future tests, such as tests that employ clinical simulations or standardized patients, may be able to accurately assess competence, as a factor beyond knowledge, more accurately than the methods of today.

The Availability of Credentialing for Oncology Nurses in Genetics

Several methods of credentialing now are available for oncology nurses who work in the field of genetics. The Institute for Clinical Evaluation (ICE) was the first organization to offer a credentialing exam specifically for healthcare professionals working in the area of clinical cancer genetics. Eligibility requirements for nurses include an advanced degree, valid nursing license, continuing education in the area of familial cancer-risk assessment and management, and practical experience in the provision of care related to familial cancer-risk assessment and management. Successful completion of the ICE examination demonstrates competence in a specific, well-circumscribed body of knowledge, and ICE credentialing lasts for seven years. Unfortunately, ICE stopped offering the exam after the first year it began awarding the credential, in 2001. Those individuals who took and passed the ICE exam in familial cancer-risk assessment and management will remain credentialed for seven years.

The International Society of Nurses in Genetics (ISONG) offers credentialing for the advanced practice nurse in genetics. ISONG's credentialing process involves the approval of a portfolio that documents educational requirements and clinical practice experiences. Passing an examination is not part of the ISONG credential. ISONG and the American Nursing Credentialing Center collaborated in the development of this credential, with the goal of making the credentialing process through the portfolio mechanism as credible, standardized, and sound as possible. In 2001, ISONG awarded the first credentials to successful candidates.

Questions about genetics appear on nursing credentialing examinations that are not specific to the genetics specialty. Several years ago, the licensing exam for registered nurses began including questions related to genetics. The fact that the genetics questions appeared relatively recently means that only recent nursing graduates have had to answer them. Few, if any, of the questions are specific to cancer genetics. ONCC's examinations relative to the OCN® and AOCN® credentials—for the general and advanced oncology nurse, respectively—comprise questions related specifically to cancer genetics. In fact, genetics items have been a part of both test blueprints for some time.

Does passing an ONCC or ICE examination or earning an ISONG credential indicate competence in each of the nursing roles this manual describes? Because the ONCC exams are psychometrically valid and reliable assessments of the roles to which they pertain, it is safe to say that OCN® and AOCN® certification acknowledge competence specific to the role of the general oncology nurse and advanced practice oncology nurse (APON), but not for the APON specializing in genetics. The ISONG portfolio acknowledges the competence of the advance practice nurse in genetics, but it is not specific to cancer genetics. However, it is possible to earn the ISONG credential by developing a portfolio relating to clinical cancer genetics education and experience.

An APON with a specialty in cancer genetics could demonstrate competence by successfully completing the ICE examination, even though that examination was not specific to nursing practice. States that require a second license for the APON usually require passing an advanced practice certification exam that meets requirements established by a state board. In many states, the AOCN examination meets the board's requirements for a licensing test for advanced practice nurses.

Whether any state will accept the ICE examination or the ISONG portfolio as measures that equal a licensing test for advanced practice nurses remains to be seen.

Summary

The risks of human disease result from the interactions between inherited genetic components and environmental factors. In the 21st century, cancer care requires that nurses be competent in some components of genetic counseling and that they comprehend cancer as a genetic disease. Validating clinical competence is a requirement in today's competitive and complex healthcare environment. Fortunately, nurses working at all settings and levels—in clinical cancer care and at the advanced practice level—have the opportunity to demonstrate competence in clinical cancer genetics.

References

American Nurses Association. (1992). *Preliminary report of the blue ribbon committee on credentialing in advanced practice to ANA board of directors.* Washington, DC: Author.

Finocchio, L.J., Dower, C.M., McMahon, T., Gragnola, C.M., & the Taskforce on Health Care Workforce Regulation. (1995). *Reforming health care workforce regulation: Policy considerations for the 21st century.* San Francisco: Pew Health Professions Commission.

Glassock, R.J., Benson, J.A., Copeland, R.B., Godwin, H.A., Johanson, W.G., Point, W., et al. (1991). Time-limited certification and recertification: The program of the American Board of Internal Medicine. *Annals of Internal Medicine, 114,* 59–62.

Jorde, L.B., Carey, J.C., Bamshad, M.J., & White, R.L. (1999). *Medical genetics* (2nd ed.). St. Louis: Mosby.

Kassirer, J.P. (1997). The new surrogates for board certification: What should the standards be? [Editorial]. *New England Journal of Medicine, 337,* 43–44.

Lea, D., Jenkins, J., & Monsen, R. (1999). Incorporating genetics into nursing practice. *Nurse Educator, 24,* 4–5.

McCartney, R.D. (1997). Accreditation and certification [Letter to the editor]. *New England Journal of Medicine, 337,* 858.

Monsen, R., Anderson, G., New, F., Ledbetter, S., Frazier, L., Smith, M., & Wilson, M. (2000). Nursing education and genetics: Miles to go before we sleep. *Nursing Health Care Perspectives, 21,* 34–37.

Murphy, C.M. (1996, December). Assessing continued competence. *ONCC News* [Special issue], p. 8.

Murphy, C.M., & Story, K.T. (1998). *Oncology Issues, 13*(1), 21–25.

National Council of State Boards of Nursing. (1996). *Assuring competence: A regulatory responsibility. A proposed position statement.* Chicago: Author.

Oncology Nursing Society. (2000). Oncology Nursing Society position on the role of the nurse in cancer genetic counseling. Retrieved October 25, 2001, from http://www.ons.org/xp6/ONS/Information.xml/Journals_and _Positions.xml/ONS_Positions.xml

Reengineering a mature credentialing program: Established strengths and evolutionary vision. (1994, May/June). *Association Educator* [Suppl.], pp. 1–4.

Scanlon, C., & Fibison, W. (1995). *Managing genetic information: Implications for nursing education.* Washington, DC: American Nurses Association.

Volpintesta, E.J. (1997). Accreditation and certification [Letter to the editor]. *New England Journal of Medicine, 337,* 859.

12

Recommendations for Education

Editor's note: In three sections, this chapter presents recommendations regarding the education of nurses at three levels of practice: the general oncology nurse in practice, the advanced practice oncology nurse in practice, and the advanced practice oncology nurse with a subspecialty in genetics. References immediately follow the section to which they pertain. A list of suggested readings appears at the end of this chapter.

Introduction

Jean Jenkins, PhD, RN, FAAN

The proposition that nurses lack an adequate background in human genetics is not a novel one. Anderson (1996) conducted a search of the literature and identified nine studies from 1976 through 1994 that supported the proposition. Despite the fact that more than 20 years have elapsed since researchers first made efforts to identify the adequacy of nurses' training in human genetics, recent evidence suggests that training has changed little in that time (Hetteberg, Prows, Deets, Monsen, & Kenner, 1999). In 1995, Scanlon and Fibison completed a national survey for the American Nurses Association (ANA) to determine the state of nurses' knowledge of genetic testing, counseling, and referral (Scanlon & Fibison, 1995). The researchers studied 1,000 ANA members whose education and experience varied but who were all currently involved in direct patient care. Nearly 70% of the respondents reported that they were either not too knowledgeable or not at all knowledgeable about genetics, although they considered themselves knowledgeable in other areas of nursing practice. Interestingly, although only 14% of the nurses reported completing a course in human genetics, 80% stated that they would be willing to take continuing education courses about the subject.

Additionally, the researchers of the Human Genome Education Model Project completed a survey of 329 healthcare professionals, including physicians, nurses, social workers, and psychologists. Only 54% of physicians and 26% of nurses surveyed reported having completed some genetics education (Kozma, Lapham, & Weiss, 1996).

The work of Scanlon and Fibison and the Human Genome Education Model Project researchers indicates that nurses in general lack sufficient education in human genetics. This chapter will present recommendations about cancer genetics education for oncology nurses at every level of practice.

A nurse may not immediately recognize the fact that an understanding of genetics is important to his or her professional role as a healthcare provider. However, as increasing numbers of individuals seek advice about genetic testing and other applications of the evolving science of genetics, nurses will find it necessary to integrate genetics information into oncology nursing practice. Introducing an individual to new information is the first step of the innovation-diffusion process, a step that may motivate the person to obtain more information (Rogers, 1995). Knowing does not mean using; after learning about a topic, an individual must be persuaded that incorporating new knowledge as an innovation in daily practice is a worthy goal.

The Core Competency Working Group of the National Coalition for Health Professional Education in Genetics proposed that all healthcare professionals be responsible for extracting the essence of this evolving body of knowledge so they can better explain genetic information and facilitate consumer decision making (Collins, 1997; Donaldson, 1997; Guttmacher, Jenkins, & Uhlmann, 2001; Jenkins et al., 2001). Unfortunately, there has been limited recognition of the importance of genetics information for future nurses (Anderson, 1996). Cohen (1979), Monsen (1984), and Hetteberg et al. (1999) reported that the genetics content in basic nursing curricula was sparse. As a result, most nurses' genetics knowledge is sparse as well.

A study that assessed oncology nurses' knowledge, practice, and educational needs regarding cancer genetics found that the oncology nurses surveyed viewed cancer genetics as important to their specialty practice (Peterson, Rieger, Marani, deMoor, & Gritz, 2001). Almost half (48%) of respondents indicated that patients or family members had inquired about cancer genetic counseling or testing during the previous year. However, knowledge deficits existed at the basic, intermediate, and advanced levels of practice.

Although the preparation of future nurses is crucial, the need to provide currently practicing nurses with information about genetics is even more challenging because their education, specialization, work settings, and responsibilities vary (ANA, 1995). What is more, training opportunities for nurses who want to improve their understanding of genetics are limited. All these factors make it hard for most nurses to apply leading-edge genetics concepts as part of holistic patient care.

Recommendations Regarding the Education of the General Oncology Nurse in Practice

Jean Jenkins, PhD, RN, FAAN

Defining a Core Curriculum

In July 1996, the need to develop genetics education was the focus of a two-day meeting at the National Institutes of Health (NIH). Attending the meeting—which the National Human Genome Research Institute, the National Cancer Institute (NCI), and the National Institute for Nursing Research sponsored—were nurses, physicians, and genetic counselors who were experts in the field of genetics. Their goal was to develop the objectives and content of a core curriculum in basic genetics for the practicing nurse.

Through a review of literature, program evaluations, and personal reports of program outcomes, the group developed recommendations regarding a core curriculum that can provide the needed foundation for all nurses in any practice setting, with any specialty, and in regard to all types of patient care. The group designed the curriculum to allow educators within each specialty to tailor additional content to the needs of their students. For example, case examples illustrating the implications of genetic discoveries for cancer prevention, detection, treatment, and care are useful curriculum enhancements for nurses in oncology practice and education. Educators can adapt a general-purpose genetics resource list to the needs of oncology nurses by adding information about oncology-specific resources, such as the Oncology Nursing Society (ONS).

Validating and Expanding Curriculum Recommendations

By using a survey, researchers gathered nurses' opinions about the core genetics curriculum. Respondents included members of the International Society of Nurses in Genetics (ISONG), other invited genetics experts, and the ONS Cancer Genetics Special Interest Group (SIG). ISONG members and other invited respondents were considered experts in genetics because of their publications, presentations, or work experience. The SIG members were considered potential consumers of genetics education—people with a professional interest but not necessarily expertise in genetics. Of the 356 contacted, 162 (45.5%) agreed to participate in the study by completing the survey. Table 12-1 shows how the respondents rated the importance of each item in the core curriculum (Jenkins, Dimond, & Steinberg, 2001).

Overall analysis of the main objective categories resulted in little controversy about primary content items; experts and nonexperts gave similar ratings regarding the level of importance of subject matter in each major competency category.

One survey question asked respondents to state the format in which they thought the core curriculum in genetics should be presented. Table 12-2 shows the respondents' format preferences.

Peterson et al. (2001) proposed a targeted specialty educational approach for oncology nurses. A study of 656 oncology nurses' knowledge of basic genetics, cancer biology, cancer genetics, and cell biology identified suggested content areas that should be included in nurses training. Those surveyed were most knowledgeable about cancer biology but had deficits in the areas of cell biology, basic genetics, and cancer genetics. This study found a significant need for cancer genetics education for those who worked in nursing staff positions, those with a bachelor's degree or less, and those who had not had cancer genetics continuing education.

All oncology nurses need a basic foundation in genetics. Only with such a foundation can nurses expand their specialty knowledge to include cancer-specific applications. The core genetics curriculum provides the foundation upon which specialty organizations can build to individualize content to reflect their needs. Oncology nursing is an example of a specialty in need of an expanded curriculum.

A cancer genetics education program designed by the American Society of Clinical Oncology (ASCO) (1997) used specific examples of hereditary cancers to illustrate each of the general content areas; this teaching strategy promotes critical thinking and the application of knowledge to clinical practice situations.

The National Action Plan on Breast Cancer (1998) provided an oncology-specific genetics curriculum about hereditary breast and ovarian cancer that would be useful for all healthcare professionals.

An Australian model of education for oncology nurses in cancer genetics offers a 16-week course for nurses already in practice (Gaff, Aittomaki, & Williamson, 2001). This course is designed to enable oncology nurses to assess a person's inherited cancer risk, facilitate referral, and identify psychosocial issues. Syllabus, learning goals, and content were designed to address counseling skills, knowledge of the science and genetics of cancer, and practice and

Table 12-1. Recommended Basic Core Curriculum in Genetics

Item	Mean Level of Importance[a]
Indications for a genetic referral Competency: recognizes indications for a genetic referral	8.85
Knowledge of basic human genetics Competency: demonstrates knowledge of basic human genetics and current applications to practice	8.67
Ethical and societal issues of genetics Competency: identifies ethical and societal issues related to genetic information and technology	8.42
Identifies appropriate resources Competency: able to identify appropriate resources (professionals and patient)	8.38
Psychological effect of genetics Competency: describes the psychological effects of genetic information and technology on individuals and families	8.37
Genetic evaluation and counseling Competency: describes the essential components of genetic evaluation and counseling	8.22
Relevance of genetics to practice Competency: able to identify the relevance of genetics to nursing practice	8.19
Awareness of new genetic methods Competency: demonstrates an increased awareness of the genetic methods and technologies	7.71
Ethnocultural factors Competency: recognizes the effect of ethnocultural differences as they relate to genetics	7.38
Awareness of own attitudes and values Competency: evaluates effects of one's own attitudes, self-awareness, and values related to genetics science and services	6.78

[a] Importance is ranked on a 1–10 scale, with 0 being least important and 10 being most important.

Note. From "Preparing for the Future Through Genetics Nursing Education," by J. Jenkins, E. Dimond, and S. Steinberg, 2001, Journal of Nursing Scholarship, 33(2), pp. 193–194. Copyright 2001 by Sigma Theta Tau International. Adapted with permission.

Table 12-2. Responses Regarding Formats Preferred for the Core Curriculum in Genetics

Format	Percentage of Respondents Who Preferred the Cited Format Over Other Formats
Modules	39
Manual	29
Slides with script	16
Teleconferencing, interactive CD-ROM, videos, or courses	7

Note. Based on information from Jenkins, 2001.

perspective. Completion of this module format course improved assessment and appropriate referral of at-risk individuals.

Summarizing Core Curriculum Recommendations

Based on the 1996 core curriculum recommendations and subsequent research to test and expand the recommendations, education in genetics should enable the general oncology nurse to, at minimum,
- Identify the relevance of genetics to oncology care.
- Demonstrate an understanding of the basic mechanisms of genetic change that relate to carcinogenesis.
- Understand the components of basic cancer-risk assessment.
- Demonstrate assessment skills that permit risk identification.
- Describe the issues involved in cancer-susceptibility testing.
- Identify resources to which patients can be referred.

Summary

The general oncology nurse must be able to recognize new terminology, develop new skills and tools, and know when to refer patients to others. The expectations of the general oncology nurse require a baseline foundation of genetics so that application to oncology diagnosis, prevention, and treatment is enhanced. Knowing when to collaborate with other genetic specialists, including advanced practice oncology nurses (APONs) and APONs with a subspecialty in genetics, to enhance client services and care provided is an important outcome of education of all oncology nurses. The summarized examples provide a starting point for educational planning for programs appropriate for the general oncology nurse in practice.

References

American Nurses Association. (1995). *Today's registered nurse: Numbers and demographics.* Washington, DC: Author.

American Society of Clinical Oncology. (1997). Resource document for curriculum development in cancer genetics education. *Journal of Clinical Oncology, 15*, 2157–2169.

Anderson, G.W. (1996). The evolution and status of genetics education in nursing in the United States 1983–1995. *Image: Journal of Nursing Scholarship, 28*(2), 101–106.

Cohen, F. (1979). Genetic knowledge possessed by American nurses and nursing students. *Journal of Advanced Nursing 4*, 493–501.

Collins, F.S. (1997). Preparing health professionals for the Genetic Revolution. *JAMA, 278*, 1285–1286.

Donaldson, S. (1997). The Genetic Social Revolution and the professional status of nursing. *Nursing Outlook, 45*, 278–279.

Gaff, C., Aittomaki, K., & Williamson, R. (2001). Oncology nurse training in cancer genetics. *Journal of Medical Genetics, 38*, 691–695.

Guttmacher, A., Jenkins, J., & Uhlmann, W. (2001). Genomic medicine: Who will practice it? A call to open arms. *American Journal of Medical Genetics, 106*, 216–222.

Hetteberg, C.G., Prows, C.A., Deets, C., Monsen, R.B., & Kenner, C.A. (1999). Survey of genetics content in basic nursing preparatory programs in the United States. *Nursing Outlook, 47*, 168–180.

Jenkins, J. (2001). *Diffusion of innovation: Genetics nursing education.* Unpublished doctoral dissertation, George Mason University, Fairfax, VA. *Dissertation Abstracts International, 60*, B2608.

Jenkins, J., Blitzer, M., Boehm, K., Feetham, S., Gettig, B., Johnson, A., et al., for the Core Competency Working Group of the National Coalition for Health Professional Education in Genetics. (2001). Recommendations of core competencies in genetics essential for all health professionals. *Genetics in Medicine 3*(2), 155–158.

Jenkins, J., Dimond, E., & Steinberg, S. (2001). Preparing for the future through genetics nursing education. *Journal of Nursing Scholarship, 33*(2), 191–195.

Kozma, C., Lapham, V., & Weiss, J. (1996). Health professionals' knowledge of the Human Genome Project and genetic issues: The need for continuing education. *American Journal of Human Genetics, 59*, A169.

Monsen, R. (1984). Genetics in basic nursing program curricula: A national survey. *Maternal-Child Nursing Journal, 13,* 177–185.

National Action Plan on Breast Cancer. (1998). *Hereditary susceptibility to breast and ovarian cancer: An outline of fundamental knowledge needed by all healthcare professionals.* Retrieved April 13, 2002, from http://www.4woman.gov/napbc/napbc/hsedcurr.htm

Peterson, S., Rieger, P., Marani, S., deMoor, C., & Gritz, E. (2001). Oncology nurses' knowledge, practice, and educational needs regarding cancer genetics. *American Journal of Medical Genetics, 98,* 3–12.

Rogers, E. (1995). *Diffusion of innovations* (4th ed.). New York: Free Press.

Scanlon, C., & Fibison, W. (1995). *Managing genetic information: Implications for nursing practice.* Washington, DC: American Nurses Association.

Recommendations Regarding the Education of an Advanced Practice Oncology Nurse in Practice

Kathleen A. Calzone, RN, MSN, APNG(c), and Jean Jenkins, PhD, RN, FAAN

Genetic information is rapidly moving into the primary care community, where nurses will play a major role in the provision of genetic services. All practicing nurses, at both the basic and advanced practice levels, will require a foundation in genetics to practice in today's healthcare environment. Genetics knowledge will be especially critical for the advanced practice oncology nurse (APON) already in clinical practice. An APON must have expanded genetics knowledge and skills competencies to ensure quality outcomes in cancer care.

Researchers from the University of Pennsylvania Cancer Center and the NCI/Navy Medical Oncology Branch began to develop a curriculum in cancer genetics for the APON already in practice in 1997. This project was built on the basic nursing core curriculum developed at the National Human Genome Research Institute and NCI (Jenkins, Prows, Dimond, Monsen, & Williams, 2001).

The Goals of the Curriculum Development Process

The two goals of the process to develop a cancer genetics curriculum for APONs were to

- Establish the skills and competencies in cancer genetics that should be expected of an APON in practice.

- Determine the knowledge the APON in practice needs to have to demonstrate the competencies.

The Methods and Steps of Curriculum Development

To develop the curriculum for APONs, the researchers used the Delphi technique to enhance the basic nursing core curriculum shown in Table 12-1 and make it specific to oncology nursing practice. The Delphi technique involves a panel of experts that respond anonymously to questions posed on a questionnaire. The researchers tabulate the responses, and each panel member receives a copy of all members' responses to review, refine, and rank. The process continues until all members reach consensus about the answers to the questions (Williams & Webb, 1994). This form of consensus building enhances communication between different groups and facilitates thoughtful, honest responses that are not subject to peer judgment.

Members of the Panel of Experts

The goal in forming the panel of experts was to include nurses with expertise in clinical practice, coordination, nursing research, education, administration, and health policy. The panelists included
- 9 members who were nurse educators or nurse researchers
- 9 general genetic experts
- 9 genetics experts who specialized in oncology
- 10 APONs who were potential consumers of genetics information.

Panel members were selected based on the type and breadth of their professional experience, their clinical specialty, and the geographic area in which they practiced. The experts included members of ISONG, the ONS Cancer Genetics SIG, and other genetics and academic experts. Several of the participants were nurses who participated in both the core curriculum development meeting in 1996 and the ONS Think Tank on Cancer Genetics meeting (ONS, 2000). The APON consumers were graduates of the University of Pennsylvania School of Nursing's oncology advanced practice nursing degree program. They were selected because, as a group, they had experience in all aspects of oncology nursing care but were novices in genetics.

The Questionnaires

The curriculum development process involved two Delphi questionnaires. The questionnaires, which will be detailed later in this section, were independent, self-contained tools that reflected existing materials about the role of the nurse as defined at the ONS Think Tank on Cancer Genetics meeting.

The major domains of competency that the questionnaires cited were those cited in the ONS publication *Standards of Advanced Practice in Oncology Nursing* (ONS, 1990). The domains were direct caregiver, coordinator, consultant, educator, researcher, and administrator. Given the unique nature of genetic information, the researchers added a sixth domain of competency, a domain associated with professional attitudes.

The instructions the panel of experts received asked the panelists to relate their responses to skills, competencies, and attitudes specific to genetics, especially if existing practice standards did not encompass these skills, competencies, and attitudes. The overall response rate for both questionnaires was 73%.

The first Delphi questionnaire: Along with the first Delphi questionnaire, the experts received the ONS publication *Standards of Advanced Practice in Oncology Nursing* (ONS, 1990). The first questionnaire consisted of three parts.

- **Part I—Skills:** This part contained six questions regarding the skills that should be expected of an APON in practice in the area of cancer genetics.
- **Part II—Attitudes:** This part contained one question regarding the attitudes that should be expected of an APON in practice in the area of cancer genetics.
- **Part III—Other Competencies:** Part III consisted of one question about other areas of genetics competency that an APON should master.

Each question was open-ended.

The second Delphi questionnaire: The second questionnaire comprised a compilation of the competencies and knowledge items respondents identified by means of the first questionnaire. The second questionnaire consisted of two parts.

- In Part I, the respondent ranked each identified competency according to importance as rated on a scale of 1–4 (1 being least important, 4 being most important). Competencies were grouped according to the practice domains identified by ONS professional practice standards: direct caregiver, coordinator, consultant, educator, researcher, and administrator. Respondents also ranked knowledge items by importance on a scale of 1–4.
- Part II asked the respondents to further define the knowledge the nurse must have to be competent in the areas they ranked as important.

Table 12-3 summarizes the results of the curriculum development process, establishing competencies in cancer genetics. The table includes only those items that respondents ranked higher than 3.0 in importance. In each domain of competency, Table 12-3 presents the criteria to be used to measure competency in that domain. Each skill is ranked according to the degree of importance on a scale of 1–4, with 4 being the most important. The knowledge items that respondents determined to be necessary to achieve each competency are not included; study groups are continuing to refine the list of items.

APON Education: A Summary

The primary purpose of this project was to determine the competencies expected of all practicing APONs in the field of cancer genetics. Unfortunately, very few nurses have had genetics in their academic preparation and are therefore not currently prepared to understand the implications or meet the needs of patients utilizing genetic services or therapeutics (Scanlon & Fibison, 1995). The competencies identified in this study provide a valuable foundation and direction for the development of continuing education programs for APONs already in practice. These competencies also provide a foundation of information that may be useful to academic nurse educators integrating genetics into the advanced practice oncology nursing curriculum.

References

International Society of Nurses in Genetics. (1998). *Statement on the scope and standards of genetics clinical nursing practice.* Washington, DC: American Nurses Publishing.

Jenkins, J., Prows, C., Dimond, E., Monsen, R., & Williams, J. (2001). Recommendations for educating nurses in genetics. *Journal of Professional Nursing, 17*, 283–290.

Lashley, F.R. (1997). Nursing and genetics: The past and the future. In F.R. Lashley (Ed.), *The genetics revolution: Implications for nursing* (pp. 5–7). Washington, DC: American Academy of Nursing.

Oncology Nursing Society. (1990). *Standards of advanced practice in oncology nursing.* Pittsburgh: Author.

Oncology Nursing Society. (2000). ONS position on the role of the oncology nurse in cancer genetic counseling. *Oncology Nursing Forum, 27*, 1348.

Scanlon, C., & Fibison, W. (1995). *Managing genetic information: Implications for nursing practice.* Washington, DC: American Nurses Association.

Williams, P.L., & Webb, C. (1994). The Delphi technique: A methodological discussion. *Journal of Advanced Nursing, 19*(1), 180–186.

Table 12-3. Core Competencies in Cancer Genetics for the Advanced Practice Oncology Nurse Already in Practice

Competency	Mean Level of Importance[a]
Direct caregiver	
Facilitates informed decision making associated with genetic testing and/or therapeutics	3.87
Facilitates genetic therapeutic options	3.84
Performs a nursing assessment from a genetic perspective	3.80
Provides support services specific to genetic issues	3.71
Based on the genetic assessment, interprets the data and establishes a plan	3.70
Provides education about cancer genetics	3.68
Coordinator	
Facilitates health-promotion behaviors associated with genetic conditions	3.90
Provides supportive care associated with the delivery of genetics services	3.90
Creates communication links between oncology and genetic healthcare providers	3.84
Provides coordination of care associated with the delivery of genetics services	3.69
Refers patients to appropriate cancer genetics research studies	3.47
Participates in genetic program development and monitoring	3.22
Consultant	
Provides referral and resources information on where to obtain genetics services	4.00
Incorporates genetics into oncology nursing care	3.78
Collaborates and consults with all members of the genetic multidisciplinary team	3.71
Facilitates the diffusion of genetic knowledge	3.53
Assists and serves as a mentor in the provision of cancer genetics services	3.33
Provides expert knowledge on cancer genetics	3.30
Provides input to committees or groups establishing policies regarding genetics services	3.14
Educator	
Identifies genetics learning needs for both clients and professionals	3.94
Utilizes appropriate adult learning principles in the delivery of complicated genetics information	3.65
Participates in cancer genetics-related professional activities	3.60
Provides education about cancer genetics	3.34
Plans and implements genetic-focused educational activities	3.29
Evaluates effectiveness of genetic education provided	3.17

(Continued on next page)

298

Table 12-3. Core Competencies in Cancer Genetics for the Advanced Practice Oncology Nurse Already in Practice *(Continued)*

Competency	Mean Level of Importance[a]
Researcher	
Modifies practice based on current genetic research findings	3.91
Collaborates with all members of the interdisciplinary team on cancer genetics research initiatives	3.67
Recognizes the unique features of conducting genetics research	3.54
Promotes participation in cancer genetics research	3.42
Serves as a mentor to other nurses regarding the research process applied to cancer genetics	3.24
Identifies research questions in cancer genetics	3.22
Participates in and facilitates cancer genetics research initiatives	3.18
Participates in establishing cancer genetics research priorities	3.10
Administrator	
Participates in cancer genetics program planning	3.67
Ensures the competency of the staff delivering genetics services	3.44
Evaluates the quality of cancer genetics care and provision of cancer genetics services	3.38
Participates in cancer genetics program implementation	3.29
Professional Attitudes	
Respects autonomous genetic decision making	3.96
Handles genetic information responsibly	3.96
Recognition that genetics impacts the family and not just the individual	3.96
Recognizes the advanced skills required to deliver cancer genetics services	3.92
Pursues ongoing cancer genetics education	3.91
Recognizes the uncertainty associated with genetic information	3.88
Aware of the unique aspects of genetic information	3.88
Sensitive to the complex psychosocial issues associated with genetic information	3.83
Open and positive regarding new ideas and information associated with genetics	3.83
The APN in oncology is aware of his or her own beliefs, biases, and capabilities.	3.81
Willing to collaborate with all members of the genetics healthcare team	3.77
Values and maintains a research-based practice associated with genetic services	3.70
Avoids making assumptions about genetics without research findings	3.67

(Continued on next page)

Table 12-3. Core Competencies in Cancer Genetics for the Advanced Practice Oncology Nurse Already in Practice (Continued)

Competency	Mean Level of Importance[a]
Believes the nurse has a responsibility to advocate for the patient in regard to cancer genetics	3.67
Views critical thinking as an essential component of cancer genetics practice	3.66
Other	
Participates in professional activities that enhance genetic nursing	3.60

[a] Importance is ranked on a 0–4 scale, with 0 being least important and 4 being most important.

Recommendations Regarding the Education of an Advanced Practice Oncology Nurse With a Subspecialty in Genetics

Rita S. Wickham, PhD, RN, AOCN®, and Mira Lessick, PhD, RN

The nursing literature offers few resources that discuss the specific educational needs of advanced practice nurses in cancer genetics. Most articles on the topic focus on the needs of pediatric nurses who care for children with congenital conditions or nurses in reproductive genetics (Anderson, 1996; Forsman, 1988; George, 1992; Kenner & Berling, 1990; McElhinney & Lajkowicz, 1994). In addition, as of 1998, few schools of nursing offered graduate-level nursing options in genetics (see Table 12-4), although the number ber is growing. Because genetics has not been integrated into basic or continuing nursing education, Lashley (1997b) believed that most nurses were not interested in or committed to incorporating genetics into practice.

If you are looking for programs leading to an advanced degree in oncology nursing with a subspecialty in cancer genetics, check the ISONG Web site at http://nursing.creighton.edu/isong and ONS Online at www.ons.org. These sites often list programs that may be of interest.

This belief is changing, however, as oncology nurses find themselves in the midst of a torrent of phenomenal advances in scientific and clinical applications related to the Human Genome Project and new knowledge regarding the molecular biology of cancer. The identification and sequencing of human genes that play roles in the initiation, promotion, and progression of malignancies are having a major impact on diagnosis for individuals at risk of inheriting mutated cancer-susceptibility genes as well as all people with cancer. As we learn more about how these genes are expressed and how their protein products function, genetic knowledge will be increasingly applied in general cancer therapy and in the prevention and early detection of cancer. Nurses thus need to recognize a new paradigm, a paradigm in which genetics moves from a tangential concept to a central underpinning of nursing practice (George, 1992; Lashley, 1997a). Furthermore, oncology nurses in clinical practice and in education must be proactive in articulating the necessity to incorporate genetics into undergraduate and graduate courses, with the ultimate goals of enhancing oncology nursing practice and establishing oncology nurses as leaders in the area of cancer genetics.

> The explosion of knowledge regarding human genetics and the molecular biology of cancer will have major implications for cancer diagnosis, prevention, and treatment. This, in turn, will change oncology nurses' education and practice.

This paradigm shift will most dramatically affect the preparation of advanced practice oncology genetics nurses (oncology/genetics APNs) who focus their studies and practice (clinical, education, or research) on both cancer and genetic health nursing. Few nursing resources are available to guide the development of the specialized oncology/genetics APN curriculum at this time, but physicians and genetic counselors have recognized that nurses *must* play a key role in the multidisciplinary management of individuals and families at risk of genetically based diseases (Collins, 1997; McKinnon et al., 1997). For instance, ASCO has addressed the need to develop courses and educational materials related to cancer genetics and cancer-predisposition testing for physicians *and* nurses. The ASCO guidelines (1997) stated that cancer genetics education should include four broad categories—information about

- Basic concepts and principles of genetics
- The role of genetics in the etiology, diagnosis, and management of different malignancies
- The ethical, legal, and social issues surrounding predisposition testing
- The multidisciplinary approach to the long-term management of individuals at high risk for developing cancer.

In addition, the ONS position on the role of the oncology nurse in cancer genetic counseling (ONS, 2000) and the ISONG (1998) *Statement on the Scope and Standards of Genetics Clinical Nursing Practice* list genetics nursing interventions that should be performed by genetics APNs only.

Cancer genetics subspecialists may be prepared as clinical nurse specialists (CNSs), nurse practitioners (NPs), or nurse scientists educated at the

Table 12-4. Academic Programs That Offered Graduate-Level Nursing Education in Genetics in 1998

University	Comments
University of Washington School of Nursing Box 357266 Seattle, WA 98195-7266 Web site: www.washington.edu Betty Gallucci, PhD, RN Telephone: 206-616-1961 Fax: 206-543-4771 E-mail: gallucci@u.washington.edu	Options/focus: MN in advanced practice genetics nursing and genetics nursing minor (certificate program) Majors: Students take genetics courses based in Colleges of Nursing, Medicine, and Public Health. Didactic (required and elective) and clinical genetics courses include, at minimum, 25 quarter-hours. Minors: Students take selected didactic and clinical genetics courses (nursing genetics certificate).
Columbia University School of Nursing 630 W. 168th St. Box 6 New York, NY 10032 Web site: http://cpmcnet.columbia.edu/ dept/nursing Sara Sheets Cook, PhD, RN Professor of Clinical Nursing, Vice Dean Telephone: 212-305-3582 E-mail: ssc3@columbia.edu	Major: Genetics is a subspecialization (may be taken with MS curriculum for any specialty major, or by nonmatriculated BS- or MS-prepared nurses). Genetics content: 3 courses (7 semester hours) and practicum in genetics (in area of didactic specialty)
Rush University College of Nursing 600 S. Paulina St., Suite 1080 Chicago, IL 60612 Web site: www.rushu.rush.edu Mira Lessick, PhD, RN Telephone: 312-942-6996 Fax: 312-942-2549 E-mail: mlessick@rushu.rush.edu	Options: MSN, ND, DNSc Major: Genetics health nursing (clinical nurse specialist, nurse practitioner, pediatrics). Options: combine with other major (e.g., women's health, oncology). Genetics content: 4 courses (11 quarter-hours), clinical practicum (12–16 hours); oncology and cancer genetics focus.
University of Cincinnati 3110 Vine St. Cincinnati, OH 45221-0038 Web site: www.nursing.uc.edu Carole Kenner, DNS, RNC, FAAN Department Head, Parent Child Health Nursing Telephone: 513-558-5228 Fax: 513-558-7523 E-mail: Carole.Kenner@UC.edu	Options: MSN, genetics counseling focus or dual major (adult health; community health; family nurse practitioner; neonatal, pediatric, women's health practitioner) plus genetics content (focus: molecular genetics, genetic counseling from an interdisciplinary perspective, clinical applications); hours vary with area of interest. Postmaster's, pre- and postdoctoral options.

(Continued on next page)

Table 12-4. Academic Programs That Offered Graduate-Level Nursing Education in Genetics in 1998 (Continued)

University	Comments
University of Iowa College of Nursing Iowa City, IA 52242 www.nursing.uiowa.edu Janet Williams, PhD, RN, FAAN Associate Professor Telephone: 319-335-7079 Fax: 319-335-9990 E-mail: janet-williams@uiowa.edu	MSN, dual major. MSN and advanced practice genetics nursing (APGN). Didactic courses in genetics, counseling, and advanced practice nursing. More than 500 hours of clinical experience supervised by an interdisciplinary team of APGNs and genetic specialists. Post-master's degree certificate as APGN available.

doctoral level. Each type of practitioner requires a broad knowledge base to be able to provide cancer genetics services to individuals and families; to mentor other oncology nurses in the area of cancer genetics; and to advance the science of cancer genetics, particularly as it relates to nursing care (Jenkins, 1997). At this time, most oncology/genetics APNs fill direct-care roles and function as members of cancer-predisposition risk teams or in cancer-risk clinics. Thus, the focus of their practice differs from that of APNs in other areas of cancer care. The tasks of cancer genetics subspecialists include providing psychosocial support and counseling to individuals seeking information about their genetic susceptibility to cancer and those undergoing genetic testing, identifying individuals who may need genetic screening to determine risk, obtaining comprehensive health and family histories, constructing detailed family pedigrees, obtaining information to confirm reported malignancies in a family; ensuring informed consent regarding genetic testing, and teaching and counseling family members about follow-up and the implications of test results.

Sources that may aid in evaluating oncology/genetics education include "The Oncology Nursing Society Position on the Role of the Oncology Nurse in Cancer Genetic Counseling" (ONS, 2000), *Statement on the Scope and Standards of Genetics Clinical Nursing Practice* (ISONG, 1998), and "Resource Document for Curriculum Development in Cancer Genetics Education" (ASCO, 1997).

Oncology/genetics APNs may function as clinical nurse specialists, nurse practitioners, or nurse scientists and in clinical, administrative, educational, and/or research roles.

Accordingly, the education of oncology/genetics APNs must provide a broad background in oncology, including education about physical care and psychosocial needs, and offer the student an opportunity to develop in-depth knowledge and skills specific to cancer-risk genetic counseling. The education of oncology/genetics APNs also must prepare them for leadership and administrative roles in the development of cancer genetics programs, in current and future clinical trials (e.g., trials involving chemoprevention or gene therapy), in the formal or informal education of other oncology professionals, and in the development of or participation in oncology genetic nursing research.

An important role for many oncology/genetics APNs is the role of cancer genetic-risk counselor on a multidisciplinary team. APNs in clinical or other roles must develop broad knowledge regarding psychosocial and physical care and the principles, skills, and ramifications of genetic-risk counseling.

Figure 12-1 lists the potential activities of oncology/genetics APNs in practice. No program is likely to prepare oncology nurses for all the activities, but the list can serve as a means of evaluating programs designed to prepare nurses for practice in the cancer-genetics field.

A program of study leading to an advanced degree as an oncology/genetics APN would be rigorous. It would include required core and cognate courses relating to oncology specialization as well as courses relating to the genetic

---

Figure 12-1. Activities of Advanced Practice Oncology Nurses Subspecializing in Cancer Genetics

- Provide genetic counseling interventions to individuals and families who are considering and/or undergoing genetic testing, including pedigree construction, taking comprehensive disease-specific health and family histories, interpreting the rationale for and the results of cancer genetic-risk testing, and interpreting genetics laboratory data.
- Address the emotional and psychosocial stress experienced by people who learn they have a potential or actual risk of inheriting a mutated cancer-susceptibility gene or a related malignancy.
- Collaborate with a multidisciplinary team to provide or facilitate case management for patients, which includes comprehensive assessment of health needs; development of diagnoses; and planning, managing, and evaluating complex care.
- Monitor and evaluate clients with genetic cancer-susceptibility problems and provide comprehensive health teaching related to cancer genetics.
- Act as a consultant to interdisciplinary team members regarding family or patient care issues, to nurses, and to others to clinically evaluate clients and to guide nursing care.
- Participate in the development of recommendations addressing the ethical, legal, and social consequences of existing and predicted genetics services and technologies.
- Participate in the planning, implementation, and evaluation of screening programs that incorporate cancer genetic-risk testing.
- Develop and conduct genetic nursing research, and/or evaluate and incorporate such research into practice.
- Coordinate or participate in medical or multidisciplinary cancer genetics research studies.

Note. Based on information from ISONG, 1998; Lashley, 1997b; ONS, 2000.

health subspecialty. The clinical practicum component should include both general oncology nursing and specialized oncology genetic health nursing clinical experiences.

To provide broad-based understanding, the program should include genetic health classes that outline the scientific concepts underlying general human genetics, classes about genetically influenced syndromes and conditions, and course work in cancer genetics. In such a program, courses and clinical practicums would present the advanced concepts and principles of genetic health and the critical ethical, legal, policy, and psychosocial issues relating to the advanced nursing care of individuals and families with potential or diagnosed cancer related to cancer-susceptibility genes. The program would offer a cancer genetics course and the content recommended by ASCO (1997). Such a curriculum would discuss how oncology/genetics APNs can incorporate cancer-risk assessment, counseling, psychological issues, and gene therapy into practice (Biesecker, 1997; ISONG, 1998; Jenkins & Lea, 1997; Lea, 1997; MacDonald, 1997; ONS, 2000).

> Other roles for oncology/genetics APNs include leadership and administration, cancer genetics education, and cancer genetics nursing science.

As scientific advances are applied to clinical practice, the need for oncology/genetics APNs will increase and schools of nursing will develop programs to prepare APNs for the subspecialty. Figure 12-2 shows current and planned courses in the curriculum of Rush University College of Nursing, Chicago.

> A program of study leading to an oncology/genetics APN degree should include both oncology and genetics (general human genetics and cancer-specific genetics); discussion of the ethical, legal, and social implications involved in cancer genetics; and consideration of the current and future implications of cancer genetics for APNs.

The need for oncology/genetics APNs is illustrated by the fact that, of the approximately 1,300 genetic counselors in the United States today, only one-third focus on cancer genetics (Farmer & Chittams, 2000). Several oncology APNs already are recognized pioneers in cancer genetics nursing practice, and they provide models for others. These recognized nurses, for the most part, have worked in research-based programs where they play key roles in clinics dedicated to genetic cancer risk (Fraser, Calzone, & Goldstein, 1997). Up to this time, many clients were referred to such clinics for predisposition screening. As cancer-susceptibility gene tests become commercially available, however, testing will occur with increasing frequency in community settings, and the need for oncology/genetics APNs will increase.

Figure 12-2. Suggested Cognate Courses for the APON Genetics Subspecialty

Cell Biology/Molecular Biology (2 quarter-hours)
This science course underpins both the oncology MSN and the oncology/genetics MSN curriculum.

Course Objectives
1. Describe the structural and biochemical features of eukaryotic cells.
2. Discuss basic concepts related to genetic mechanisms and the regulation of gene expression.
3. Describe approaches to evaluate structural, biochemical, and functional parameters of eukaryotic cells.
4. Discuss the processes involved in cell division and growth, and the mechanisms of cell-to-cell communication (i.e., signaling and adhesion).

Course Content
1. Review of biochemistry
2. Laboratory approaches to the study of cells
3. Basic genetic mechanisms: DNA, RNA, and protein synthesis
4. Regulation of gene expression
5. Cell signaling
6. Cell division and growth
7. Cell adhesion

Scientific Basis of Genetic Health (3 quarter-hours)
This course focuses on the integration and beginning application of genetics concepts and principles to clinical practice situations in a broad spectrum of settings.

Course Objectives
1. Examine basic concepts and principles of genetics and their application across the lifespan.
2. Explain the role of genetics in the etiology, diagnosis, and management of inherited health problems in individuals and families.
3. Describe concepts and principles of genetic counseling.

Course Content
1. Clinical genetics and advanced nursing practice
2. Basic concepts of genetics
   a. The nature of genes: DNA structure, function, and expression
   b. Distribution of genes within a population
   c. Genetic variation: organization of the human genome, chromosomes, and gene mutations
   d. Genetic replication: meiosis and mitosis
   e. Genetic expression: penetrance and expressivity
3. Teratogenesis and mutagenesis
4. Inherited disorders, single gene
   a. Autosomal inheritance patterns
   b. X-linked patterns of inheritance
5. Nonclassical patterns of single gene inheritance
6. Multifactorial inheritance
7. Clinical cytogenetics
   a. Autosomal abnormalities

(Continued on next page)

Figure 12-2. Suggested Cognate Courses for the APON Genetics Subspecialty
(Continued)

---

     b. Chromosome analysis and clinical applications
  8. Gene mapping and genetic engineering
  9. Prenatal diagnosis and reproductive technologies
10. Genetic counseling and screening
     a. Principles of genetic counseling
     b. Stages of counseling
     c. Risk estimation and Bayes' theorem
     d. Carrier screening
     e. Prenatal and newborn screening
     f. Presymptomatic and predictive screening
11. Treatment of genetic diseases

Advanced Concepts in Genetic Health Nursing (3 quarter-hours)
The second genetics course focuses on analyzing and integrating advanced concepts and principles of clinical genetics as the foundation for advanced nursing practice in a variety of settings.

Course Objectives
1. Analyze concepts and principles relevant to selected models of genetic health problems.
2. Consider how concepts of genetic assessment and counseling may be applied to particular genetic health conditions.

Course Content
1. The foundation of genetic assessment: comprehensive family history, pedigree construction
2. Human variation and genes in populations
3. Models of genetically influenced diseases
     a. Mental retardation and developmental disabilities
     b. Genetics of pregnancy loss
     c. Genetic orthopedic disorders
     d. Genetic disorders of metabolism
     e. Cancer genetics
     f. Cardiovascular disorders
     g. Neuromuscular disorders
     h. Neurologic disorders
     i. Genetics of the immune system
     j. Craniofacial anomalies and hereditary hearing and visual disorders
     k. Skin and connective tissue disorders
     l. Endocrine disorders
     m. Renal disorders
     n. Respiratory disorders
     o. Hematologic disorders
     p. Cancer cytogenetics

Critical Issues for Genetic Health Nurses (2 quarter-hours)
This course focuses on integration and application of issues related to advanced nursing care in genetic health, specifically ethics, law, health policy, and psychosocial responses.

(Continued on next page)

Figure 12-2. Suggested Cognate Courses for the APON Genetics Subspecialty
(Continued)

Course Objectives
1. Analyze ethical and genetic healthcare issues.
2. Interpret the impact of federal regulations on access to genetic/biotechnological discoveries.
3. Debate the positive and negative implications of utilizing expanding genetic technology on clients across the life span.
4. Discuss patient and family interactions and responses that may result from making difficult case-related decisions.

Course Content
1. Ethical issues and decision making
2. Social policy issues
3. Issues of justice in genetic health care
4. Legal issues in genetics
    a. Implications of counseling
    b. Duty to warn
5. Issues in predisposition testing
    a. Important considerations prior to testing
    b. Informed-consent considerations
    c. Ethical, legal, and social aspects of genetic testing
    d. Impact of culture and ethnicity
6. Application of genetic counseling principles (mock genetic counseling sessions)
7. Ethics committees and consultations (mock ethics committee exercise)
8. Hot topics (e.g., cloning)

Cancer Genetics and Applications for Nurses (3 quarter-hours)
This course focuses specifically on cancer genetics, the issues surrounding the care of individuals at increased risk for having a cancer predisposition gene mutation, and implications for advanced oncology/genetics practice.

Course Objectives
1. Apply concepts and principles of genetics to malignant disease (familial and sporadic).
2. Explain the role of genetics in the etiology, diagnosis, and management of different malignancies.
3. Address specific ethical, legal, and social issues surrounding cancer genetic predisposition-risk testing.
4. Identify the oncology/genetics APN's role in the multidisciplinary approach to long-term management issues for individuals at high risk for developing cancer.

Course Content
1. The basis for practice: Incorporating the ["ONS Position Regarding Cancer Genetic Testing and Risk Assessment Counseling"] and ISONG's *Statement on the Scope and Standards of Genetics Clinical Nursing Practice* into advanced nursing practice
    a. Eliciting a comprehensive family medical history to identify genetic risk
    b. Explaining risk estimates for cancers for which screening (laboratory or pedigree construction) is available

(Continued on next page)

Figure 12-2. Suggested Cognate Courses for the APON Genetics Subspecialty (Continued)

---

   c. Interpreting risk information for individuals and families
   d. Identifying resources for genetic referrals and services
2. The interaction of genes and the environment in the onset of cancer
   a. The roles of genes in cancer: oncogenes, suppressor genes, DNA-mismatch repair genes
   b. Germline mutations versus somatic mutations
   c. Models for the genetic basis of cancer
   d. Genetic changes in cancer
   e. Contribution of environmental factors
3. Laboratory methods in cancer genetics
   a. Methods to identify genes
   b. Methods to identify unknown mutations in genes
   c. Methods to identify known mutations in genes
   d. Cancer cytogenetics
4. Predisposition testing: clinical applications and process
   a. Important considerations prior to testing
   b. Laboratory considerations
   c. Informed-consent considerations
   d. Ethical, legal, and social aspects of genetic testing
5. Specific hereditary cancer syndromes
   a. Breast and ovarian (*BRCA1, BRCA2, BRCAX,* and other)
   b. Colon cancer syndromes (FAP, HNPCC genes)
   c. Multiple endocrine neoplasia (*MEN1, MEN2A, MEN2B, FMTC*)
   d. Pediatric tumors: retinoblastoma, Wilms' tumor
   e. Other adult-onset syndromes: neurofibromatosis, Li-Fraumeni syndrome, melanoma, prostate cancer, etc.
6. Other current and future applications of cancer genetics
   a. Chemoprevention trials
   b. Gene therapy trials
   c. Therapies that capitalize on cancer genetics knowledge

Clinical Practicum in Oncology/Genetics Nursing
The clinical practicum (12–18 quarter-hours) is designed to complement the student's didactic course work. Ideally, clinical hours commence after the basic oncology and genetics health courses have been taken and occur over two or three quarters. Clinical practice hours for oncology nursing and cancer genetics nursing care are negotiated between the adviser and the student, based upon the student's needs. In addition to clinical hours, students attend seminars in which clinical activities are discussed, constructed pedigrees are shared, and students present specific case studies, review a counseling situation, and review research-based articles relevant to genetic nursing practice.

References

American Society of Clinical Oncology. (1997). Resource document for curriculum development in cancer genetics education. *Journal of Clinical Oncology, 15,* 2157–2169.

Anderson, G.W. (1996). The evolution and status of genetics education in nursing in the United States 1983–1995. *Image: Journal of Nursing Scholarship, 28*(2), 101–106.

Biesecker, B.B. (1997). Psychological issues in cancer genetics. *Seminars in Oncology Nursing, 17,* 129–134.

Collins, F.S. (1997). Preparing health professionals for the Genetic Revolution [Editorial]. *JAMA, 278,* 1285–1286.

Farmer, J.M., & Chittams, J. (2000). Professional status survey 2000. *Perspectives in Genetic Counseling, 22*(Suppl. 4), S1–S12.

Fraser, M.C., Calzone, K.A., & Goldstein, A.M. (1997). Familial cancers: Evolving challenges for nursing practice. *Oncology Nursing Updates, 4*(3), 1–18.

Forsman, I. (1988). Education of nurses in genetics. *American Journal of Human Genetics, 43,* 552–558.

George, J.B. (1992). Genetics: Challenges for nursing education. *Journal of Pediatric Nursing, 17,* 5–8.

International Society of Nurses in Genetics. (1998). *Statement on the scope and standards of genetics clinical nursing practice.* Washington, DC: American Nurses Publishing.

Jenkins, J. (1997). Educational issues related to cancer genetics. *Seminars in Oncology Nursing, 13,* 141–144.

Jenkins, J., & Lea, D.H. (1997). Cancer genetics for nurses. Part II: Integrating genetics into oncology nursing practice. *Oncology Nursing Updates, 4*(6), 1–16.

Kenner, C., & Berling, B. (1990). Nursing in genetics: Current and emerging issues for practice and education. *Journal of Pediatric Nursing, 5,* 370–374.

Lashley, F.R. (1997a). Nursing and genetics: The past and the future. In F.R. Lashley (Ed.), *The genetics revolution: Implications for nursing* (pp. 5–7). Washington, DC: American Academy of Nursing.

Lashley, F.R. (1997b). Thinking about genetics in new ways. *Image: Journal of Nursing Scholarship, 29,* 202.

Lea, D.H. (1997). Gene therapy: Current and future implications for oncology nursing practice. *Seminars in Oncology Nursing, 13,* 115–122.

MacDonald, D.J. (1997). The oncology nurse's role in cancer risk assessment and counseling. *Seminars in Oncology Nursing, 13,* 123–128.

McElhinney, T., & Lajkowicz, C. (1994). The new genetics and nursing education. *Health Care, 15,* 528–531.

McKinnon, W.C., Baty, B.J., Bennett, R.L., Magee, M., Neufeld-Kaiser, W.A., Peters, K.F., et al. (1997). Predisposition genetic testing for late-onset disorders in adults. A position paper of the National Society of Genetic Counselors. *JAMA, 278,* 1217–1220.

Oncology Nursing Society. (2000). The role of the oncology nurse in cancer genetic counseling. *Oncology Nursing Forum, 27*, 1348.

Conclusion

Most nurses question the introduction of genetic information: "Why do I need to know about genetics? I'm an *oncology* nurse." Patient care is the main justification for the oncology nurse to become knowledgeable about genetics. Cancer care can only benefit if there is mainstreaming of genetics discoveries into the practice of every healthcare provider (Collins & Mansoura, 2001). There is a definite need for expertise in genetics to facilitate training in all healthcare disciplines. Only with training can there be a redesign of the infrastructure of the healthcare system to effectively and efficiently integrate genetics into all services provided.

The need to communicate cancer-risk information challenges nurses to address the potential for health problems, forecasted on the basis of medical and family history as well as individual genetic profiling (Bottorff, Ratner, Johnson, Lovato, & Joab, 1998). Already, direct consumer advertising about genetic testing is appearing (Hull & Prasad, 2001). Healthcare providers must gain sufficient expertise to answer consumers' questions, which are driven by Internet and media information (Taylor, Alman, & Manchester, 2001). For healthcare providers, learning and understanding new tests, new terminology, and new ways of doing business will be constant. Recognition of factors influencing client decisions about preventive care and health promotion must be the focus of ongoing research. Through better understanding of the psychological and physical consequences of genetic information, factors influencing client decisions can be addressed proactively (Broadstock, Michie, & Marteau, 2000).

Ongoing advances in the understanding of genetic changes that predict cancer risk, response, and prognosis will expand options in cancer care. Simultaneously, these scientific advances create new concerns as new genetic technology revolutionizes human capabilities (Zajtchuk, 1999). New capabilities and technologies—such as genetic targeted therapy, genetic engineering, gene therapy, cloning, and DNA chips—will transform health care during the coming decade. Oncology nurses who have a clear understanding of the value of genetic technologies can take the lead in introducing potential life-saving changes across the cancer continuum. These nurse leaders will be able to head off problems and expand ethical discussion regarding genetics in oncology practice.

References

Bottorff, J., Ratner, P., Johnson, J., Lovato, C., & Joab, A. (1998). Communicating cancer risk information: The challenges of uncertainty. *Patient Education and Counseling, 33,* 67–81.

Broadstock, M., Michie, S., & Marteau, T. (2000). Psychological consequences of predictive genetic testing: A systematic review. *European Journal of Human Genetics, 8,* 731–738.

Collins, F., & Mansoura, M. (2001). The Human Genome Project: Revealing the shared inheritance of all humankind. *Cancer Supplement, 91,* 221–225.

Hull, S., & Prasad, K. (2001). Reading between the lines: Direct-to-consumer advertising of genetic testing. *Hastings Center Report, 31,* 33–35.

Taylor, M., Alman, A., & Manchester, D. (2001). Use of the Internet by patients and their families to obtain genetics-related information. *Mayo Clinical Proceedings, 76,* 772–776.

Zajtchuk, R. (1999). New technologies in medicine: Biotechnology and nanotechnology. *Disease-a-Month, 45,* 449–495.

Suggested Readings

Alberts, B., Bray, D., Johnson, A., Lewis, J., Raff, M., Roberts, K., et al. (1998). *Essential cell biology: An introduction to the molecular biology of the cell.* New York: Garland Publishing.

Bartels, D.M., LeRoy, B.S., & Caplan, A.L. (Eds.). (1993). *Prescribing our future: Ethical challenges in genetic counseling.* New York: Aldine D. Gruyter.

Connor, J.M., & Ferguson-Smith, M.A. (Eds.). (1993). *Essential medical genetics* (4th ed). Oxford: Blackwell Scientific Publications.

Eeles, R.A., Ponder, B.A.J., Easton, D.F., & Horwich, A. (Eds.). (1996). *Genetic predisposition to cancer.* New York: Chapman & Hall Medical.

Emery, A., & Rimoin, D. (Eds.). (1996). *Emery and Rimoin's principles and practice of medical genetics* (3rd ed.). New York: Churchill Livingstone.

Gert, B., Berger, E.M., Cahill, G.F., Clousser, K.D., Culver, C.M., Moeschler, J.B., et al. (1996). *Morality and the new genetics: A guide for students and health care providers.* Boston: Jones and Bartlett.

Goodman, S.R. (1994). *Medical cell biology.* Philadelphia: J.B. Lippincott.

Jorde, L., Carey, J., & White, R. (1995). *Medical genetics.* St. Louis: Mosby.

Korf, B.R. (1996). *Human genetics: A problem-based approach.* Cambridge, MA: Sinauer Associates.

Lashley, F. (1998). *Clinical genetics in nursing practice* (2nd ed.). New York: Springer.

Lea, D., Jenkins, J., & Francomano, C. (1998). *Genetics in clinical practice: New directions for nursing and health care*. Boston: Jones and Bartlett.

Lewis, R. (1997). *Human genetics. Concepts and applications* (2nd ed.). Chicago: William C. Brown.

MacDonald, F., & Ford, C.H.J. (1997). *Molecular biology of cancer*. Oxford, England: BIOS Scientific Publishers.

Offit, K. (1998). *Clinical cancer genetics: Risk counseling and management*. New York: Wiley-Liss.

Yarnold, J.R., Stratton, M., & McMillan, T.J. (Eds.). (1996). *Molecular biology for oncologists* (2nd ed.). New York: Chapman & Hall.

Glossary

Some of the definitions in this glossary are based on definitions developed by the National Human Genome Research Institute (NHGRI). The editors of this text gratefully acknowledge the contributions of the NHGRI authors and refer the reader to the full version of the NHGRI glossary, which is available on the Internet at www.genome.gov/glossary.cfm.

absolute risk In regard to cancer, the measure of the occurrence of cancer, whether incidence (new cases) or mortality (deaths), in the general population.

accuracy The degree to which a measurement represents the true value of the characteristic being measured.

adenine (A) One of the four bases in DNA. The others are guanine (G), cytosine (C), and thymine (T). Adenine always pairs with T.

allele One of the variant forms of a gene at a particular locus, or location, on a chromosome. Different alleles produce variation in inherited characteristics (e.g., hair color, blood type). In an individual, one form of the allele (the dominant one) may be expressed more than another form (the recessive one).

amino acid One of 20 different kinds of small molecules that link in long chains to form proteins. Amino acids are often called the building blocks of proteins.

antisense Refers to the noncoding strand in double-stranded DNA. The antisense strand serves as the template for mRNA synthesis.

apoptosis Programmed cell death, the body's normal method of disposing of damaged, unwanted, or unneeded cells.

attributable risk In regard to cancer, the amount of cancer within a population that could be prevented by altering a risk factor.

autosomal dominant A pattern of Mendelian inheritance whereby an affected individual possesses one copy of a mutant allele and one normal allele. (In contrast, recessive diseases require that the individual have two copies of the mutant allele.) Individuals with autosomal-dominant diseases have a 50-50 chance of passing the mutant allele (hence, the disorder) to their children. Examples of autosomal-dominant diseases include Huntington's disease, neurofibromatosis, and polycystic kidney disease.

autosome Any chromosome other than a sex chromosome. Humans have 22 pairs of autosomes.

base pair A set of two bases that form a "rung" of the DNA "ladder." The bases are adenine (A), thymine (T), guanine (G), and cytosine (C). A DNA nucleotide is made of a molecule of sugar, a molecule of phosphoric acid, and a base. In base pairing, A always pairs with T, and G always pairs with C.

315

BRCA1, BRCA2 The first breast cancer genes to be identified. Mutated forms of these genes are believed to be responsible for about half the cases of inherited breast cancer, especially those that occur in younger women. Both are tumor suppressor genes.

cell The basic unit of any living organism. A cell is a small, watery compartment filled with chemicals and a complete copy of the organism's genome.

chromosome One of the threadlike "packages" of genes and other DNA in the nucleus of a cell. Different kinds of organisms have different numbers of chromosomes. Humans have 23 pairs of chromosomes, 46 in all: 44 autosomes and two sex chromosomes. Each parent contributes one chromosome to each pair, so a child gets half his or her chromosomes from the mother and half from the father.

codon Three bases, in a DNA or RNA sequence, that specify a single amino acid.

cytosine (C) One of the four bases in DNA. The others are adenine (A), guanine (G), and thymine (T). C always pairs with G.

deletion A particular kind of mutation: loss of a piece of DNA from a chromosome. Deletion of a gene or part of a gene can lead to a disease or abnormality.

DNA replication The process by which the DNA double helix unwinds and makes an exact copy of itself.

DNA sequence The specific order of the bases arranged along one strand of the sugar-phosphate backbone.

DNA sequencing Determining the exact order of the base pairs in a segment of DNA.

dominant In regard to a gene, a gene that almost always results in a specific physical characteristic (e.g., a disease), even though the patient's genome possesses only one copy. With a dominant gene, the chance of passing the gene (therefore, the disease) to children is 50-50 in each pregnancy.

enzyme A protein that encourages a biochemical reaction, usually speeding it up. Organisms could not function if they had no enzymes.

exon The region of a gene that contains the code for producing the gene's protein. Each exon codes for a specific portion of the complete protein. In some species (including humans), a gene's exons are separated by long regions of DNA that have no apparent function. These regions are called introns or junk DNA.

false negative (FN) A test result indicating that the tested person does not have cancer, but he or she actually does have cancer.

false positive (FP) A test result indicating that the tested person has cancer, but he or she does not have cancer.

fibroblast A type of cell found just underneath the surface of the skin. Fibroblasts are part of the support structure for tissues and organs.

fluorescence in situ hybridization (FISH) A process that involves painting chromosomes or portions of chromosomes with fluorescent molecules. This technique is useful for identifying chromosomal abnormalities and for gene mapping.

gene The functional and physical unit of heredity passed from parent to offspring. Genes are pieces of DNA, and most genes contain the information for making a specific protein.

gene expression The process by which proteins are made from the instructions encoded in DNA.

gene therapy An evolving medical procedure, used to treat inherited diseases, that involves replacing, manipulating, or supplementing nonfunctional genes with healthy genes.

genetic code The instructions in a gene that tell the cell how to make a specific protein. The instructions are sequences of the chemicals adenine (A), thymine (T), guanine (G), and cytosine (C). Each gene's code combines the four chemicals in various ways to spell out three-letter "words" that specify which amino acid is needed at every step in making a protein.

genome All the DNA contained in an organism or cell, including the chromosomes within the nucleus and the DNA in mitochondria.

genotype Genetic identity that is not manifested as outward characteristics.

germ line Inherited material that comes from eggs or sperm and that offspring inherit.

guanine (G) One of the four bases in DNA. The others are adenine (A), cytosine (C), and thymine (T). G always pairs with C.

heterozygous Possessing two different forms of a particular gene, one inherited from each parent.

Human Genome Project An international research project to map each human gene and to completely sequence human DNA.

incidence In regard to cancer, the number of cancers that develop in a population during a defined period (e.g., one year).

inherited Transmitted through genes from parents to offspring.

insertion A type of chromosomal abnormality in which a DNA sequence is inserted into a gene, disrupting the normal structure and function of that gene.

karyotype The chromosomal complement of an individual, including all the chromosomes and any abnormalities. The term also refers to a photograph of an individual's chromosomes.

messenger RNA (mRNA) The template for protein synthesis. Each set of three bases, called codons, specifies a certain protein in the sequence of amino acids that composes the protein. The sequence of a strand of mRNA is based on the sequence of a complementary strand of DNA.

microarray A new way of studying how large numbers of genes interact with each other and how a cell's regulatory networks control vast batteries of genes simultaneously. The method uses a robot, which precisely applies tiny droplets containing functional DNA to glass slides. Researchers then attach fluorescent labels to DNA from the cell they are studying. The labeled probes are allowed to bind to complementary DNA strands on the slides. The slides are put into a scanning microscope that can measure the brightness of each fluorescent dot; brightness reveals how much of a specific DNA fragment is present, an indicator of how active it is.

microsatellite A repetitive short sequence of DNA that is used as a genetic marker to track inheritance in families.

mitosis The type of cell division that occurs in the replication of somatic cells.

mortality rate In regard to cancer, the number of people who die of a particular cancer during a defined period.

mutation A permanent structural alteration in DNA. In most cases, DNA changes either have no effect or cause harm. Occasionally, however, a mutation improves an organism's chance of surviving.

nonsense point mutation A single DNA base substitution resulting in a stop codon.

nucleotide One of the structural components, or building blocks, of DNA and RNA. A nucleotide consists of a base (one of four chemicals: adenine, thymine, guanine, and cytosine) plus one molecule of sugar and one molecule of phosphoric acid.

nucleus The central cell structure that houses the chromosomes.

oligo Oligonucleotide.

oligonucleotide A short sequence synthesized to match a region where a mutation is known to occur and then used as a probe.

oncogene A gene that is capable of causing the transformation of normal cells into cancer cells.

outcome A benefit, harm, or cost of screening or testing or a diagnostic evaluation that results from screening or testing.

peptide Two or more amino acids joined by a peptide bond.

phenotype The observable traits or characteristics of an organism (e.g., hair color, weight, the presence or absence of a disease). Phenotypic traits are not necessarily genetic.

ploidy The status of multiplication of chromosome sets (e.g., aneuploidy, diploidy, haploidy).

polymerase An enzyme that catalyzes the breakdown of nucleotides to polynucleotides.

polymerase chain reaction (PCR) A fast, inexpensive technique for making an unlimited number of copies of any piece of DNA. Sometimes called molecular photocopying, PCR has had an immense impact on biology and medicine, especially genetic research.

population In regard to cancer, the number of people in a defined group who are capable of developing cancer. It may refer to the general population or a specific group of people defined by geographic, physical, or social characteristics.

prevalence In regard to cancer, the actual number of cancers in a defined population at a given time. Usually expressed as the number of cancers per 100,000 individuals.

primary cancer prevention Measures to avoid carcinogen exposure and improve health practices. In some cases, primary cancer prevention includes the use of chemopreventive agents or prophylactic surgery.

promoter The part of a gene that contains the information to turn the gene on or off. The process of transcription is initiated at the promoter.

protease A protein that digests other proteins.

protein A large, complex molecule made up of one or more chains of amino acids. Proteins perform a wide variety of activities in the cell.

proteolytic enzyme Matrix metalloproteinases, or MMPs.

proto-oncogene A gene involved in regulating cell growth. When transformed through mutation, a proto-oncogene becomes an oncogene involved in unregulated or uncontrolled cell growth.

recessive A genetic disorder that appears only in patients who have received two copies of a mutant gene, one from each parent.

relative risk (RR) In regard to cancer, a comparison of the incidence of a risk factor or the number of deaths among those with the risk factor compared to those without the risk factor.

ribonucleic acid (RNA) A chemical whose composition is similar to a single strand of DNA. In RNA, however, uracil (U) replaces thymine (T) in the genetic code. RNA delivers DNA's genetic message to the cytoplasm of a cell where proteins are made.

ribosome Cellular organelle that is the site of protein synthesis.

risk factor A trait or characteristic associated with a statistically significant increased likelihood of developing a disease.

secondary cancer prevention Identifying people at risk of malignancy and implementing appropriate screening recommendations.

sensitivity In regard to cancer, the ability of a screening test to detect individuals with cancer. It is calculated by dividing the total number of true positives by the total number of cancer cases.

single locus The site of a gene on a chromosome.

somatic cells All body cells, except the reproductive cells.

specificity In regard to cancer, the ability of a test to identify individuals who do not have cancer. Specificity is calculated by dividing the total number of true negatives by the sum of the number of true negative and false positive results.

tertiary cancer prevention Monitoring for and preventing recurrence of a previously diagnosed cancer and screening for second primary cancers.

thymine (T) One of the four bases in DNA. The others are adenine (A), guanine (G), and cytosine (C). T always pairs with A.

TP53 A gene that normally regulates the cell cycle and protects a cell from damage to its genome. Mutations in this gene cause cells to develop cancerous abnormalities.

transcription The process of transforming information from DNA into a single-stranded RNA molecule.

translation The synthesis of amino acids, which then become proteins, from the mRNA template.

translocation Breakage and removal of a large segment of DNA from one chromosome, followed by the segment's attachment to a different chromosome.

true negative (TN) A test result indicating that the tested person does not have cancer and, indeed, the person neither has nor develops cancer within a defined period.

true positive (TP) A test result indicating that the tested person has cancer and, indeed, the person does have cancer.

tumor suppressor gene A protective gene that normally limits the growth of tumors. When a tumor suppressor is mutated, it may fail to keep a cancer from growing. *BRCA1* is a well-known tumor suppressor gene.

uracil (U) One of the four bases in RNA. The others are adenine (A), guanine (G), and cytosine (C). Like thymine (T), U always pairs with A.

validity A measure of how well a test measures what it is supposed to measure.

Index

Page locators in **boldface** indicate definitions found in Glossary. The letter *f* after a page number indicates a figure; the letter *t* indicates a table.